Bayer-Symposium VIII

The Pathogenesis of Bacterial Infections

Edited by

G. G. Jackson · H. Thomas

In Collaboration with

V. Braun · Z. A. McGee · W. Opferkuch
Ph. Y. Paterson

With 141 Figures and 69 Tables

Springer-Verlag
Berlin Heidelberg New York Tokyo

Bayer-Symposium VIII
held at Schloss Gracht, Germany, May 29 – June 2, 1984

Dr. GEORGE GEE JACKSON
Department of Medicine, Section of Infectious Diseases
The University of Illinois at Chicago College of Medicine
Box 6998, Chicago, IL 60680, USA

Privatdozent Dr. HERBERT THOMAS
Bayer AG, Pharma-Forschungszentrum,
Institut für Chemotherapie
Postfach 101709, D-5600 Wuppertal 1

ISBN-13: 978-3-642-70353-9 e-ISBN-13:978-3-642-70351-5
DOI: 10.1007/978-3-642-70351-5

Library of Congress Cataloging in Publication Data. Bayer-Symposium (8th: 1984: Schloss Gracht, Germany) The pathogenesis of bacterial infections. "Bayer-Symposium VIII held at Schloss Gracht, Germany" – T.p. verso. Held in 1984. Includes bibliographies. 1. Bacterial diseases – Congresses. 2. Host-parasite relationships – Congresses. I. Jackson, George Gee, 1920–. II. Thomas, Herbert, 1938–. III. Title. [DNLM: 1. Bacteria – pathogenicity – congresses. 2. Bacterial Infections – etiology – congresses. W3 BA266 8th 1984p/WC 200 B357 1984p]
QR201.B34B39 1984 576'.165 85-2883
ISBN-13: 978-3-642-70353-9 (U.S.)

2127/3130-543210

Contents

List of Contributors

The names of the participants at the eighth Bayer Symposium are underlined.

ABRAHAM, S.N.	VA Medical Center, University of Tennessee Center for the Health Sciences, Memphis, TN 38104, USA
ANDERSON, P.W.	The University of Rochester School of Medicine and Dentistry, Rochester, NY 14642, USA
BARBOUR, A.G.	Department of Health and Human Services, National Institutes of Health, National Institute of Allergy and Infectious Diseases, Laboratory of Microbial Structure and Function, Rocky Mountain Laboratories, Hamilton, MT 59840, USA
BEACHEY, E.H.	VA Medical Center, University of Tennessee Center for the Health Sciences, Memphis, TN 38104, USA
BHAKDI, S.	Institut für Medizinische Mikrobiologie, Klinikum der Justus-Liebig-Universität Gießen, Schubertstr. 1, D-6300 Gießen
BLAKE, M.S.	The Rockefeller University, Laboratory of Bacteriology and Immunology, 1230 York Avenue, New York, NY 10021, USA
BRAUN, V.	Institut für Biologie II, Lehrstuhl Mikrobiologie II, Universität Tübingen, Auf der Morgenstelle 28, D-7400 Tübingen 1
BROWN, T.A.	Department of Microbiology, Institute of Dental Research, Comprehensive Cancer Center, The University of Alabama in Birmingham, University Station, Birmingham, AL 35294, USA
BUCHANAN, TH.M.	Division of Infectious Diseases, University of Washington School of Medicine, Pacific Medical Center, 1200 12th Avenue South, Seattle, WA 98144, USA

BURGER, D.R.	Surgical Research Laboratory, Veterans Administration Medical Center, Portland, OR 97201, USA
CLARKE, J.	European Molecular Biology Laboratory, Postfach 10 22 40, D-6900 Heidelberg
COSTERTON, J.W.	Department of Microbiology, University of Calgary, Calgary, Alberta, Canada
DELIUS, H.	European Molecular Biology Laboratory, Postfach 10 22 40, D-6900 Heidelberg
DEVEY, M.E.	Department of Medical Microbiology, London School of Hygiene and Tropical Medicine, London, Great Britain
DUNCAN, Jr., R.L.	Department of Microbiology and Immunology, Emory University School of Medicine, 502 Woodruff Memorial Building, Atlanta, GA 30322, USA
DYER, D.W.	Department of Microbiology and Immunology, University of North Carolina School of Medicine, Chapel Hill, NC 27514, USA
FARIS, A.	Department of Bacteriology, Biomedicum, Box 583, S-751 23 Uppsala
FRANK, M.M.	Laboratory of Clinical Investigation, National Institute of Allergy and Infectious Diseases, National Institutes of Health, Bethesda, MD 20205, USA
FRÖMAN, G.	Connective Tissue Laboratory, Diabetes Hospital, University of Birmingham in Alabama, Birmingham, AL 35294, USA
GOODMAN, S.A.	Department of Microbiology and Immunology, Emory University School of Medicine, Atlanta, GA 30322, USA
HAAS, R.	Max-Planck-Institut für Medizinische Forschung, Abteilung Molekulare Biologie und Zentrum für Molekulare Biologie der Universität, Jahnstr. 29, D-6900 Heidelberg
HAHN, H.	Institut für Medizinische Mikrobiologie, Freie Universität Berlin, D-1000 Berlin 45
HALTER, R.	Max-Planck-Institut für Medizinische Forschung, Abteilung Molekulare Biologie und Zentrum für Molekulare Biologie der Universität, Jahnstr. 29, D-6900 Heidelberg

HAMMOND, M.E.	Department of Pathology, University Utah School of Medicine, Salt Lake City, UT 84132, USA
HANCOCK, R.E.W.	Department of Microbiology, The University of British Columbia, Vancouver, British Columbia, V6T 1W5, Canada
HÖÖK, M.	Connective Tissue Laboratory, Diabetes Hospital, University of Birmingham in Alabama, Birmingham, AL 35294, USA
IGLEWSKI, B.H.	Department of Microbiology and Immunology, Oregon Health Sciences University, 3181 S.W. Sam Jackson Park Road, Portland, OR 97201, USA
INZANA, TH.	University of Rochester Medical Center, Rochester, NY 14642, USA
JOINER, K.A.	Laboratory of Clinical Investigation, National Institute of Allergy and Infectious Diseases, National Institute of Health, Bethesda, MD 20205, USA
KARNOVSKY, M.L.	Department of Biological Chemistry, Harvard Medical School, Boston, MA 02115, USA
KIYONO, H.	Department of Oral Biology, The University of Alabama in Birmingham, University Station, Birmingham, AL 35294, USA
LARK, D.L.	Departments of Medicine and Medical Microbiology, Stanford University Medical Center, Stanford, CA 94305, USA
LEVINE, R.P.	James S. McDonnell Department of Genetics, Washington University School of Medicine, St. Louis, MO 63110, USA
LINDBERG, M.	Biomedicum, Department of Bacteriology, Box 583, S-751 23 Uppsala
MAYRAND, D.	Groupe de Recherche en Ecologie Buccale, Ecole de Médecine Dentaire, Université Laval, Quebec, G1K 7P4, Canada
McGEE, Z.A.	Center for Infectious Diseases, Diagnostic Microbiology and Immunology, University of Utah School of Medicine, Salt Lake City, UT 84132, USA

McGHEE, J.R. — Department of Microbiology, Institute of Dental Research, Comprehensive Cancer Center, The University of Alabama in Birmingham, University Station, Birmingham, AL 35294, USA

MESTECKY, J. — Department of Microbiology, Institute of Dental Research, Comprehensive Cancer Center, The University of Alabama in Birmingham, University Station, Birmingham, AL 35294, USA

MEYER, TH.F. — Max-Planck-Institut für Medizinische Forschung, Abteilung Molekulare Biologie und Zentrum für Molekulare Biologie der Universität, Jahnstr. 29, D-6900 Heidelberg

MICHALEK, S.M. — Department of Microbiology, Institute of Dental Research, Comprehensive Cancer Center, The University of Alabama in Birmingham, University Station, Birmingham, AL 35294, USA

MORRISON, D.C. — Department of Microbiology and Immunology, Emory University School of Medicine, Atlanta, GA 30322, USA

MOXON, E.R. — Department of Paediatrics, University of Oxford, John Radcliffe Hospital, Headington, Oxford OX3 9DU, Great Britain

MURPHY, P.A. — Department of Medicine, The Johns Hopkins University School of Medicine, Baltimore, MD 21205, USA

NÄHER, H. — Institut für Medizinische Mikrobiologie, Freie Universität Berlin, D-1000 Berlin 45

NICAS, T.I. — Department of Microbiology and Immunology, Oregon Health Sciences University, 3181 S.W. Sam Jackson Park Road, Portland, OR 97201, USA

NICKEL, P. — Max-Planck-Institut für Medizinische Forschung, Abteilung Molekulare Biologie und Zentrum für Molekulare Biologie der Universität, Jahnstr. 29, D-6900 Heidelberg

OPFERKUCH, W. — Lehrstuhl für Medizinische Mikrobiologie und Immunologie, Ruhr-Universität Bochum, Universitätsstr. 150, D-4630 Bochum 1

PATERSON, PH.Y. — Department of Microbiology-Immunology, Northwestern University Medical School, 303 E. Chicago Avenue, Chicago, IL 60611, USA

PICHICHERO, M.	University of Rochester Medical Center, Rochester, NY 14642, USA
POHLNER, J.	Max-Planck-Institut für Medizinische Forschung, Abteilung Molekulare Biologie und Zentrum für Molekulare Biologie der Universität, Jahnstr. 29, D-6900 Heidelberg
POOLMAN, J.T.	Laboratory of Medical Microbiology, University of Amsterdam, Meibergdreef 15, NL-1105 AZ Amsterdam
QUIE, P.G.	Department of Pediatrics, Division of Infectious Diseases, University of Minnesota Medical School, Minneapolis, MN 55455, USA
ROBINSON, Jr., E.N.	Center for Infectious Diseases, Diagnostic Microbiology and Immunology, University of Utah School of Medicine, Salt Lake City, UT 84132, USA
ROTHBARD, J.B.	Departments of Medicine and Medical Microbiology, Stanford University Medical Center, Stanford, CA 94305, USA
RUBIN, K.	Department of Bacteriology, Biomedicum, Box 583, S-751 23 Uppsala
RYDÉN, C.	Department of Bacteriology, Biomedicum, Box 583, S-571 23 Uppsala
SCHOOLNIK, G.K.	Departments of Medicine and Medical Microbiology, Stanford University Medical Center, Stanford, CA 94305, USA
SEEGER, W.	Zentrum für Innere Medizin, Universität Gießen, D-6300 Gießen
SO, M.	Scripps Clinic and Research Foundation, Department of Molecular Biology, 10666 North Torrey Pines Road, La Jolla, CA 92037, USA
SPARLING, P.F.	Department of Microbiology, The University of North Carolina, 804 Faculty Laboratory Office Bldg. 231H, Chapel Hill, NC 27514, USA
SPEZIALE, P.	Institute of Biochemistry, University of Pavia, I-Pavia
STERN, A.	Max-Planck-Institut für Medizinische Forschung, Abteilung Molekulare Biologie und Zentrum für Molekulare Biologie der Universität, Jahnstr. 29, D-6900 Heidelberg

STEWARD, M.W.	Department of Medical Microbiology, London School of Hygiene and Tropical Medicine, London, Great Britain
SUTTORP, N.	Zentrum für Innere Medizin, Universität Gießen, D-6300 Gießen
SWITALSKI, L.	Connective Tissue Laboratory, Diabetes Hospital, University of Birmingham in Alabama, Birmingham, AL 35294, USA
TRANUM-JENSEN, J.	Anatomy Institute C, University of Copenhagen, The Panum Institute, Blegdamsvej 3C, DK-2200 Copenhagen
VETTO, R.M.	Department of Microbiology and Immunology, Oregon Health Sciences University, Portland, OR 97201, USA
VUKAJLOVICH, S.W.	Department of Microbiology and Immunology, Emory University School of Medicine, Atlanta, GA 30322, USA
WADSTRÖM, T.	Department of Bacteriology, Biomedicum, Box 583, S-751 23 Uppsala
WAGNER, C.R.	Department of Microbiology and Immunology, Oregon Health Sciences University, Portland, OR 97201, USA
WEST, S.E.H.	Department of Microbiology and Immunology, The University of North Carolina School of Medicine, Chapel Hill, NC 27514, USA
WILLIAMSON, S.I.	Department of Microbiology, Institute of Dental Research, Comprehensive Cancer Center, The University of Alabama in Birmingham, University Station, Birmingham, AL 35294, USA
WOLLENWEBER, H.-W.	Department of Microbiology and Immunology, Emory University School of Medicine, Atlanta, GA 30322, USA
YOUNG, L.S.	Division of Infectious Diseases, University of California Medical Center, Los Angeles, CA 90024, USA

Welcome

H. Thomas

Ladies and Gentlemen, it is a great pleasure for me to welcome you on behalf of Bayer to Schloss Gracht. I would like to thank all of you very much for accepting our invitation to the eighth Bayer Symposium and for your interest in discussing among colleagues the latest scientific findings on mechanisms of microbial virulence and host factors in the pathogenesis of bacterial infections. My special thanks go to Dr. George G. Jackson, the Chairman of our Symposium, who has performed a great task not only in designing an ambitious program, but also in selecting the most interesting personalities with the greatest knowledge in their field.

Bayer Symposia already have a 16-year-old tradition. We started in 1968 with *Current Problems in Immunology*. The third Symposium dealt with *Bacterial Infections*. It was held in 1970 and was organized by Finland, Marget and Bartmann. Our general idea behind these Symposia is to bring together a small, selected group of scientists and to give them a stimulating environment for discussing current topics in modern biology and medicine.

We have chosen Schloss Gracht as the place for our Symposium because it combines tradition with progress, a combination of factors which may influence the quality of our meeting and which may also determine good science and personality.
Furthermore, Schloss Gracht reminds us of the long and lively tradition and the exchange of ideas and people between Germany and North America. Here in Schloss Gracht, Carl Schurz was born, a German-American statesman who emigrated to the United States in 1852. He served as Senator for Missouri and Secretary of the Department of the Interior. Another important reason to meet here is that Schloss Gracht represents one famous and typical form of German castle in the northern Rhine area, namely a moated castle. During your stay we will help you to complete your knowledge of German castles by visiting Schloss Augustusburg at Brühl for a concert and Schloss Vollrads at the end of our Symposium.

When we first met in London with Dr. Jackson in September 1982 to set up the program of our Symposium we were aware of the fact that a topic like ours represents a very fascinating area for physicians involved in infectious diseases, medical microbiologists, molecular and cell biologists, geneticists, and biochemists. Therefore, this subject has already induced exciting meetings during the last decade. Nevertheless, we stayed with our idea of discussing mechanisms involved in the pathogenesis of bacterial infections, because this field is in an extremely active state of growth and the availability of new techniques in molecular biology, biochemistry, biophysics, and immunology provides the means for rapid and profound advances.

Multiple factors are involved in the pathogenesis of bacterial infections. Bacterial attachment mechanisms, interactions between pathogens and host defense mechanisms, dissemination, tissue invasion, and immunopathologic mechanisms play an important role. Because it is not possible to discuss all important aspects in detail in a two-and-a-half-day meeting, we will concentrate on those which provide the greatest insights into this multifactorial process of bacterial infections and those where we need more information for the basic understanding of bacterial pathogenesis. We have also selected some non-Enterobacteriaceae like *Neisseria*, *Hemophilus*, *Pseudomonas*, *Bacteroides*, and *Staphylococcus*, which in some of the scientific disciplines mentioned have been pushed into the background by *Escherichia coli*.

I am sure our discussion during the next two and a half days will provide a better understanding of bacterial virulence and pathogenesis, but it will also help to define or discover those factors and mechanisms which have to be investigated more deeply. I also hope that the Symposium may help to identify new leads for applied research with respect to new therapeutics against bacterial diseases *and* that it may turn out to be as rewarding as everyone is anticipating.

Last, but not least, I would like to express my deepest gratitude to our ladies. Thank you very much for attending. I think you are the best guarantee that we will not forget other important, interesting, and stimulating aspects of such a meeting which retain their significance even in the face of science. We will help you in this respect with organizing the social events, may we ask you to help us to make this meeting a scientific as well as a social success.

Introduction

G. G. Jackson

The pathogenesis of bacterial infection defines the dynamics at an interface of ecologic association of bacteria and host. First, it occurs at the portal of initial contact with a permissive target cell. The infected cell provides either a passive or a specific receptor for the bacterium or its products, together with ligands and an environment of helper and inhibiting factors. The result is bacterial replication to produce an imbalance of a potentially commensal relation which, under other defined conditions, would be optimal for the survival of both the host and bacterial cells. Virulence and pathogenesis are both absolute and relative terms. They must be interpreted strictly according to the circumstances of site-specific interactions of bacterial and host cells, membrane composition, structure, characteristics, and environmental substances.

The bacteria themselves may have, acquire, or switch on or off under certain conditions, the products or properties that produce cellular damage that we recognize as virulence. Another result of bacterial infection may be to stimulate a normal host cell function to perform at a pathophysiologic level, causing illness that we recognize as virulence. A third marker of virulence may be the ability to invade a cell or tissue barrier and produce a pathologic effect at a site that is remote from the portal of commensal association or pathologic entry. These markers of virulence: (a) tissue damage; (b) specific pathophysiologic dysfunction; and (c) spread of infection, may result from dynamic properties of bacteria that are present by endowment or acquisition through gene transfer of different biologic capabilities. They are variably expressed as electrical charge, hydrophobicity, or surface antigens. The pathogenic process of bacterial virulence may proceed with little regard for the host response to the local events of bacterial replication. In other circumstances, the bacterial replicative imbalance may be from the absolute or relative susceptibility of the host owing to age, genetic constitution, or a failure of the host defense system to stem the measures of virulence. This battleground, involving the selection of susceptible host sites by bacteria, host confinement of infection, or invasive bacterial infection and disease, is one of high kinetic activity with the outcome determined by many humoral, cellular, and environmental components acting in complementary or anticomplementary fashion and sequences.

Thus, the problem in pathogenesis is one of recognizing strain selection of clones of bacteria with capabilities of overcoming normal host defense mechanisms and the differentation of a process from the dyskinesis (congenital, acquired, or temporal) in the number of permissive host cells, and/or number and function of host defense mechanisms. Ubiquitous and usually commensal microorganisms may be permitted to produce the pathophysiologic state of virulence from either limb of the host-parasite balance.

From still another viewpoint, a proper, biologically programmed sequence of host reponses to infection may cause disease, using the endowed capacity to produce and release factors to kill invasive bacteria, and in the process fail to control the detrimental effect on host tissues as well. Further along this viewpoint, the host reponse may be inordinately strong through recognition of a foreign antigen for which genetic incompatibilities, prior experience, or molecular presentation cause the host pathologically to alter a part or the whole tissue, organ, or system. The stimulated host may even provide the pathogenesis of the condition by perpetuating an abnormal process through such mechanisms as variable presentation of antigen or anti-idiotypic antibody that elicits a renewed pathogenic stimulation of the host.

So, in examing the absolute mechanisms of pathogenesis, the relativity of virulence must always be emphasized and the conditions well circumscribed. We can not, and do not, propose to develop simple or consensus definitions of virulence – instead our task is to identify mechanisms, some of which may have generic importance in understanding the pathogenesis of bacterial infections. But we will not assume the legitimacy of transfer to other species and hosts without justification. To complete our task, we must ask questions of increasing sophistication about why and how the intermembrane and product reactions between parasite and host occur, determining molecular and biophysical as well as biologic explanations. To do so we have limited the target to a group of common bacteria with a large reservoir in humans, usually in nonenteric sites. And we have posed the questions of pathogenesis in a chronological sequence of contact, bacterial selection, replication, and invasion of bacteria; as well as deficient, regulatory, overwhelmed, or pathologic host defense systems.

We have provided a group of selected skilled scientists from many disciplines, each of whom knows a piece of the puzzle. Because others can not be here, but have a keen interest in the topic and discussions, it is our responsibility while we are together, to ask those questions of one another that would be asked by other investigators, so that we can extract the maximum, both the data base and perceptions of it, from the expert group.

Finally, opportunities for practical applications toward the goal of preventing or modifying disease, although not a necessity of scientific experimentation, are a natural desire and result of the achievement of a better understanding of the processes that are involved in the pathogenesis of bacterial infection. That goal provides some encouragement and additional justification for the broad interest and importance of the papers and discussions that are scheduled. If we educate one another with a spirit of inquiry and free exchange of knowledge and thought, we can define the forefront of new areas of information and serve as a stimulus for us and for others to accelerate the development of understanding and promote the prospects of control measures in the pathogenesis of bacterial infections.

Session 1

Infection of Mucosal Surfaces

Chairman: Z. A. McGee

Bayer-Symposium VIII
The Pathogenesis of Bacterial Infections, 8-16 (1985)

Molecular Mechanisms by Which Pathogenic Bacteria Interact with Host Mucosal Cells

Z. A. McGee and E. N. Robinson, Jr.

Summary

Current strategies in the use of antibiotics force bacteria to evolve mechanisms of antimicrobial resistance. These mechanisms, in addition to making the organisms antibiotic resistant, may also enhance acquisition of genetic factors which increase virulence. To evolve new strategies which do not rely on antimicrobials for prevention and management of infections, it is necessary to improve our understanding of the molecular mechanisms by which bacteria cause disease. The first step in the disease process caused by many bacteria is interaction with host mucosal surfaces. Studies using pathogenic *Neisseria*, *N. gonorrhoeae*, and *N. meningitidis*, have shown a complex series of events by which these human pathogens attach to, damage, and cross mucosal cells. The bacteria utilize pili and perhaps other surface structures to attach to mucosal cells. Damage is effected by lipopolysaccharide and peptidoglycan monomers. Organisms appear to invade mucosal cells, but are actually phagocytized by these cells and transported to the base of the cells where they appear to undergo multiplication. They are then exocytosed into the subepithelial tissues where they may cause local disease or enter the bloodstream to cause disseminated disease. Further understanding of the molecular mechanisms involved in these processes may help in the development of new immunologic or other means of intervening in the disease process.

Introduction

The production of disease by many bacterial species requires the successful completion of an obstacle course comprised of various physical barriers and other host defense factors. In the first of the series of steps that comprise the pathogenic process, the bacterium must attach to the surface of mucosal cells. It then must transgress the mucosal barrier and enter the bloodstream. After avoiding phagocytosis and bacteriolysis in the bloodstream, the bacterium must identify and invade the target tissue, e.g., the meninges or a joint space. Finally, the bacterium must avoid host defenses in the target tissue and cause disease. The contributions to this Symposium are arranged in approximately this sequence of events and are designed to elucidate the molecular mechanisms by which various pathogens are able to effect the different steps in the pathogenic process. The molecular mechanism used by the bacterium in one step may be entirely different from those utilized in subsequent steps. This paper will focus on those factors that determine the nature of the initial interaction of the bacterium with host mucosal cells and its subsequent transgression of the mucosal barrier. For the sake of continuity, studies of pathogenic *Neisseria* will be emphasized.

Attachment of Bacteria to Epithelial Cells

The major pathogens that attach to mucosal cells have surface structures, called ligands or adhesins, that interact with specific receptors on host cells and anchor the bacteria to these cells. For most of these pathogens the surface structures that mediate attachment are pili [1] (Fig. 1). Elsewhere in this volume, Schoolnik and Rothbard discuss the structure and organization of pili as well as the probable biochemical mechanisms of the interaction between pili and their receptors.

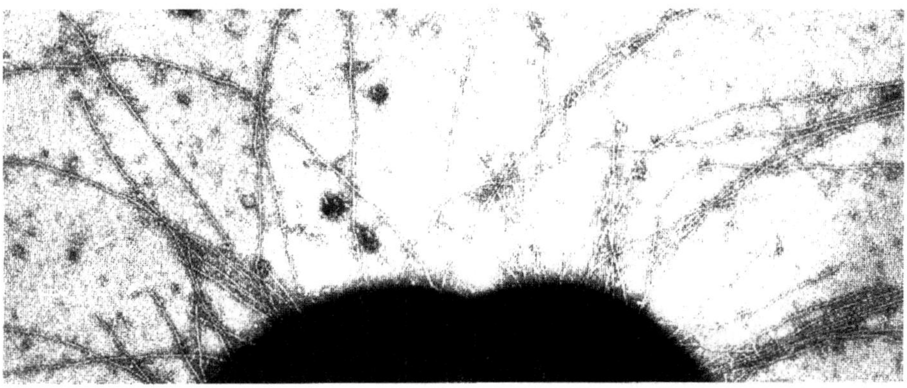

Fig. 1. Transmission electron micrograph of *Neisseria gonorrhoeae* showing pili, hair-like protein appendages, emanating from the surface of the organism (negative stain, × 40 000)

There is great diversity of the amino acid sequences of pili from different species of bacteria [2]. Pili may differ among different strains of the same species, and even from time to time in the same strain [3, 4]. Structural differences in pili appear to determine the types of cells to which the bacteria attach and thus which cells will play a role in or be targets of the disease process. For instance, gonococci simultaneously isolated from different sites in the same patient have been shown to be derived from the same strain, yet have pili with different subunit molecular weights [5]. In addition, the pili with different subunit molecular weights were shown to have affinity for different cell types. It is likely that the other bacterial pathogens that use pili as a means of attachment [1] exhibit similar diversity in pilus structure and function.

Another type of receptor-ligand interaction is employed by microorganisms that elaborate long-chain carbohydrates. These carbohydrates may interact with similar polymers on host cells and form a glycocalyx network in which other bacteria may become enmeshed. Such polysaccharide networks appear to be important in colonization of the gut by normal flora [6].

Bacterial surface structures other than pili have been demonstrated to mediate attachment to the surface of host mucosal cells. For instance, lipoteichoic acid of *Streptococcus pyogenes* appears to mediate the specific attachment of streptococci to erythrocytes, lymphocytes, and oral epithelial cells. Recent evidence indicates that fibronectin on the surface of epithelial cells may serve as a receptor for lipoteichoic acid [7]. Therefore, variation in the amount of fibronectin present on the surface of epithelial cells might influence the likelihood of streptococcal colonization and resultant active streptococcal disease or postinfectious disease (i.e., rheumatic fever).

Receptors may be found on the surface of host cells in only certain locations. There, the receptors demonstrate a high degree of specificity for the ligands with which they interact. For instance, the development of isogenic piliated and nonpiliated clones of *N. meningitidis* enabled Stephens and McGee [8] to examine the distribution of receptors for meningococcal pili as well as the effect of pili on meningococcal attachment. Meningococci which lacked pili attached in only low numbers to cells from a variety of mucosal surfaces. In contrast, piliated meningococci attached in large numbers to cells of the nasopharynx and posterior pharynx, but attached in only low numbers to cells from the bladder and anterior nares, even though the latter cells reside only a centimeter or two from the nasopharynx. These findings suggest that the distribution of receptors for meningococcal pili may be a major factor in determining the selective colonization of the nasopharynx by meningococci.

The distribution of receptors may be specific not only to a given location, but even to particular cell types within that location. The epithelium of the human fallopian tube is comprised of ciliated cells and nonciliated cells. Piliated gonococci attach to nonciliated cells of the fallopian tube mucosa, but not to ciliated cells [9]. The epithelium of the human nasopharynx is also comprised of ciliated cells and nonciliated cells. Piliated meningococci do not attach to ciliated cells of the human nasopharyngeal mucosa and attach to only certain of the nonciliated cells.

Receptors on certain mucosal cell types in one host species may be absent on the analogous cells in other species. For example, piliated gonococci that attach to nonciliated cells of human fallopian tube mucosa fail to attach to nonciliated cells of fallopian tubes from a variety of primate and nonprimate animals [10]. Thus, the presence or absence of mucosal receptors for pathogenic microorganisms may be the determining factor in the species specifity of those pathogens. Even the same cell type may vary in its interaction with piliated microorganisms from time to time in the same individual. Forslin et al. [11] have shown that piliated gonococci attach to vaginal cells in greater numbers during certain phases of the menstrual cycle. These differences may result from hormonal modulation of receptor site number, affinity, or specificity.

Damage to Epithelial Cells by Bacteria

Although attachment of microorganisms to mucosal surfaces is almost certainly important in the pathogenesis of a variety of infections in humans, the molecules which mediate attachment are not, per se, likely to cause tissue damage. Rather, it is likely that attachment facilitates the interaction of other molecules located on or elaborated by the bacteria and that these molecules are responsible for consummating the disease process.

Toxic Factors

In studies of the sequential events of infection of human fallopian tube mucosa in organ culture by gonococci, attachment of the organisms to the mucosal surface was followed shortly by damage to the epithelial cells [9]. This damage was manifest primarily by sloughing of ciliated cells from the epithelium (Fig. 2). In a series of studies performed by Melly et al. [12], supernatant fluid removed from gonococcal infected organ cultures and filter sterilized was found to reproduce the damage to human fallopian tube mucosa by active gonococcal infection. The toxic activity was heat stable and not substantially diminished by dialysis. These characteristics were compatible with the hypothesis that either or both of two products elaborated by gonococci, lipopolysaccharide (LPS) and peptidoglycan monomers, were responsible for the damage.

Lipopolysaccharide

The likely involvement of gonococcal LPS in damage to human fallopian tube mucosa was suggested by several observations. Absorption of toxic supernatant fluid with *Limulus* amoebocyte lysate reduced substantially the concentration of LPS in the fluid and reduced substantially the toxicity of the fluid for genital mucosa [12]. When highly purified gonococcal LPS was added to human fallopian tube organ cultures in concentrations as low as 0.015 μg/ml, a value less than the concentration of LPS in toxic supernatant fluid, the damage produced was indistinguishable from the damage that occurred during active gonococcal infection. Polymyxin B, an antibiotic that combines with the lipid A portion of the LPS molecule, neutralized the toxic effect of LPS [13]. The LPS which was toxic for human fallopian tubes was not toxic for the fallopian tubes of a variety of animals (e.g., rabbits, pigs, cows [14]). These two latter observations suggested the possibility that the LPS molecule is comprised of two functional domains: a carbohydrate portion which acts as a haptophore to mediate recognition of the target mucosa and the lipid A portion which acts as a toxophore to mediate damage of the target mucosal cells.

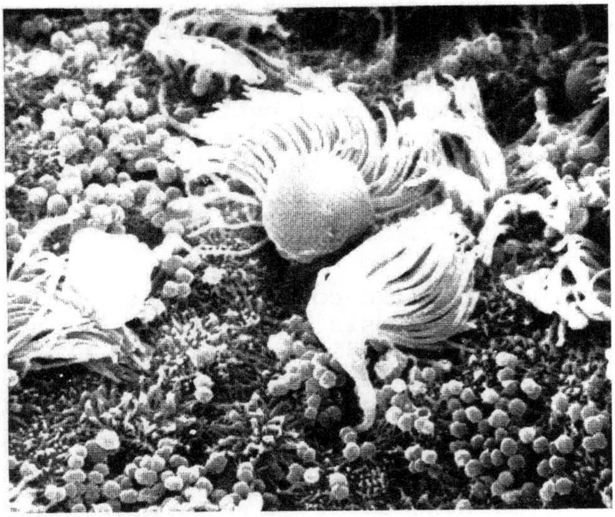

Fig. 2. Gonococcal infection of human fallopian tube mucosa in organ culture. Scanning electron micrograph of mucosa 20 h after inoculation with a piliated clone of *Neisseria gonorrhoeae*. Note gonococci attached almost exclusively to nonciliated cells. Intact ciliated cells are seen at right and top. Ciliated cells sloughing from the surface of the mucosa are seen at center and left (× 3 126). Reprinted with permission from the *Journal of Infectious Diseases* [9]

It is not necessary for gonococci and at least some other bacteria to die in order to release LPS or endotoxin. These organisms actively form outer membrane blebs which they elaborate into their milieu (Fig. 3). Robinson et al. [15] have developed a technique for complexing electron-dense gold spheres with specific antibody. By using such gold sphere-anti-protein I antibody complexes as immunoprobes, it has been shown that a majority of the blebs contain protein I in the same orientation as on the surface of the organisms (Fig. 3). The blebs therefore appear to present to the host cell the same array of molecules as is present on the surface of the organism itself. The blebs have the potential for serving as surrogate microorganisms in their interaction with host cells.

Fig. 3. Distribution of accessible outer membrane protein I on the surface of a pair of gonococci and the outer membrane blebs elaborated by them. The gonococci were exposed to gold spheres complexed with monoclonal antibody against protein I. The gold spheres appear as *black dots* on the electron micrograph. Note heavy marking of both the organisms and the outer membrane blebs elaborated by them (negative stain, × 68 400)

Peptidoglycan Monomers

Studies were also performed to evaluate the possible role of peptidoglycan monomers in damage to human fallopian tube mucosa. Two forms of gonococcal peptidoglycan monomers might play a role in the disease process. Growing gonococci elaborate a nonreducing anhydromuramyl-containing monomer. Gonococcal peptidoglycan acted on by human lysozyme yields an analogous reducing monomer. Both forms of peptidoglycan monomers produced sloughing of ciliated cells from human fallopian tube mucosa in a manner indistinguishable from active gonococcal infection. In an effort to determine the functional parts of the peptidoglycan molecule, *N*-acetylglucosamine and muramyldipeptide, both components of the peptidoglycan monomer, were tested for their ability to produce damage. Neither did so [16]. A soluble toxin produced by *Bordetella pertussis* which damages tracheal epithelial cells was found to contain a peptidoglycan subunit with additional amino acids [17].

None of these studies has documented that the toxic compounds act directly on ciliated cells, even though the sloughing of these ciliated cells may be the end result of the toxic action of the compounds. It is notable that both LPS and peptidoglycan are immunoregulatory molecules. It is possible that they stimulate the production of compounds such as prostaglandins which may secondarily effect the damage to ciliated cells. Further information is needed about these reactions so that means of protecting mucosal surfaces from damage may be developed.

Transgression of the Mucosal Barrier by Bacteria

Invasion of Epithelial Cells

Light microscopic studies of gonococcal infected human fallopian tube organ cultures showed gonococci entering nonciliated cells of the mucosa, beginning about 24 h after infection. Although this phenomenon has been termed "invasion", the major activity resulting in entry of gonococci into the epithelial cells is on the part of the nonciliated epithelial cells themselves. During the "invasion" phase of the infection, the microvilli of nonciliated cells to which gonococci were attached (see Fig. 2) began to retract, pulling the gonococci to the surface of the cell. Other microvilli appeared to surround the gonococci, entrapping them against the cell surface (Fig. 4). This surface then retracted, pulling gonococci into membrane-bound vesicles in a manner similar to phagocytosis of bacteria by polymorphonuclear leukocytes. The available evidence suggests that the phagocytosis step is not simply the result of passive circumferential adhesion of host cell membranes initiated by attachment, but rather is the result of initiation by gonococci of an active process of phagocytosis by host mucosal epithelial cells.

Transport to the Base of Cells

The phagocytic vesicles containing gonococci were seldom seen between the luminal surface of the cells and the base of the cells. Thus, the phagocytic vesicles were apparently transported

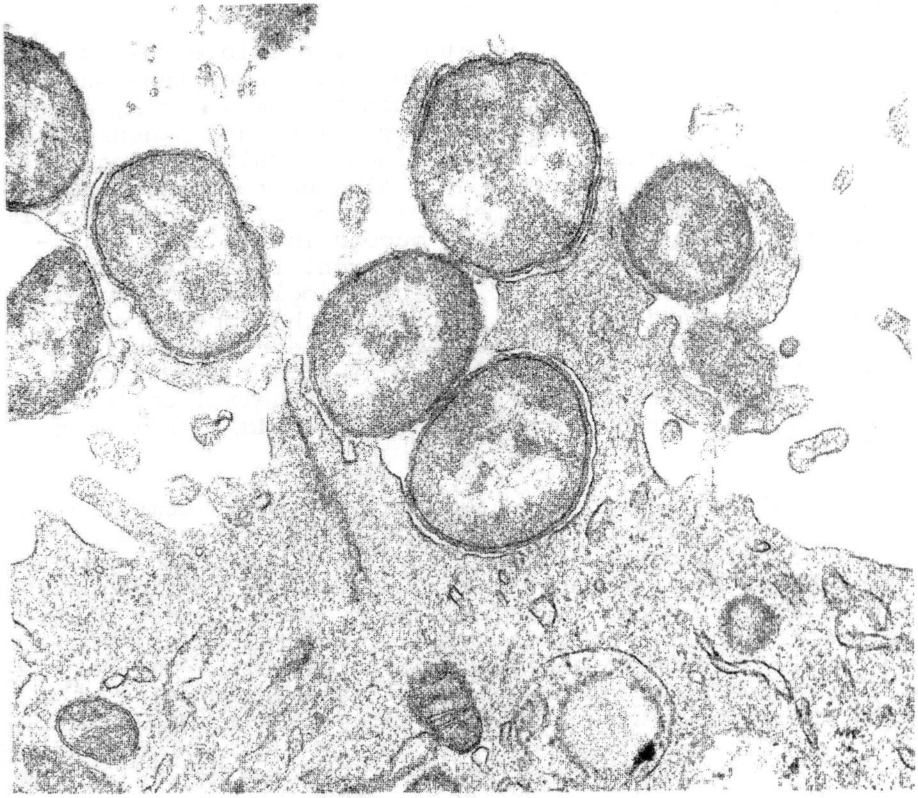

Fig. 4. Interaction of *Neisseria gonorrhoeae* with surface structures of nonciliated cells of human fallopian tube mucosa in organ culture. Note microvilli conforming to the shape of gonococci (right and left of center) and almost complete engulfment of a gonococcal pair (center) (× 24 700)

rapidly to the base of the cells following their formation. At the base of the cells either the microorganisms multiplied with enlargement of the vesicles fusion of multiple vesicles occurred, or both.

Exocytosis of Bacteria into the Subepithelial Tissues

Beginning about 40 h after infection, the membranes of vesicles at the base of the nonciliated cells appeared to fuse with the basilar cell membranes in that area, forming channels through which gonococci were exocytosed into the subepithelial tissues. Gonococci were occasionally seen in between epithelial cells, but only at a level below the nucleus. These gonococci appeared to have been phagocytized, transported part way down the cell, and then exocytosed into the intercellular space near the basement membrane. The available morphological and cultural evidence suggests that the gonococci in the vesicles and subepithelial tissues are viable.

Thus, phagocytosis and transport of bacteria across the mucosal barrier is of particular interest because of the relatively long intracellular phase of the infection and because the whole process results from host epithelial cells acting as Trojan horses, aiding gonococci in their transgression of the mucosal barrier. If this process takes place in vivo, as is suggested by pathologic studies on tissues from naturally occurring gonococcal disease [18, 19], it results in delivery of gonococci to subepithelial tissues where they might cause local inflammation (acute salpingitis) or might invade blood vessels to cause disseminated gonococcal infection. Virtually nothing is known of the mechanisms that induce or modulate this "invasion" process.

A similar process of attachment, interaction with microvilli, phagocytosis, and possible multiplication within phagocytic vesicles occurs as *N. meningitidis* interact with the nonciliated cells of human nasopharyngeal mucosa [20]. Studies to determine whether exocytosis of meningococci into the subepithelial tissues occurs have not been completed. This method of crossing mucosal barriers may be a more general phenomenon than is usually appreciated. The intestine also contains specialized cells that transport microorganisms across the mucosal barrier [21, 22]. A more complete understanding of the molecular mechanisms by which microorganisms attach to, damage, and cross the mucosal barrier should provide new strategies for preventing and more successfully managing a variety of diseases of humans and animals.

Acknowledgments. These studies were supported in part by research grant AI-20265 from the National Institute of Allergy and Infectious Diseases, U.S. Public Health Service. Dr. Robinson is the recipient of a Venereal Diseases Research Fellowship from the American Social Health Association.

References

1. Beachey EH (1981) Bacterial adherence: adhesin-receptor interactions mediating the attachment of bacteria to mucosal surfaces. J Infect Dis 143:325-345
2. Schoolnik GK, Tai JY, Gotschlich EC (1983) A pilus peptide vaccine for the prevention of gonorrhea. Prog Allergy 33:314-331
3. Svanborg Eden C, Freter R, Hagberg L, Hull R, Leffler H, Lomberg H, Schoolnik G (1982) Role of surface proteins involved in surface adhesion: Adherence to uroepithelia in vitro and in vivo. In: Schlessinger D (ed) Microbiology 1982, American Society for Microbiology, Washington, pp 286-291
4. Duckworth M, Jackson D, Zak K, Heckles JE (1983) Structural variations in pili expressed during gonococcal infections. J Gen Microbiol 129: 1593-1596
5. Zak K, Diaz J-L, Jackson D, Heckles JE (1984) Antigenic variation during infection with *Neisseria gonorrhoeae*: detection of antibodies to surface proteins in sera of patients with gonorrhea. J Infect Dis 149:166-174
6. Costerton JW, Cheng KJ (1982) Autochthonous populations: Colonization of tissue surfaces by autochthonous bacteria. In: Schlessinger D (ed) Microbiology 1982, American Society for Microbiology, Washington, pp 266-273

7. Beachey EH, Simpson WA, Ofek I, Hasty DL, Dale JB, Whitnack E (1983) Attachment of *Streptococcus pyogenes* to mammalian cells. Rev Infect Dis 5:S670-677
8. Stephens DS, McGee ZA (1981) Attachment of *Neisseria meningitidis* to human mucosal surfaces: influence of pili and type of receptor cell. J Infect Dis 143:525-532
9. McGee ZA, Johnson AP, Taylor-Robinson D (1981) Pathogenic mechanisms of *Neisseria gonorrhoeae*: observations on damage to human fallopian tubes in organ culture by gonococci of colony type 1 or type 4. J Infect Dis 143:413-422
10. Johnson AP, Taylor-Robinson D, McGee ZA (1977) Species specificity of attachment and damage to oviduct mucosa by *Neisseria gonorrhoeae*. Infect Immun 18:833-839
11. Forslin L, Danielsson D, Falk V (1979) Variations in attachment of *Neisseria gonorrhoeae* to vaginal epithelial cells during the menstrual cycle and early pregnancy. Med Microbiol Immunol 167:231-238
12. Melly MA, Gregg CR, McGee ZA (1981) Studies of toxicity of *Neisseria gonorrhoeae* for human fallopian tube mucosa. J Infect Dis 143:423-431
13. Gregg CR, Melly MA, Hellerqvist CG, Coniglio JG, McGee ZA (1981) Toxic activity of purified lipopolysaccharide of *Neisseria gonorrhoeae* for human fallopian tube mucosa. J Infect Dis 143:432-439
14. Gregg CR, Johnson AP, Taylor-Robinson D, Melly MA, McGee ZA (1981) Host species-specific damage to oviduct mucosa by *Neisseria gonorrhoeae* lipopolysaccharide. Infect Immun 34:1056-1058
15. Robinson EN, McGee ZA, Kaplan J, Hammond ME, Larson JK, Buchanan TM, Schoolnik GK (1984) Ultrastructural localization of specific gonococcal macromolecules: use of antibody-gold-sphere immunologic probes. Infect Immun 46:361-366
16. Melly MA, McGee ZA, Rosenthal RS (1984) Ability of monomeric peptidoglycan fragments from *Neisseria gonorrhoeae* to damage human fallopian-tube mucosa. J Infect Dis 149:378-386
17. Goldman WE, Klapper DG, Baseman JB (1982) Detection, isolation, and analysis of a released *Bordetella pertussis* product toxic to cultured tracheal cells. Infect Immun 36:782-794
18. Harkness AH (1948) Pathology of gonorrhea. Br J Vener Dis 24:137-147
19. Pollock CE, Harrison LW (1912) Gonococcal infections. Oxford University Press, London
20. Stephens DS, Hoffman LH, McGee ZA (1983) Interaction of *Neisseria meningitidis* with human nasopharyngeal mucosa: attachment and entry into columnar epithelial cells. J Infect Dis 148:369-376
21. Bockman DE, Cooper MD (1973) Pinocytosis by epithelium associated with lymphoid follicles in the bursa of fabricus, appendix, and Peyer's patches: an electron microscopic study. Am J Anat 136:455-478
22. Wolf JL, Rubin DH, Finberg R, Kauffman RS, Sharpe AH, Trier JS, Fields BN (1981) Intestinal M cells: a pathway for entry of reovirus into the host. Science 212:471-472

Bayer-Symposium VIII
The Pathogenesis of Bacterial Infections, 17-29 (1985)

Antigen Expression Influencing Tissue Invasion of *Hemophilus influenzae* Type B

E. R. Moxon

Summary

The majority of episodes of invasive *Hemophilus influenzae* infections are caused by capsulated, type b strains. The invasive potential of *H. influenzae* was investigated in an experimental rat model. Genetically similar type a and type b strains, constructed by DNA transformation, were inoculated intranasally to investigate the contribution of these capsular antigens, or linked determinants, with respect to the stages of colonization, translocation of organisms into the blood and intravascular survival. Both the type a and type b strains colonized the nasopharynx and entered the bloodstream efficiently. In contrast, the type b transformant survived significantly more efficiently than the type a transformant in the bloodstream. In addition to the differences in their capsular antigens, the transformants differed in their lipopolysaccharide composition. In separate experiments, independently obtained type b transformants which differed in their lipopolysaccharide composition, but not capsule or outer membrane proteins, were shown to be significantly different in virulence. Further studies, using cloned DNA derived from a λ gene library, provided further evidence of the independent contribution of capsular antigen and lipopolysaccharide to the pathogenicity of *H. influenzae*.

Introduction

Studies of bacterial pathogenicity involve issues of extreme biological complexity, a special consideration being the interactive nature of microbe and host. This mutuality is of the essence; the analysis of virulence requires, as an obligatory and reciprocal substrate, a susceptible host. Yet it is important to emphasize that pathogenicity must be viewed in the context of the "co-evolutionary trajectory followed by any particular host-parasite association" [1]. The genotype of both bacterium and host display extensive and widespread polymorphism among the genes whose products mediate these encounters. As a consequence of this versatile, dynamic, relationship a particular bacterium may display a spectrum of pathogenic potential for its host which ranges from the negligible to the lethal. The past decade has made available analytic tools which make it possible to study the pathogenesis of bacterial infections at

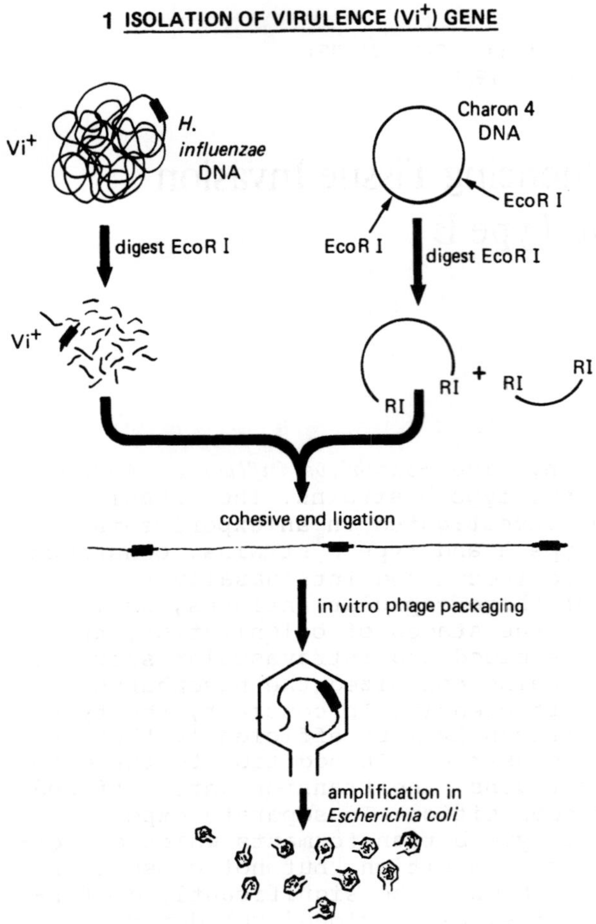

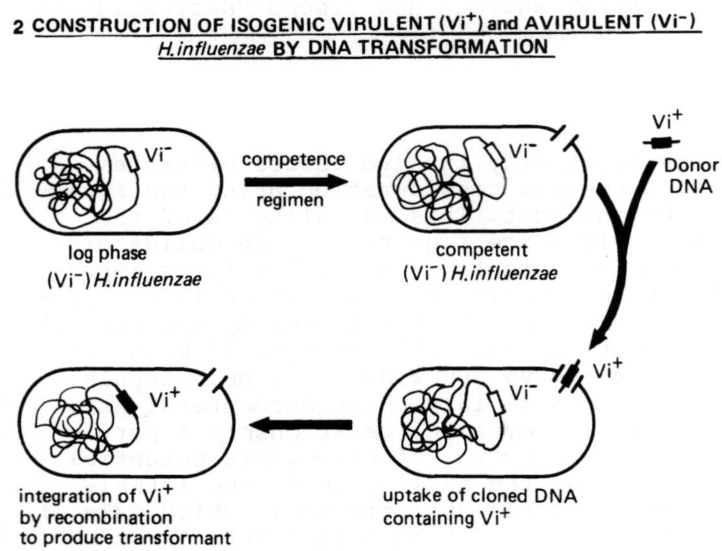

Fig. 1. General scheme for studying pathogenicity of *H. influenzae*. Fragments of chromosomal DNA are cloned into a suitable vector to isolate virulence genes (*Panel 1*). These genes can be introduced by DNA transformation into *H. influenzae* strains which lack the specific virulence determinant (*Panel 2*). Transformed and untransformed *H. influenzae* are then compared in a suitable animal model, e.g., infant rats (*Panel 3*) to allow an unambiguous analysis of the role of specific genes in pathogenicity

3 VIRULENCE ASSAY IN EXPERIMENTAL MODEL INFECTION

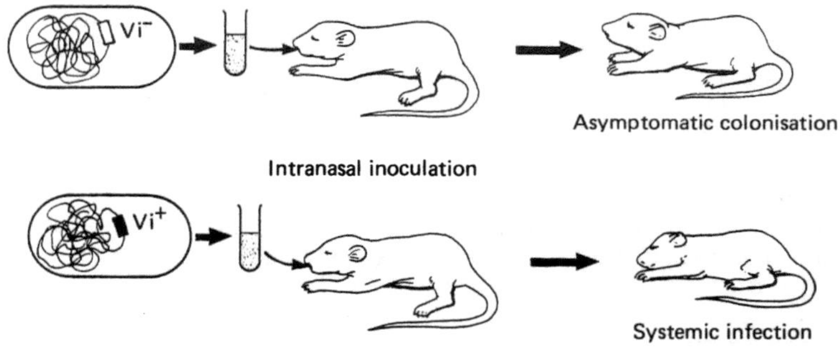

the molecular level. For example, the mechanisms by which microbial genes impose themselves upon their host are now accessible through the use of recombinant DNA technology. Virulence genes can be isolated from the bacterial genome (or extrachromosomal elements) and introduced in active or inactive states into suitable strains. In this manner, an unambiguous analysis of this gene, or a set of genes, can be undertaken using suitable animal models, cell cultures, or other in vitro systems. Thus, such studies necessarily involve a critical integration of microbial genetics and biologically relevant model systems for assaying virulence. Fig. 1 is a general scheme indicating how this kind of approach has been exploited to investigate the virulence mechanisms which determine tissue invasion by the human pathogen *Hemophilus influenzae*.

H. influenzae causes a spectrum of infections in humans, the most serious being associated with bloodstram dissemination of organisms [2]. These systemic infections occur most commonly in young children and include meningitis, septic arthritis, epiglottitis, cellulitis, and pneumonia. These bacteraemic infections are usually, but not exclusively, caused by encapsulated type b strains. The type b capsule (PRP) is a polymer of alternating ribosyl and ribitol residues joined by a phosphodiester linkage. Strains making any one of five other polysaccharide capsules have been described for *H. influenzae*, but such strains are rarely associated with haematogenous infections. The propensity of *H. influenzae* type b, but not other encapsulated or nonencapsulated strains, to cause invasive infections raises important issues as to the basic mechanisms involved. Indeed, the problem might be considered prototypic; the principles involved could shed light on the mechanisms by which other encapsulated pathogens result in invasive infection, such as meningitis. To this end the availability of an experimental model of *H. influenzae* bacteraemia and meningitis in infant rats [3] has proved extremely useful. It shares many similarities with the naturally occurring infection in humans. For example: age, serum anti-PRP antibodies, complement, and phagocytic clearance have been shown to be critical host determinants underlying host susceptibility in both the natural and experimental infection [4]. Furthermore, type b strains display a significantly greater potential for causing invasive infection of the rat than do strains expressing any of the five other capsular polysaccharides or strains lacking capsule. This review will summarize several recent studies which were conducted with André Zwahlen, MD, Lorry Rubin, MD, Susan Hoiseth, PhD, and Carla Connelly, BSc. These investigations indicate that type b strains are endowed with a significantly greater capacity to survive and replicate in the intravascular compartment. As a consequence, sustained and high level bacteraemia ensues. This, in turn, increases the probability of central nervous system infection, since the duration and magnitude of bacteraemia are important determinants of the occurrence of meningitis [5]. The enhanced pathogenicity of *H. influenzae* type b is determined, inter alia, by both the chemical composition of its capsula and its lipopolysaccharide (LPS).

H. influenzae Pathogenicity

General Considerations

The hypothetical scheme depicted in Fig. 2 indicates that the pathogenesis of *H. influenzae* meningitis can be considered as a sequence of mutually dependant, sequential steps. However, the determinants of each event are likely to be polygenic – for both bacterium and host. Furthermore, bacterial determinants critical for the consummation of one step may be redundant at the next, or perhaps counterproductive with respect to bacterial survival. This genotypic and phenotypic variation of the bacterial population together with its high rates of replication, has the potential for generating great versatility thus encouraging survivors in the face of the biological gauntlet of host defences. Dr. Anderson has already discussed factors which mediate mucosal colonization by *H. influenzae* and has emphasized the many facets bearing on this stage in the pathogenesis. With respect to the next stage in the pathogenesis of systemic infection, it should also be emphasized that the term "invasive" is often used to describe those properties of a microorganism which endow it with both the potential to penetrate a mucosal barrier and to survive in the new location. However, since different determinants may be involved in each of these events, a distinction between translocation (or penetration) and subsequent survival must be made. If, for example, a strain of *H. influenzae* can translocate from the nasopharynx to the blood, but there lacks the capacity to survive, the first event might be considered, in a sense, abortive. Furthermore, it is difficult in the experimental setting to distinguish such a strain from one that lacks those properties required for translocation since experimental demonstration of "invasiveness" requires both properties. In experimental infection of rats, haematogenous dissemination does not occur in the absence of sustained and heavy nasopharyngeal colonization with *H. influenzae*. Although this observation might imply the mutual interdependence of colonization and bloodstream dissemination (as was assumed in Fig. 2), it should be explained that this is not necessarily so. For example, organisms capable of prolonged survival in the nasopharynx of the host may also possess attributes required for systemic survival and haematogenous

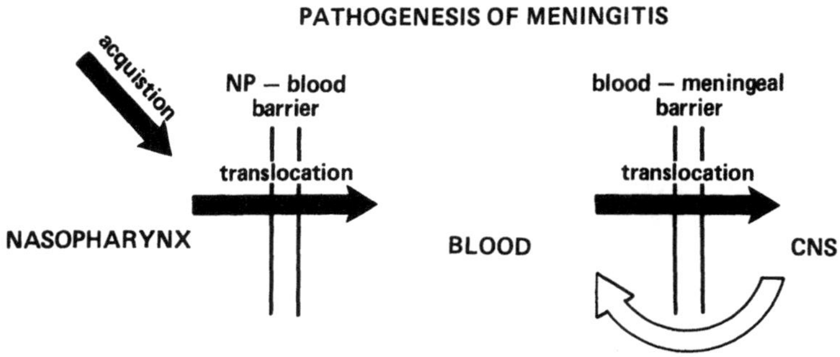

Fig. 2. Pathogenesis of *H. influenzae* meningitis. The scheme indicates sequential, but potentially independent stages in the evolution of meningitis. At each stage, either host or bacterium may prevail, resulting in termination or progression of infection. Outcome at each stage may be affected by the interaction of several host and bacterial gene products

dissemination, but as independent (although coexisting) phenotypic characteristics. The mechanisms by which *H. influenzae* reach the bloodstream from the respiratory tract are poorly understood. *H. influenzae* are nonmotile; it is possible that penetration into or between epithelial cells of the respiratory mucosa occurs. Alternatively, transport on or in host cells, perhaps phagocytes, is another possibility. If a ligand-receptor interaction between the bacterial surface and the mucous or epithelium of the host is involved in lodgement, one wonders how this adherence effects the likelihood (or not) of systemic spread as opposed to local containment of *H. influenzae*. The ability of encapsulated (type b) and nonencapsulated strains of *H. influenzae* to cause loss of ciliary activity and sloughing of epithelial cells was recently demonstrated using an organ culture system [6] (Fig. 3). Similar, if not identical results were reproduced when the organ culture system was exposed to purified LPS extracted from *H. influenzae* (A.P. Johnston, personal communication). These results suggested that the mucosal changes associated with extrusion of ciliated epithelial cells could provide a mechanism by which organisms might penetrate the respiratory mucosa, enter the vascular system and produce bacteraemia. Since strains of *H. influenzae*, with or without capsule, cause similar changes in the respiratory epithelium, both share this potential mechanism for tissue penetration. Therefore, since type b organisms possess a substantially greater propensity for causing systemic diseases, it follows that they must have additional virulence factors to promote their pathogenicity. As a further question, one needs to determine at which stage (or stages) in the pathogenetic sequence type b organisms display this greater virulence.

Use of DNA Transformation to Study Role of Capsule

In order to investigate the role played by the different capsular polysaccharides mediating invasiveness, a series of genetically similar strains were obtained using DNA transformation [7]. The recipient was the avirulent, capsule-deficient *H. in-*

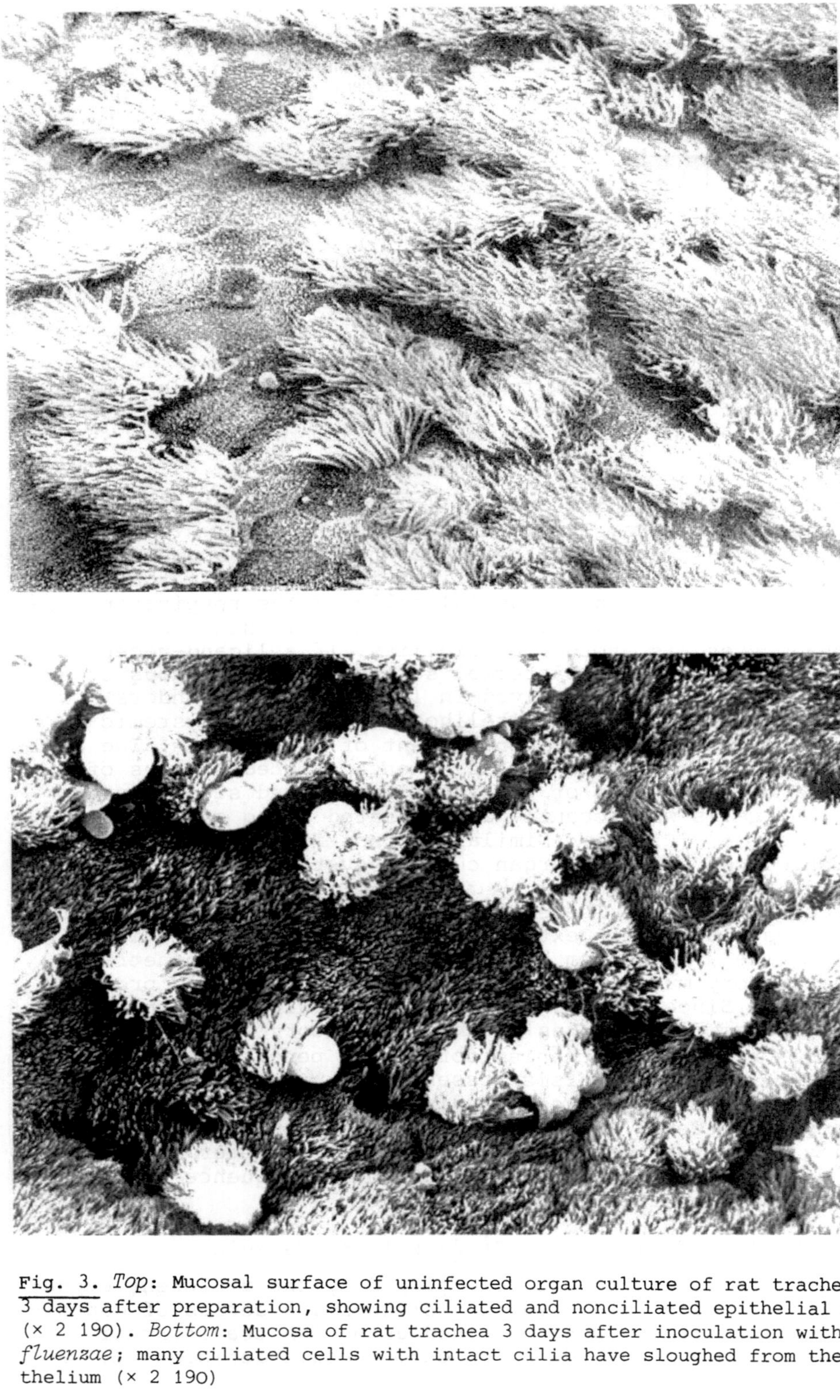

Fig. 3. *Top*: Mucosal surface of uninfected organ culture of rat trachea 3 days after preparation, showing ciliated and nonciliated epithelial cells (× 2 190). *Bottom*: Mucosa of rat trachea 3 days after inoculation with *H. influenzae*; many ciliated cells with intact cilia have sloughed from the epithelium (× 2 190)

fluenzae, strain Rd. Donor DNA was extracted from encapsulated strains representing the six capsular types [8]. Satisfactory transformants for each capsular type, with the exception of type e, were obtained. Strain Rd and each of its transformants colonized the rat nasopharynx. Furthermore, the type b transformant seemed no more efficient in this respect than did the other capsular polysaccharides [9]. These data are consistent with information gained from surveys of respiratory carriage of *H. influenzae* in humans [10, 11]. Thus, the substantially higher incidence of systemic infections caused by type b strains does not seem to reflect a capacity for relatively more efficient nasopharyngeal colonization.

The next logical question is whether or not the type b organism can penetrate the nasopharyngeal tissues more efficiently compared with transformants elaborating the other capsular polysaccharides. The type b transformant resulted in a significantly greater incidence and magnitude of bacteraemia; however, these data did not clarify whether or not type b strains translocate more efficiently from the nasopharynx to the blood. Therefore, blood cultures were obtained within minutes of the intranasal inoculation of the type a and type b transformants. We selected the type a transformant for comparison since its capsular polysaccharide is also a ribitol phosphate diester, but the ribitol moiety alternates with a glucosyl, as opposed to a ribosyl, residue. Both type a and type b transformants were recovered from the blood within minutes of inoculation, the number of organisms being similar. Although more episodes of bacteraemia were observed for the type b transformant, too few animals were studied to evaluate the significance of this observation. Nonetheless, the occurrence of early bacteraemia with the type a transformant provided evidence that it had the potential to enter the bloodstream as quickly and efficiently as did the type b transformant. In separate experiments, no difference in the early clearance of the type a and type b transformant was observed following intravenous inoculation. However, major differences in the numbers of organisms recovered from the blood were observed several hours later. Whereas the numbers of the type a organisms tended to decrease, there was a dramatic increase in the number of type b transformants recovered from blood cultures after a latent period of several hours [9]. Thus, the type b transformant is endowed with a distinctive capacity for survival and there is a critical stage – several hours into the infection – during the course of the bacteraemia when this enhanced virulence becomes manifest. The determinants of this enhanced survival of type b organisms are clearly vital to understanding the potential of the type b organism to generate sustained, high level bacteraemia. The pivotal role of this phase in the pathogenesis becomes clear when one appreciates that the probability of meningitis is directly related to the duration and magnitude of bacteraemia [8] (Table 1). Furthermore, since these differences in virulence were observed between genetically related strains, it can be inferred that the greater virulence of the type b transformant was mediated through the uptake and recombination of genes situated on a single molecule of DNA. It would seem reasonable to propose that the critical genes include those

Table 1. Correlation of meningitis with magnitude of bacteraemia after intraperitoneal challenge of normal rats with *H. influenzae* transformants of type c, d, or f [8]

Magnitude of bacteraemia (cfu/ml)	Meningitis status of rats[a]	
	Present	Absent
$>10^3$	50	18
$\leq 10^3$	1	11

[a]Results are numbers of rats in each category. These figures include only those rats with detectable bacteraemia ($\geq 10^2$ cfu/ml), since none of the 26 animals with sterile blood cultures had meningitis. The correlation between the presence of meningitis and bacteraemia of $>10^3$ cfu/ml is statistically significant ($\chi^2 = 18.07$; $p < 0.001$). Among rats without meningitis, only three had $>10^4$ cfu/ml of blood and none had $>10^5$ cfu/ml.

necessary for the polyribosylribitol phosphate capsule, but might also include one or more genes linked to the cap b region. Since the donor DNA molecules had an average size of 40 000 base pairs, there would be ample potential for the transformants to acquire linked genes distinct from those directing capsule expression. To examine this possibility further, we analysed the outer membrane proteins (OMP) and LPS composition of the transformants. The major and minor OMP were found to be similar to each other. In contrast, the LPS patterns of the transformants were distinctly different [8].

Thus, transformation of strain Rd had indeed resulted in altered expression, not only of capsular polysaccharide, but also LPS. The data indicate that one or more genes involved in LPS biosynthesis are either shared or linked to capsule genes. The findings raise a predictable, but important issue with respect to the analysis of virulence. DNA transformation evidently resulted in the altered expression of at least two major surface antigens. Thus, the precise basis for the greater virulence of the type b transformant requires more stringent analysis. However, before describing such experiments, some additional discussion of the biological significance of these results is required to place them in appropriate perspective.

It has been reported previously that the sustained bacteraemia which results from intranasal inoculation of rats with *H. influenzae* b, consists of organisms which were derived from replication of a few organisms, perhaps a single bacterium [12]. Thus, although many bacteria enter the circulation from the nasopharynx, the progeny of only a very few of these organisms ultimately prevail. An analysis of the organisms present in the blood following inoculation of a 50-50 mixture of streptomycin-sensitive and resistant *H. influenzae* b revealed that blood cultures commonly yielded mixtures of the two phenotypes for up to 10 h after inoculation, but thereafter one or other (but not both) of the phenotypes predominated (Table 2). These data fit well with the concept that most of the organisms entering the circulation are removed; however, an occasional bacterium replicates with extreme efficiency and may generate progeny which ultimately constitute all, or the vast majority, of the population responsible for the systemic infection. This seems to be the only reasonable way of explaining the occurrence of pure blood cultures of one or other phenotype among the majority of bacteraemic rats. However, whether these organisms were the result of intravascular replication or, alternatively, the result of replication in an extravascular focus and secondary seeding of the blood was not clear. Further studies indicated that prior to the emergence of sustained bacteraemia the only tissues consistently containing viable *H. influenzae* were the respiratory tract and the blood [13]. Since the respiratory tract was colonized with both phenotypes, and in approximately equal numbers, the selective seeding of the blood with only one of them made it probable that the sustained bacteraemia resulted from intravascular replication. In fact, the capacity for *H. influenzae* b to replicate intravascularly with extreme efficiency has been demonstrated by inoculating small numbers of organisms intravenously and observing an exponential increase in the number of organisms recovered from the blood over the ensuing several hours [14]. A critical question concerns the nature of the occasional, germinal organism which gives rise to the high density, sustained bacteraemia characteristic of the type b, but not the type a transformant. Although this virulence potential clearly exists within the population of type b organisms, it seems important to know whether the expansion of a particular bacterial clone is a random event or, alternatively, whether a rare type b organism possesses special characteristics which are denied to the majority of the other organisms in the infectious inoculum. If the latter hypothesis pertains, it would be critical to iden-

Table 2. Proportion of *H. influenzae* variants in blood following intranasal inoculation [12]

Cultures scored[a]	Time after inoculation 5 min	30 min	3 h	6 h	10 h	20 h	54 h
Indeterminate	0	0	1	5	0	1	0
Pure Sm^S	0	0	0	0	2	9	9
Pure Sm^R	0	0	0	0	1	1	6
Mixed	3	2	0	1	4	4	5

[a]Number of blood cultures containing one or both variants at different times after intranasal inoculation of 10^8 *H. influenzae* type b (strain Eagan). The inoculum consisted of an approximately 50-50 mixture of streptomycin-sensitive and streptomycin-resistant organisms.

tify and characterize the basis of this critical variation. Dr. Anderson has already indicated that *H. influenzae* organisms undergo phenotypic modulation with respect to their susceptibility to lysis when exposed to serum anti-LPS antibodies and complement. However, it has been shown that this shift may occur at the stage of colonization (i.e., prior to tissue penetration [15]) and is therefore unlikely to be an adequate explanation for differences in the intravascular survival of the type a and type b transformants.

Use of Molecular Genetics to Study Role of Capsule

As indicated previously, the results of comparative virulence studies using transformants suggested a critical role for type b capsule, but these transformants showed differences in LPS in addition to capsule. Thus, PRP might be merely associated with or one of several determinants mediating enhanced virulence characteristics of the type b transformant. In order to investigate the role of PRP as an independent variable, we constructed a λ (Charon 4) library of chromosomal DNA from a virulent type b transformant of strain Rd [16]. This genomic library was screened for recombinants which contained cloned inserts capable of transforming an *H. influenzae* mutant, deficient in PRP expression, so that it regained the virulent, type b, phenotype. A recombinant, designated Ch.4:48, was isolated and shown to contain a 13.4-kilobase insert containing *H. influenzae* sequences necessary for expression of type b capsule. After restriction enzyme digestion of Ch.4:48, two Eco Rl fragments of 9 and 4.4 kilobases were gel purified and subcloned into pBR328 [17]. Each of these subcloned DNA fragments was then used as donor DNA for transformation experiments. By using a number of independently obtained capsule-deficient mutants, we were able to show that both the 9 and 4.4-kilobase Eco Rl fragments contained independent sequences necessary for type b capsule expression. The mutation in strain Rd/b^-:O2 maps to a 1-kilobase region within the 4.4-kilobase subclone [17], and involves a change in so few bases that its Southern hybridization pattern was identical to its b^+ parent when each was probed with the intact 4.4-kilobase Eco Rl fragment. This suggested strongly that Rd/b^-:O2 has a mutation in one of its genes essential for PRP expression. Since Rd/b^-:O2 is avirulent, but its b^+transformant (obtained with cloned DNA) is fully virulent, there is now very strong genetic evidence to support the critical role of PRP in virulence.

Genetic Studies on Role of LPS

The virulence studies using transformants indicated a possible role for both capsule and LPS in mediating the greater pathogenicity of the type b transformant. As shown in Fig. 4, we obtained independent b^+ transformants of Rd designated O1 and O2. SDS-PAGE analysis indicated that the major and minor outer membrane proteins were similar, but the LPS patterns were different. Each elaborated identical amounts of PRP as measured by ELISA. Comparative virulence studies in rats showed that the O2 transformant was significantly more virulent than the closely related O1 transformant [18]. Further evidence suggesting the independent contribution of LPS to virulence was obtained by transforming Rd/b^+:O2 with the recombinant Ch.4:I69 obtained from the λ gene library. The transformant thus produced, designated Rd/b$^+$:I69, was shown to have a distinctly different LPS pattern from that of Rd/b$^+$:02, while retaining a similar outer membrane protein profile and type b capsule expression. However, Rd/b$^+$:I69 proved relatively avirulent for rats when inoculated intranasally or intravenously [19]. In fact, following intravenous inoculation the I69 transformants were rapidly cleared from the bloodstream. Thus, in addition to its potential role in damaging respiratory tract epithelium [6], the LPS composition of *H. influenzae* apparently plays a critical role in determining the intravascular survival of *H. influenzae* type b organisms.

In summary, we have used a biologically relevant rat model of meningitis in conjunction with classical microbial genetics and recombinant DNA technology to investigate the molecular basis of *H. influenzae* pathogenicity. Understanding the genetic basis of *H. influenzae* pathogenicity should contribute basic knowledge relevant to the better treatment and the prevention of *H. influenzae* systemic disease.

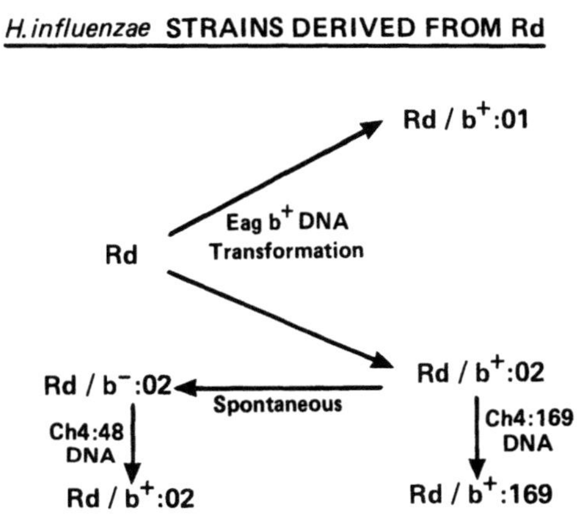

Fig. 4. Scheme to show the derivation and relationship of several strains genetically related to Rd

Acknowledgments. This work was supported by NS 12254 and by a Research Career Development Award (KO4 Al 00300) from the National Institutes of Health. I am greatly indebted to Dr. Hamilton O. Smith (Johns Hopkins University, Baltimore) and his colleagues for advice and encouragement. I am grateful to Mrs. Sheila Hayes for her help in the preparation of this manuscript. Fig. 3 is reproduced by kind permission of Dr. A.P. Johnston and the editors of the *Journal of Medical Microbiology*. Table 1 is reproduced by kind permission of the editors of the *Journal of Infectious Diseases*, and Table 2 by kind permission of the editors of the *Proceedings of the National Academy of Sciences*.

References

1. Anderson RM, May RM (1979) Population biology of infectious diseases: I. Nature 280:361-367
2. Turk DC (1982) Clinical importance of *Haemophilus influenzae*. In: Sell SH, Wright PW (eds) Biologoy of *Haemophilus influenzae*. Epidemiology, immunology, and prevention of disease. Elsevier North Holland, New York, pp 3-9
3. Moxon ER, Smith AL, Averill DR, Smith DH (1974) *Haemophilus influenzae* meningitis in infant rats after intranasal inoculation. J Infect Dis 129:154-162
4. Moxon ER (1982) Experimental study of *Haemophilus influenzae* in a rat model. In: Sell SH, Wright P (eds) Biology of *Haemophilus influenzae*. Elsevier, New York, p 59
5. Moxon ER, Ostrow PT (1977) *Haemophilus influenzae* meningitis in infant rats: The role of bacteraemia in the pathogenesis of the age-dependent inflammatory responses. J Infect Dis 135:303-307
6. Johnson AP, Clark JB, Osborn MF (1983) Scanning electron microscopy of the interaction between *Haemophilus influenzae* and organ cultures of rat trachea. J Med Microbiol 16:477-482
7. Moxon ER, Vaughn KA (1981) The type b capsular polysaccharide as a virulence determinant of *Haemophilus influenzae*: Studies using clinical isolates and laboratory transformants. J Infect Dis 143:517-524
8. Zwahlen A, Winkelstein JA, Moxon ER (1983) Surface determinants of *Haemophilus influenzae* pathogenicity: Comparative virulence of capsular transformants in normal and complement-depleted host. J Infect Dis 148:385-394
9. Rubin LG, Zwahlen A, Moxon ER (1983) Relative contribution of bloodstream invasiveness and intravascular survival to the pathogenicity of *Haemophilus influenzae*. Abstract No. 12: Presented at 83rd Microbiology Meeting at New Orleans, Louisiana, 6.-11.3.83
10. Turk DC, May RM (1967) Distribution of *H. influenzae* in healthy communities. In: *Haemophilus influenzae*: Its clinical importance. English Universities Press, London
11. Sell SH, Turner DJ, Federspiel CF (1973) Natural infections with *Haemophilus influenzae* in children: types identified. In: Sell SH, Karzon DT (eds) Vanderbilt Universities Press, Nashville, pp 3-12
12. Moxon ER, Murphy PA (1978) *Haemophilus influenzae* bacteraemia and meningitis resulting from survival of a single organism. Proc Natl Acad Sci USA 75:1534-1536
13. Rubin LG, Moxon ER (1983) Pathogenesis of bloodstream invasion with *Haemophilus influenzae* type b. Infect Immun 41:280-284
14. Rubin LG, Zwahlen A, Moxon ER (Submitted for publication) Role of intravascular replication in the pathogenesis of experimental *Haemophilus influenzae*, type b bacteraemia
15. Rubin RG, Moxon ER (1984) *Haemophilus influenzae* type b colonization resulting from survival of a single organism. J Infect Dis 149:278-279
16. Moxon ER, Deich RA, Connelly C (1984) Cloning of chromosomal DNA from *Haemophilus influenzae*: Its use for studying the expression of type b capsule and virulence. J Clin Invest 73:298-306
17. Hoiseth SK, Connelly C, Moxon ER (Submitted for publication) Genetics of spontaneous, high frequency loss of b capsule expression in *H. influenzae*
18. Zwahlen A, Rubin LG, Moxon ER (1983) Contribution of lipopolysaccharide to *Haemophilus influenzae* pathogenicity: Comparative virulence of genetically related strains. Abstract No. 12: Presented at the 23rd Inter-

science Conference on Antimicrobial Agents and Chemotherapy at Las Vegas, Nevada, 24.-26.10.83

19. Zwahlen A, Rubin LG, Connelly C, Inzana TJ, Anderson PW, Moxon ER (1983) Alteration of lipopolysaccharide of *Haemophilus influenzae* type b by transformation with cloned DNA is associated with attenuated virulence. Ped Res 286A

Bayer-Symposium VIII
The Pathogenesis of Bacterial Infections, 30-38 (1985)

Surface Factors and Nasopharyngeal Colonization by *Hemophilus influenzae* B

P. W. Anderson, Th. Inzana, and M. Pichichero

Summary

Although capable of systemic invasion, *Haemophilus influenzae* type b (Hib) are found mainly in asymptomatic colonization of the nasopharynx. Hib expresses extracellular factors and cell surface structures with a potential for influencing colonization, but their respective contributions have not been clarified. It has been found to release a factor inhibitory to cultured ciliated epithelium and, like several other meningeal pathogens, to elaborate an IgA_1 protease. The capsule, better known as a determinant of invasiveness, also appears to confer a slight advantage in the initial stages of colonization. Certain of the nonfimbrial outer membrane proteins appear to be surface-exposed in the presence of capsule, but none have yet been identified as adhesins. Cell-surface expression of the lipopolysaccharide is quite limited in Hib as it seems to exist in vivo; however, released fragments of membrane containing LPS have toxic activities that may influence colonization. Hib was long believed to be non-fimbriated but now is known to have a rarely expressed ability to make a pilus that promotes a mannose-resistant binding to human cells. Experiments in infant rats indicate that fimbriation may increase the ability to initiate colonization. In the rat as in man, however, the Hib recovered in culture are consistently non-fimbriated.

Introduction

The traditional classification of *Haemophilus influenzae* is based upon serotyping of the capsular polysaccharides. The most frequently isolated lack capsules and thus are nontypable. These usually are part of the normal flora of the nasopharynx (NP), but can also cause infections of mucosal surfaces such as otitis media, conjunctivitis, and exacerbations of chronic bronchitis; occasionally they also cause systemic infections in immunocompromised subjects. Understanding of the host-parasite relationships of nontypable *H. influenzae* has been assisted by a recently developed nonserological biotyping classification [8]. Capsular types a and c-f are infrequently found among the normal flora and even less frequently as pathogens. *H. influenzae* type b (Hib) can be found in the NP of healthy individuals and occasionally causes mucosal infection but, in addition, is the only member of the species that causes systemic infections at a substantial frequency in otherwise healthy subjects (primarily young children). In the USA Hib causes annually about 15 000 cases of cerebrospinal meningitis and about 9 000 cases of other invasive infections such as cellulitis, arthritis, epiglottitis, or nonfocal septicemia [1]. The organism is transmitted from one NP to another within families or by other close contact such as in nursery schools. Most encounters of children with Hib, however, are nonpathogenic – for each child succumbing to systemic infection there are perhaps 10-100 who experience asymptomatic colonization [17]. While the variables determining invasiveness of Hib have long been the object of analysis (E.R. Moxon, this volume), determinants of colonization have been less studied. This article will briefly review surface factors of Hib that are variably expressed and discuss roles they may play in colonization.

Extracellular Products

Denny [2] reported that *H. influenzae* releases a factor able to inactivate ciliated epithelium in cultured tracheal tissue; the factor has not been identified biochemically but has been surmised to be lipopolysaccharide (LPS), which is a component of shed membrane fragments. Following the discovery of IgA_1 protease in pathogenic *Neisseriae*, a similar enzyme was found in pneumococci and *H. influenzae* and postulated to be a virulence determinant for meningococcal pathogens [10]. Virulence can not be absolutely dependent upon this enzyme, for protease-negative strains are occasionally found among pathogenic isolates [6]. Unfortunately, the effect of protease expression can not be evaluated in animal models due to the insusceptibility of nonhuman IgA_1 to the enzyme.

Capsule

Since its recognition by Pittman, the capsule has been considered a critical virulence determinant due to its ability to impede phagocytosis. Whether this property of the capsule influences the persistence on NP mucosa is not known. The results of simple mucosal cell adherence assays in vitro depend upon the choice of medium (Table 1). A capsule-deficient mutant of Hib bound as well or better to human buccal epithelial cells (EC) in vitro than the capsulated parent (both nonpiliated) when assayed in saline. The addition of Ca^{2+} ions increased the binding of the parent about 10-fold to a value exceeding that of the mutant. This is a reasonable result since the phosphodiester residues of the capsular polymer poly (-3β-D-ribose [1-1] ribitol-5-phosphate-) would be "bridged" to anionic residues of the mucosal cell surface by divalent cations. Interestingly, in the presence of a sample of normal human nasal mucus (clarified by slow speed centrifugation) the binding of both capsulated and capsule-deficient bacteria was strongly reduced (Table 1). Colonization of course depends upon numerous phenomena beyond simple adherence to mucosal cells. In the most satisfactory animal model of Hib

Table 1. Binding of nonpiliated capsulated or capsule-deficient *H. influenzae* b to human buccal cells in vitro

Bacteria	Medium	Bacteria/cell
Capsulated	Saline	0.6[a,b]
	Saline + 10 m*M* $CaCl_2$	6.3[a]
	Human nasal mucus	0.1[b]
Capsule-deficient mutant	Saline	0.8[c,d]
	Saline + 10 m*M* $CaCl_2$	1.3[c]
	Human nasal mucus	0.1[d]

[a] $P = 0.02$ [b] $P = 0.001$ [c] $P = 0.05$ [d] $P = 0.01$

infection, infant rats inoculated intranasally become colonized in the NP and develop bacteraemia and meningitis [11]. Colonization can be affected by the capsulated parent in much lower challenge doses ($<10^2$) than by the capsule-deficient mutant; the latter can achieve a stable colonization but only rarely produces bacteraemia (E.R. Moxon, unpublished data).

Nonfimbrial Outer Membrane Proteins (OMP)

The OMP of Hib consists of about six (quantitatively) major and several dozen minor proteins as enumerated in one-dimensional sodium dodecyl sulfate-polyacrylamide gel electrophoresis (SDS-PAGE) [9]; among Hib strains the OMP are electrophoretically heterogeneous, a property that has been used epidemiologically by several laboratories. Certain of the OMP are surface-exposed (by the criterion of being accessible to antibody despite the capsulation) [5]. Presumably these would be accessible also to mucosal cell surface structures; however, presently none of the OMP has been found to act as an adhesin.

LPS

H. influenzae LPS has endotoxic properties similar to the more well characterized LPS of enteric bacteria [3], but structurally contains only short saccharide chains in contrast to the elongated polysaccharides of S type enteric LPS (Fig. 1, lane 3 vs. 1). Antigenic determinants of the LPS are surface-exposed in Hib as grown in the typical broth media but appear inaccessible and thus resistant to LPS antibody in the bacterial phenotype that pertains in vivo. The resistant phenotype can be reproduced in vitro by a brief exposure at 37°C to an unidentified low-molecular weight component of serum or plasma [16]. Paradoxically, the serum factor-induced decrease in accessibi-

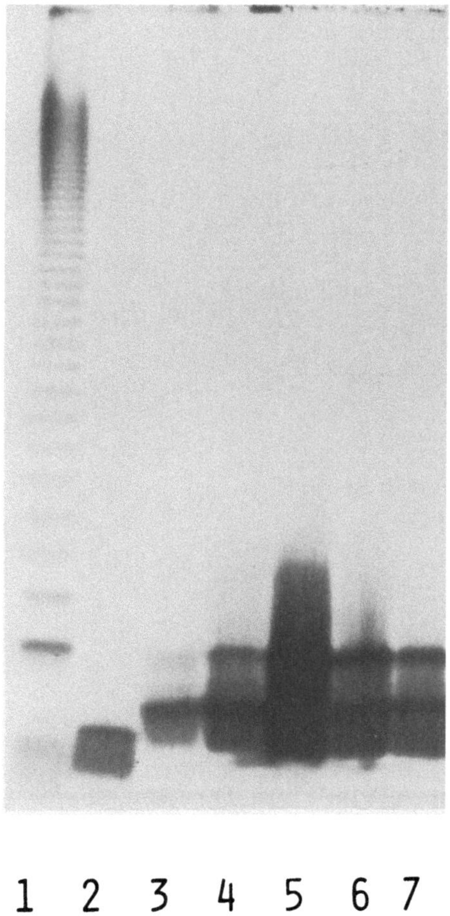

Fig. 1. Electrophoretic profiles of LPS preparations. *Lanes 1* and *2*, 10 µg of conventionally purified LPS from *S. typhimurium*, S type and R type, respectively; *lane 3*, 2 µg of conventionally purified LPS from *H. influenzae* type b (Hib) strain Eag; *lane 4*, 5 µl of crude extract from Hib Eag in the "sensitive" phenotype; *lanes 5-7*, 5 µl, 2.5 µl and 1.25 µl, respectively, of crude extract from Hib Eag in the "resistant" phenotype. Approximately 10^8 bacteria are represented by 5 µl of crude extract

lity of the LPS accompanies a rapid increase in LPS synthesis that results in a 4-fold increase in the cell's content of LPS within 30 min (Fig. 1, lanes 4-7). Conversion from the LPS antibody-sensitive to the resistant phenotype caused a 3-fold reduction in the binding of nonpiliated Hib to either human buccal or pharyngeal mucosal cells in vitro (Table 2). In the infant rat model the sensitive and resistant phenotypes are equally able to initiate colonization, but the organisms recoverable from the NP are in the resistant phenotype – indicating that NP secretions contain the factor(s) necessary for maintenance of the LPS antibody-resistant phenotype in NP colonization [15]. Thus, although the saccharide chains of LPS may have the potential for increasing the binding to mucosal cells, these may not be significantly expressed in vivo.

Table 2. Effect of the LPS antibody-sensitive or -resistant phenotypes upon the binding of nonpiliated *H. influenzae* b to human buccal or pharyngeal cells in vitro

Bacterial phenotype[c]	Bacteria bound by 2 × 10^5 cells	
	Buccal	Pharyngeal
Sensitive	245[a]	280[b]
Resistant	79[a]	92[b]

[a] $P = 0.02$
[b] $P = 0.02$
[c] Phenotype produced by incubation 30 min at 37°C at 10^7 cfu/ml in an ultrafiltrate of normal serum

Pilus

Pili or fimbriae have long been recognized on nontypable *H. influenzae*, particularly conjunctival strains, but were long sought and not found on Hib. Guerina et al. [4] and Pichichero et al. [13] reported the isolation of piliated Hib from the NP. These showed enhanced binding to human buccal and pharyngeal epithelial cells and to erythrocytes of all blood types, but not to the cells of nonhuman species; the binding is mannose resistant. These isolates proved to be rare strains in which the piliation was genetically stable. Most if not all strains of Hib as cultured in vitro contain a minority (roughly 0.1%) of piliated bacilli, and by selectively culturing those bacilli that adhere to human cells it is possible to generate highly piliated (≥98%) populations for study in vitro. The selected strains express pili with a specificity similar to the stably piliated strains [13] and have a similarly enhanced binding to human buccal cells in vitro (Table 3). Upon nonselective subculture in vitro the proportion of piliated bacilli slowly declines: hemagglutination (HA) of human erythrocytes typically became undetectable after about four additional transfers on solid medium (roughly 120 generations after selection for adherence). We have examined Hib isolates as soon as 1-2 transfers following primary isolation (thus 60-90 generations after residence in the body); of about 40 isolates from blood or cerebrospinal fluid, none has been found to be HA+ at this stage of study (although all examined have given rise to HA+ populations after subsequent selection). This finding indicates that the populations cultured from the body fluid specimens did not include a high proportion of piliated bacilli; further, it is in accord with the observation that the Hib examined by electron microscopy of freshly sampled cerebrospinal fluid from cases of suspected meningitis

Table 3. Adherence of *H. influenzae* b systemic isolates to human buccal epithelial cells in vitro

Strain	Number of bacteria attached/epithelial cell		
	Pili- variant	Pili+ variant	Rat blood reisolate[a]
(C54)	1.3[b]	9.8	3.2[c]
(C194)	1.0[b]	3.5	1.4
(S109)	0.3[b]	1.9	0.3[c]
(S113)	1.2[b]	4.8	1.4[c]
(S112)	0.8[b]	4.0	1.0[c]
(S124	0.4[b]	3.3	1.0[c]

[a]After inoculation with pili+ variant (see Table 4).
[b]$P < 0.05$, comparing attachment of pili- variant to pili+ variant for each strain.
[c]$P < 0.05$, comparing attachment of red blood isolate to pili+ variant for each strain.

displayed no pili (R. Goldstein and D.H. Smith, unpublished). Thus, if Hib are piliated upon invasion of the bloodstream, these observations imply either that pilus expression is counterselected systemically or that with a mixture of piliated and nonpiliated, only the latter are likely to be in suspension in the body fluid specimens. Investigation of the relation of pilus expression to colonization and invasion has been limited by the fact that the piliated Hib do not agglutinate the erythrocytes of nonhuman species. Presumably, the other cells of interest (mucosal, phagocytic, etc.) also lack receptors that bind the pilus; thus, animal model experiments would lack physiological relevance. Indeed, the binding of Hib to rat buccal epithelial cells in vitro was examined and found not to be significantly affected by piliation (not tabulated). However, despite the possible lack of relevance, curiosity led us to investigate the effect of piliation upon systemic infection in the infant rat model (Table 4). Nonpiliated and piliated populations of the six systemic isolates examined in Table 3 were inoculated intraperitoneally into infant rats, and bacteraemia and meningitis were scored after 48 h. The pili-negative population induced a significantly higher degree of bacteraemia than the piliated in four of the six strains and a higher frequency of meningitis in three of the six; in no strain was the piliated population more effective in induction of bacteraemia or meningitis. The colonies isolated from the blood after inoculation with piliated Hib were examined for agglutination of human erythrocytes and found uniformly to be HA-negative (not tabulated). One rat blood isolate from each of these strains was also tested for binding to human buccal epithelial cells in vitro (Table 3,

Table 4. Bacteraemia and meningitis after intraperitoneal inoculation of infant rats

Strain	Pili- variant			Pili+ variant		
	No. of rats studied	Bacteraemia (cfu/0.01 ml)	Meningitis (%)	No. of rats studied	Bacteraemia (cfu/0.01 ml)	Meningitis (%)
(C54)	5	172[a]	100[b]	5	11	0
(C194)	15	115[a]	60[b]	13	62	15
(S109)	8	626[a]	50	8	152	13
(S113)	6	295	80	6	542	50
(S112)	7	732[a]	100[b]	8	19	0
(S124)	5	283	40	8	271	25

[a] $P < 0.05$, comparing intensity of bacteraemia of the pili- variant to that of the pili+ variant.
[b] $P < 0.05$, comparing incidence of meningitis of the pili- variant to that of the pili+ variant.

last column); the binding was found to have declined to levels characteristic of the nonpiliated populations originally studied. Similar findings were recently reported from another laboratory [7]. Thus, in rats as in humans, either pilus expression was counterselected systemically or the nonpiliated progeny were selectively cultivable from body fluid specimens. We have speculated [13] that the genetic capacity for reversible expression/nonexpression of pili may be important in the pathogenesis of Hib - that piliation may be favored in NP colonization and transmission, while nonpiliated progeny might be better able to invade or persist systemically.

Conclusions

Mucosal colonization is obviously an important aspect of the host-parasite relationship of Hib, but the relevant variables have been less well studied than the other pathogens such as the *Neisseriae*. The infant rat model has some important similarities to human infection but, as mentioned above, is remiss in two valuable respects - the susceptibility of IgA_1 antibody to the *H. influenzae* protease and the apparent lack of receptors for the pilus. Human tissue culture models that have proved instructive with other bacterial pathogens have not yet been extensively applied to Hib. Studies on specific immunity have mainly focused upon circulating antibody, and only recently have secretory antibodies to Hib been examined. Mucosal antibodies to the Hib capsular polymer are present in normal humans [12] and rise in patients with systemic Hib infections [14]. Such antibodies have an obvious potential for influencing the outcome of a nasopharyngeal encounter with Hib. It is hoped that evidence bearing upon this and other questions raised here will be forthcoming in the near future.

References

1. Band JD, Fraser DW, Ajells G (1984) *Haemophilus influenzae* disease study group. Prevention of *Haemophilus influenzae* type b disease. JAMA 251: 2381-2386
2. Denny FW (1974) Effect of a toxin produced by *Haemophilus influenzae* on ciliated respiratory epithelium. J Infect Dis 129:93-100
3. Flesher AR, Insel RA (1978) Characterization of liposaccharide of *Haemophilus influenzae*. J Infect Dis 138:719-730
4. Guerina NG, Langermann S, Clegg HW, Kessler TW, Goldmann DA (1982) Adherence of piliated *Haemophilus influenzae* type b to human oropharyngeal cells. J Infect Dis 146:564-569
5. Hansen EJ, Frisch CF, Johnston KH (1981) Detection of antibody-accessible proteins on the cell surface of *Haemophilus influenzae* type b. Infect Immun 33:950-953
6. Insel RA, Allen PZ, Berkowitz ID (1982) Type and frequency of *Haemophilus influenzae* IgA 1 proteases. In: Seminars in infectious disease, volume IV: Bacterial vaccines. Thieme, New York Stuttgart
7. Kaplan SL, Mason EO, Wiedermann BL (1983) Role of adherence in the pathogenesis of *Haemophilus influenzae* type b infection in infant rats. Infect Immun 42:612-617

8. Kilian M (1976) A taxonomic study of the genus *Haemophilus*, with the proposal of a new species. J Gen Microbiol 93:9-62
9. Loeb MR, Smith DH (1980) Outer membrane composition in disease isolates of *Haemophilus influenzae*: pathogenic and epidemiologic implications.
10. Male C (1979) Immunoglobulin A1 protease production by *Haemophilus influenzae* and *Streptococcus pneumoniae*. Infect Immun 26:254-261
11. Moxon ER, Smith AL, Averill DR, Smith DH (1974) *Haemophilus influenzae* meningitis in infant rats after intranasal inoculation. J Infect Dis 129:154-160
12. Pichichero ME, Insel RA (1982) Relationship between naturally occurring human mucosal and serum antibody to the capsular polysaccharide of *Haemophilus influenzae* type b. J Infect Dis 146:243-247
13. Pichichero ME, Anderson P, Loeb M, Smith DH (1982) Do pili play a role in pathogenicity of *Haemophilus influenzae* type b? Lancet 30:960-963
14. Pichichero ME, Hall CB, Insel RA (1981) A mucosal antibody response following systemic *Haemophilus influenzae* type b infection in children. J Clin Invest 67:1482
15. Rubin LG, Moxon ER (to be published) Effect of serum factor-induced resistance upon the virulence of *Haemophilus influenzae* type b. J Gen Microbiol
16. Shaw S, Smith AL, Anderson P, Smith DH (1976) The paradox of *Haemophilus influenzae* type b bacteraemia in the presence of serum bactericidal activity. J Clin Invest 58:1019-1029
17. Turk DC, May JR (1967) *Haemophilus influenzae*: its clinical importance. English Universities Press, London

Discussion

(pp. 8-38)

Drs. McGhee and Morrison noted the similarity of the pathologic picture in human fallopian tubes infected with gonococci, human nasopharyngeal mucosa infected with meningococci, and rat trachea infected with *H. influenzae*, namely, sloughing of ciliated cells. They questioned Drs. McGee and Moxon regarding whether there was evidence for the participation of exotoxins or enzymes elaborated by these organisms that might result in sloughing of cells and whether the apparent specificity of lipopolysaccharide in producing this type of damage was related to the cabohydrate or lipid A portion of the LPS molecule.

Dr. McGee and Dr. Moxon indicated that there was no evidence of an enzyme which might, for instance, destroy intercellular bridges. Dr. McGee pointed out that the fact that filter-sterilized supernatant fluid from gonococcal infected human fallopian tube organ cultures was toxic after heating at 56°C for 30 min made it unlikely that such an enzyme was critical to the process. In addition, the damage in the respective gonococcal and *H. influenzae* models can be reproduced by highly purified LPS. Definitive experiments have not been done to determine if the apparent specificity of LPS resides in the lipid A or carbohydrate portions. Although LPS from other organisms, such as *E. coli*, does damage, it does so with considerably less specific activity.

Dr. McGhee asked about the relationship of attachment to subsequent transport across the mucosal barrier by nonciliated mucosal cells. Dr. Moxon responded by noting that *H. influenzae* very rapidly (in minutes) traverse the nasal mucosa of infant rats to cause bacteraemia. The mechanism is under study. Dr. McGee noted that transport of gonococci across the human fallopian tube mucosa is much slower; it is just beginning 24 h after infection. Nonetheless, some factor from the organisms – perhaps the protein 1 (the porin protein of gonococci) as suggested by Dr. Blake, or the LPS – seems to influence transport, since meningococci enter the cells in about half the time required for gonococcal entry. It is possible, as suggested by Dr. Moxon, that the microorganisms might spend prolonged periods in mucosal cells. Dr. McGhee suggested that Dr. Moxon's LPS mutants would be useful in addressing the possible role of LPS in the transport process.

Dr. Joiner asked Drs. Anderson and Moxon about the role of LPS in the greater resistance of some of Dr. Anderson's *H. influenzae* strains and the altered virulence of Dr. Moxon's LPS mutants as they relate to serum resistance. Dr. Anderson indicated that he had not detected differences in the LPS of more resistant strains. Dr. Moxon noted that the resurgence of *H. influenzae* in the blood after a delay might be proliferation of clones with more resistance to bactericidal activity but that that was unclear.

Dr. Sparling expressed concern that antibody to the antigen CB-2 which is common to all gonococcal and meningococcal pili had not blocked attachment and did not seem accessible in native pili when probed for by Drs. Robinson and McGee with gold particles labeled with anti-CB-2. Drs. Schoolnik and McGee pointed out that the original studies were done with purified pili which may have had some unfolding of their tertiary structure, whereas the studies in which anti-CB-2 failed to block attachment and to find its antigen were done with viable gonococci with native pili. Dr. Schoolnik pointed out that studies were underway with synthetic pilin subunit fragments which might circumvent the problem.

Bayer-Symposium VIII
The Pathogenesis of Bacterial Infections, 41-50 (1985)

The Molecular Organization of Gonococcal Pili

G. K. Schoolnik and J. B. Rothbard

Introduction

Pili are proteinaceous surface appendages of bacteria that promote infectivity by facilitating the adherence of gonococci to mucosal surfaces. Piliation is also correlated with the resistance of gonococci to phagocytosis by human polymorphonuclear leukocytes and mouse peritoneal macrophages [1, 2]. Pili are immunogenic and the anti-pili antibody elicited in humans by natural infection or systemic immunization with pili binds both strain-specific (homologous) and cross-reactive (common) antigenic determinants [3-5]. The molecular basis for the functional and antigenic properties of gonococcal pili is the subject of this paper.

Primary Structure of Gonococcal Pili

Each pilus filament is an assembly of up to 10 000 identical protein subunits, termed pilin, which polymerize to form a linear structure approximately 6 nm in diameter and 1000-4000 nm in length [6, 7]. Pili purified from different gonococcal strains possess subunit molecular weights that vary between 17 500 and 21 000 [8, 9]. The subunit molecular weights of pili from isogenic opaque (Op) and transparent (Tr) opacity variants may also differ [9-11].

Pili were purified from the transparent colonial variants of two gonococcal strains (R10 and MS11) isolated from patients with uncomplicated gonorrhea and their physicochemical and antigenic attributes compared. The subunit molecular weights of MS11 (Tr) and R10 (Tr) pilin were 17 500 and 16 400 respectively [12]. Although they competed for the same human erythrocyte receptor, they exhibited less than 5% shared antigenicity. Tryptic peptide maps of the two pilus preparations indicated that of the 22 peptides resolved by the system, 14 were identical; however, 30% of the peptides were different [12]. These observations indicate that differences in the primary structure of gonococcal pili exist and may be responsible for their physical and serologic diversity.

In order to determine regions within gonococcal pilin that mediate adherence function and antigenicity, the entire amino acid sequence of pilin from MS11 (Tr) and the sequence from constant and variable regions of R10 (Tr) pilin were determined by automated Edmund degradation of the intact protein and overlapping cyanogen bromide, citraconylated tryptic, and iodosobenzoic acid peptides [13]. The MS11 pilin sequence is comprised of 159 residues in a single polypeptide chain with two cysteines in disulfide linkage and serine-bonded phosphate residues (Fig. 1). The NH_2 terminal sequence of pilin from gonococcal strain R10 (Tr) was completed through residue 57 and found to be identical to the MS11 sequence. In contrast, NH_2 terminal amino acid sequencing of the MS11 and R10 CNBr-3 fragments (residues 93-159) revealed regions of substantial sequence heterogeneity (Fig. 2).

MePhe-Thr-Leu-Ile-Glu-Leu-Met-Ile-Val-Ile-Ala-Ile-Val-Gly-Ile-Leu-Ala-Ala-Val-Ala- 20

Leu-Pro-Ala-Tyr-Gln-Asp-Tyr-Thr-Ala-Arg-Ala-Gln-Val-Ser-Glu-Ala-Ile-Leu-Leu-Ala- 40

Glu-Gly-Gln-Lys-Ser-Ala-Val-Thr-Glu-Tyr-Tyr-Leu-Asn-His-Gly-Lys-Trp-Pro-Glu-Asn- 60

Asn-Thr-Ser-Ala-Gly-Val-Ala-Ser-Pro-Pro-Ser-Asp-Ile-Lys-Gly-Lys-Tyr-Val-Lys-Glu- 80

Val-Glu-Val-Lys-Asn-Gly-Val-Val-Thr-Ala-Thr-Met-Leu-Ser-Ser-Gly-Val-Asn-Asn-Glu- 100

Ile-Lys-Gly-Lys-Lys-Leu-Ser-Leu-Trp-Ala-Arg-Arg-Glu-Asn-Gly-Ser-Val-Lys-Trp-Phe- 120

Cys-Gly-Gln-Pro-Val-Thr-Arg-Thr-Asp-Asp-Asp-Thr-Val-Ala-Asp-Ala-Lys-Asp-Gly-Lys- 140

Glu-Ile-Asp-Thr-Lys-His-Leu-Pro-Ser-Thr-Cys-Arg-Asp-Lys-Ala-Ser-Asp-Ala-Lys (COOH)

Fig. 1. Covalent structure of P+Tr MS11 gonococcal pilin; MePhe, *N*-methylphenylalanine [13]

Receptor Binding Domain

Gonococcal pili appear to associate with epithelial cell surfaces by specific recognition of glycoconjugate receptor molecules that are stereochemically complementary to receptor binding residues in the pilin sequence. These residues are collectively termed the receptor binding domain. In order to identify receptor binding peptides of the pilus subunit, MS11 pilin was citraconylated and subjected to arginine-specific hydrolysis with trypsin (Fig. 3). ^{125}I- labeled TC-2 (residues 31-111) was employed in a radiobinding assay with human buccal cells, columnar epithelial cells aspirated from the endocervical canal of normal women of childbearing age, and HeLa cells. TC-2 exhibited saturable binding of endocervical cells, but did not bind buccal or HeLa cells [13]. These results indicate the following: (a) TC-2, a peptide derived from the conserved portion of the pilus sequence, encompasses receptor binding amino acids;

	93																	110
MS11	Leu	Ser	Ser	Gly	Val	Asn	Asn	Glu	Ile	Lys	Gly	Lys	Lys	Leu	Ser	Leu	Trp	Ala
R10	Ala	Ser	Ser	Asn	Val	Asn	Lys	Glu	Ile	Lys	Asp	Lys	(Lys)	Leu	Ser	Leu	Trp	Ala

	111																	128
MS11	Arg	Arg	Glu	Asn	Gly	Ser	Val	Lys	Trp	Phe	Cys	Gly	Gln	Pro	Val	Thr	Arg	Thr
R10	Lys	Arg	(Gln)	Ala	Gly	Ser	Val	Lys	Trp	Phe	Cys	Gly	Gln	Pro	Val	Thr	Arg	Ala

	129									138
MS11	Asp	Asp	Asp	Thr	Val	Ala	Asp	Ala	Lys	Asp
R10	Asp	(Lys)	(Asp)	(Asn)	Arg	Thr	Val	Ala	(Asp)	(Ala)

Fig. 2. Amino terminal 46 residue sequences of P+Tr MS11 and R10 CNBr-3 pilus fragments. Residues in parentheses were identified by reverse-phase HPLC of the Pth derivative, only. Identical residues are *boxed* [13]

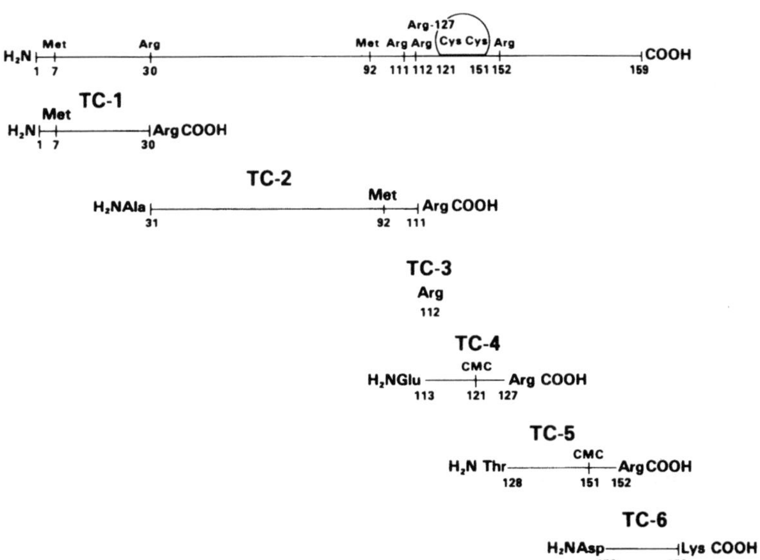

Fig. 3. Tryptic cleavage of reduced, carboxymethylated, and citraconylated MS11 pilin at arginine residues. TC-2 (residues 31-111) was purified, radiolabeled, and shown to exhibit saturable binding of human endocervical cells [13]

and (b) TC-2 can discriminate between epithelial surfaces and may thereby determine the tissue tropism and host range of gonococcal infection.

Common and Strain-Specific Antigenic Determinants

In order to identify regions of the gonococcal subunit that encompass strain-specific and common antigenic determinants, MS11 (Tr) and R10 (Tr) pilins were cleaved at methionine residues with cyanogen bromide (Fig. 4), and CNBr-2 (8-92) and CNBr-3 (93-159) were purified by reverse-phase HPLC. Antisera to MS11 and R10 pili and their CNBr-2 and CNBr-3 fragments were employed in a two-step competitive ELISA to determine their specificity (Fig. 5). Antibody to whole MS11 and R10 pili and their CNBr-3 fragments detected less than 5% shared antigenicity between heterologous undenatured pilus proteins [14]. In contrast, antibody to the MS11 and R10 CNBr-2 fragments detected more than 80% shared antigenicity. These experiments indicate that: (a) an epitope common to heterologous gonococcal pili exists in the conserved portion of the sequence between residues 8 and 92, is normally immunorecessive, but becomes immunodominant when the fragment encompassing it is cleaved from the intact subunit by cyanogen bromide cleavage of methionine residues; and (b) an immunodominant, strain-specific epitope is located in the variable portion of the sequence between residues 93 and 159. The precise location of these epitopes was sought by examining the antigenicity of synthetic peptides corresponding to regions of the MS11 pilin sequence.

Synthetic Peptide Analogs of Common and Strain-Specific Epitopes

Eight synthetic peptides corresponding to regions of sequence homology and diversity (Table 1) were prepared by the solid phase Merrifield method, conjugated to bovine serum albumin through cysteine residues with a heterobifunctional cross-linker,

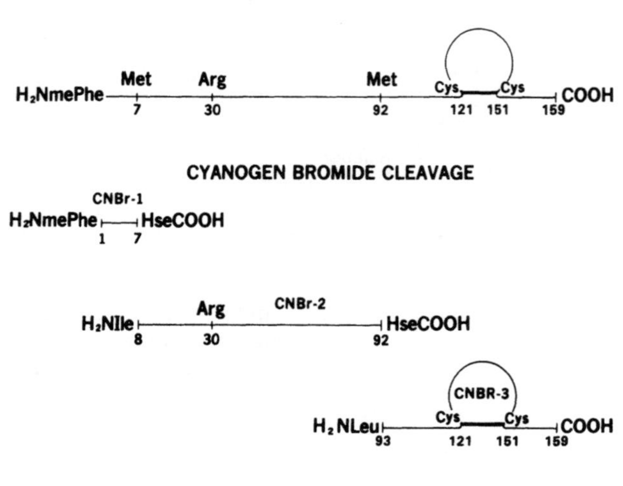

Fig. 4. Cyanogen bromide cleavage of MS11 pilin at methionine residues. CNBr-2 (8-92) and CNBr-3 (93-159) were purified by reverse-phase HPLC [13] and used as immunogens [14]

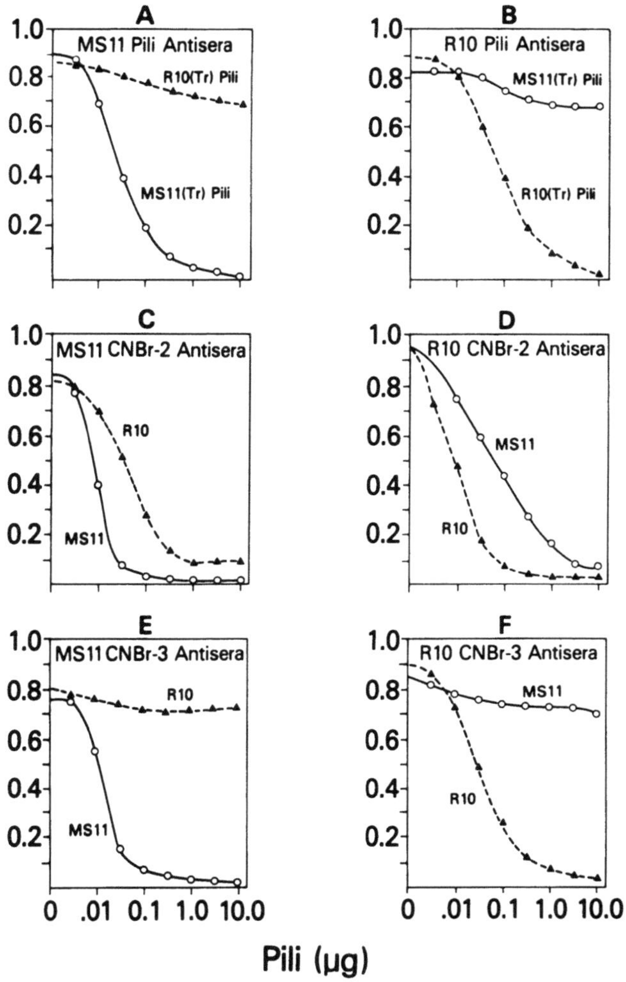

Fig. 5 A-F. The specificity of antisera generated against either intact MS11 pili, intact R10 pili, or each of their principal cyanogen bromide generated fragments, CNBr-2 (residues 8-92) and CNBr-3 (residues 93-159). Antisera against intact MS11 pili (A), MS11 CNBr-2 (C), and MS11 CNBr-3 (E) were assayed in a two-step competitive ELISA for their ability to bind wells coated with MS11 (Tr) pili in the presence of increasing amounts of either soluble R10 or MS11 pili (abscissa). Similarly, antisera against intact R10 pili (B), R10 CNBr-2 (D), and R10 CNBr-3 (F) were tested for their ability to bind wells coated with R10 (Tr) pili in the presence of increasing concentrations of soluble MS11 and R10 pili (abscissa) [14]

and employed as antigens in a solid phase binding assay with antibody to MS11 and R10 pili and their respective CNBr-2 and CNBr-3 fragments. Of the four peptides from the conserved portion of the sequence (21-35, 41-50, 48-60, and 69-84), antibody to MS11 and R10 pili bound only peptide 48-60 (Fig. 6 A,C) and both sera bound equally well [14]. In contrast, antisera to the MS11 and R10 CNBr-2 fragments (Fig. 6 B,D) bound peptides 69-84 and 48-60, and 41-50 and 69-84, respectively. These experiments indicate that an epitope common to both R10 and MS11 pili exists between residues 48-60 and that the immunogenicity of this region is determined by interactions present in intact pili, but absent from CNBr-2. Another common determinant, corresponding to residues 69-84, is exposed when CNBr-2 is used as an immunogen.

Table 1. Amino acid sequences of the eight synthetic oligopeptides and their corresponding location in MS11 pilin

Sequence	Location
L P A Y Q D Y T A R A Q V S E G C[a]	21–35
E G Q K S A V T E Y G C	41–50
T E Y Y L N H G K W P E N G C	48–60
P P S D I K G K Y V K E V E V K G C	69–84
C S G V N N E I K G K K L S	95–107
S L W A R R E N G S V K W F C	107–121
C G Q P V T R T D D D T V A	121–134
D A K D G K E I D T K H L P S T C	135–151

[a] Underlined residues do not exist in the primary structure of MS11 pilin. Additional glycine and cysteine residues were added as spacers and as a mode of attachment to carrier molecules, respectively

Of the four peptides from the variable portion of the sequence (95-107, 107-121, 121-134, and 135-151), antibody to MS11 pili and its CNBr-3 fragment bound only peptides 121-134 and 135-151 (Fig. 7A, B). Antibody to R10 pili did not bind these four peptide analogs of the MS11 sequence (Fig. 7C). These results indicate that peptides 121-134 and 135-151, which together comprise the entire intramolecular disulfide loop subtended by cysteine residues 121 and 151, encode a strain-specific epitope of MS11, but not R10 gonococcal pili [14]. In order to determine if these two peptides jointly specify a single strain-specific epitope or each specify a separate epitope, MS11 pili antiserum was absorbed with either 121-134 or 135-151 and the specificity of the absorbed serum for the heterologous peptide was determined. The absorbed and unabsorbed serum bound the heterologous peptide equally well (data not shown). These results indicate that each peptide encodes a separate, strain-specific epitope within the disulfide loop.

The structural basis by which the disulfide loop peptides determine antigenic diversity was analyzed by examining the available MS11 and R10 loop sequences for regions that might constitute unique epitopes. Variations in sequence between R10 and MS11 pilin occur within or adjacent to predicted β-turns, yet none of the substitutions affects the predicted secondary structure. Thus, both peptides that contain strain-specific determinants

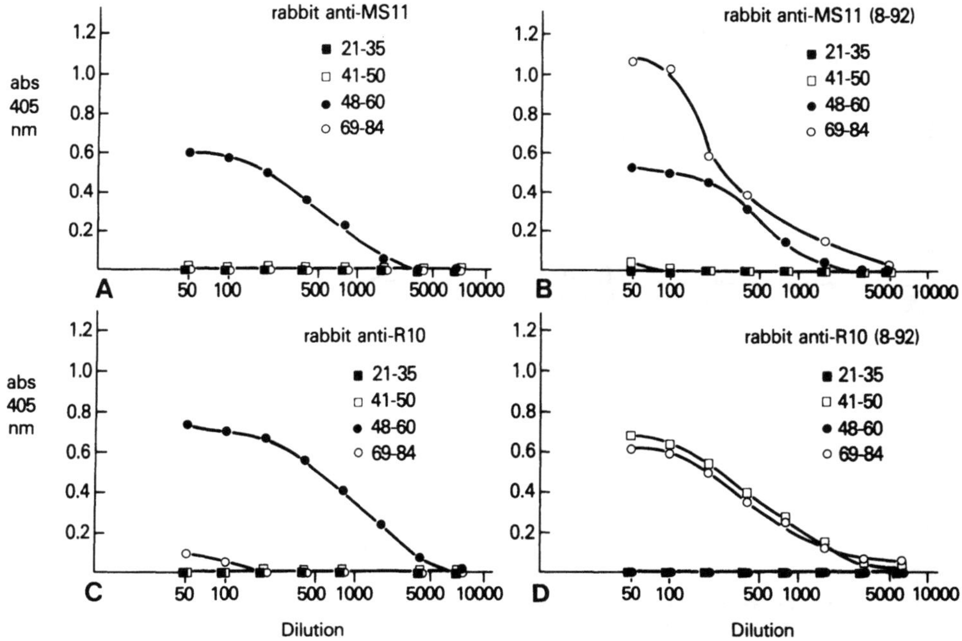

Fig. 6 A-D. Reaction of antigonococcal pili sera with peptide-BSA conjugates corresponding to regions of conserved sequence between strains. Anti-MS11 pili (A), anti-MS11 CNBr-2 (B), anti-R10 pili (C), and anti-R10 CNBr-2 (D) antisera were assayed for their ability to bind peptides corresponding to residues 21-35 (*full squares*), 41-50 (*open squares*), 48-60 (*full circles*), and 69-84 (*open circles*). The enzyme immunobinding assays were performed as described in [14]

(121-134 and 135-151) have a predicted turn around which the sequence variations are localized. Each peptide also contains a turn within which there exists a position where one strain has a lysine whereas the other contains an aspartic acid. Such a variation in sequence involving a double charge change could explain the total absence of cross-reactivity of the complementary antibody combining sites.

The location of the strain-specific determinants within the disulfide loop, a region of the protein shown not to be involved in receptor binding (as already discussed), may be part of a sophisticated molecular design that enables the organism to segregate its principal antigenic determinants in a region distinct from the residues involved in epithelial cell surface adherence [14]. By using a disulfide loop, the molecule may have evolved a domain that: (a) prominently orients the region on the surface of the molecule, perhaps even projecting out from the polymeric structure, resulting in its increased antigenicity and immunogenicity; (b) allows amino acid substitutions, additions, and deletions within the antigenic determinants, thereby maximizing antigenic variation, without disrupting areas critical for the

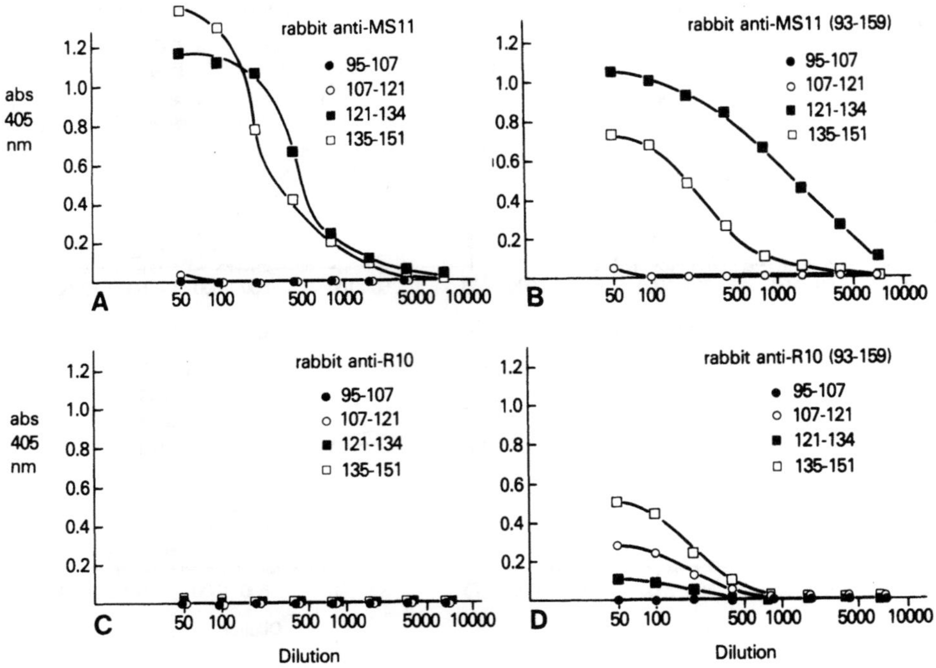

Fig. 7 A–D. Reaction of antigonococcal pili sera with peptide-BSA conjugates corresponding to regions of sequence variation between strains. Anti-MS11 pili (A), anti-MS11 CNBr-3 (B), anti-R10 pili (C), and anti-R10 CNBr-3 (D) antisera were assayed for their ability to bind peptides corresponding to residues 95-107 (*full circles*), 107-121 (*open circles*), 121-134 (*full squares*), and 135-151 (*open squares*) of the MS11 pilin sequence. The enzyme-linked immunobinding assays were performed as described in [14]

biologic role of the protein; and (c) permits an antibody to bind pili and yet not interfere with gonococcal adhesion to the mucosal cell surface.

The immunodominant character of the variable portion of the sequence can be compared with the immunorecessive character of the conserved, receptor binding segment. Less than 15% of the entire antigenicity of pili, as determined by summing the antigenicity of the eight synthetic peptide analogs of the MS11 sequence, resides in peptide 48-60 [14], a natural epitope within the receptor binding tryptic fragment, TC-2. In contrast, approximately 40% of the antigenicity resides in each of the two strain-specific epitopes of the disulfide loop [14]. These data provide a quantitative explanation for the inability of a pilus vaccine prepared from one strain to confer heterologous protection.

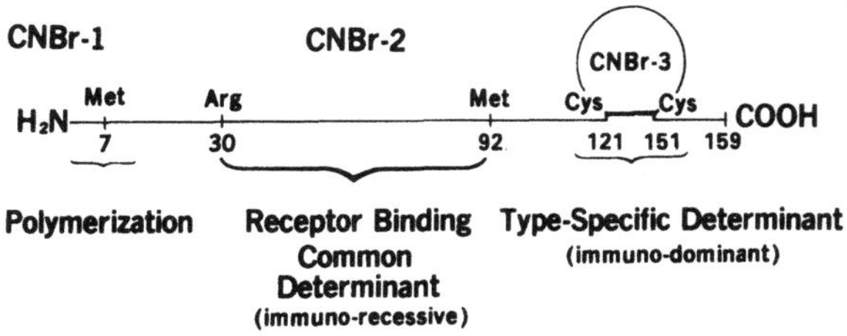

Fig. 8. Molecular organization of gonococcal pilin. CNBr-3 contains an immunodominant, variable segment within the disulfide loop that confers strain-specific antigenicity. CNBr-2 and TC-2 encompass a conserved region that contains receptor binding residues and an immunorecessive common epitope

Summary and Conclusions

The molecular organization of gonococcal pilin is depicted in Fig. 8. CNBr-3 encompasses a variable, immunodominant region that determines strain-specific antigenicity. CNBr-2 is immunorecessive and contains receptor binding residues. A common epitope is evident between residues 48 and 50, but is responsible for less than 15% of the molecule's total antigenicity. However, synthetic peptide analogs of the conserved, receptor binding region might elicit cross-reacting antibodies that block the adherence properties of pili. When included as part of a multicomponent gonorrhea vaccine, these might abrogate infectivity by inhibiting the colonization phase of pathogenesis. Studies of the immunogenicity of the synthetic peptides described in this paper are in progress.

References

1. Dilworth JA, Hendley JO, Mandell GL (1975) Attachment and ingestion of gonococci by human neutrophils. Infect Immun 11:512-516
2. Jones RB, Newland JC, Olsen DA, Buchanan TM (1980) Immune-enhanced phagocytosis of *Neisseria gonorrhoeae* by macrophages: characterization of the major antigens to which opsonins are directed. J Gen Microbiol 121:365-372
3. Buchanan TM (1975) Antigenic heterogeneity of gonococcal pili. J Exp Med 141:1470-1475
4. Novotny P, Turner WH (1975) Immunological heterogeneity of pili of *Neisseria gonorrhoeae*. J Gen Microbiol 89:87-92
5. Brinton CC, Bryan J, Dillon JA, Guerina N, Jacobson LJ, Kraus S, Labik A, Lee S, Levene A, Lim S, McMichael J, Polen S, Rogers K, To Acc, To Scm (1978) Uses of pili in gonorrhea control: role of pili in disease, purification and properties of gonococcal pili and progress in the development of a gonococcal pilus vaccine for gonorrhea. In: Brooks GF (ed) Immunobiology of *Neisseria gonorrhoeae*. American Society for Microbiology, Washington, p 155
6. Swanson J, Kraus SJ, Gotschlich EC (1971) Studies on gonococcus infection. I. Pili and zones of adhesion: their relation to gonococcal growth patterns. J Exp Med 134:886-906

7. Jephcott AE, Reyn A, Birch-Andersen A (1971) *Neisseria gonorrhoeae.* III. Demonstration of presumed appendages to cells from different colony types. Acta Pathol Microbiol Immunol Scand [B] 79:437-439
8. Hermodson MA, Chen KCS, Buchanan TM (1978) Neisseria pili proteins: aminoterminal amino acid sequences and identification of an unusual amino acid. Biochemistry 17:442-445
9. Robertson JP, Vincent P, Ward ME (1977) The preparation and properties of gonococcal pili. J Gen Microbiol 102:169-177
10. Salit IE, Blake M, Gotsclich EC (1980) Intra-strain heterogeneity of gonococcal pili is related to opacity colony variance. J Exp Med 151: 716-725
11. Lambden PR, Robertson JN, Watt PJ (1980) Biological properties of two distinct pilus types produced by isogenic variants of *Neisseria gonorrhoeae* P9. J Bacteriol 141:393-396
12. Schoolnik GK, Tai JY, Gotschlich EC (1983) A pilus peptide vaccine for the prevention of gonorrhea. Prog Allergy 33:314-331
13. Schoolnik GK, Fernandez R, Tai JY, Rothbard JB, Gotschlich EC (1984) Gonococcal pili: primary structure and receptor binding domain. J Exp Med 159:1351-1370
14. Rothbard JB, Fernandez R, Schoolnik GK (1984) Strain specific and common epitopes of gonococcal pili. J Exp Med

Bayer-Symposium VIII
The Pathogenesis of Bacterial Infections, 51-66 (1985)

Functions of the Outer Membrane Proteins of *Neisseria gonorrhoeae*

M. S. Blake

Summary

The functional aspects of purified major outer membrane proteins of *Neisseria gonorrhoeae* are described. These proteins are isolated in a novel way using calcium, zwitterionic detergent, and ethanol. By chemical analysis and amino terminal sequence, most of the proteins fall into three major families. Evidence will be given that would suggest that the protein II associated with opacity functions is in a receptor-ligand relationship with a portion of the lipopolysaccharide carbohydrate moiety. Also, evidence will be presented for the possible roles which the transfer of protein I from the gonococcal outer membrane to other membranes may have in the infectious process.

Introduction

Like that of all gram-negative organisms, the gonococcal outer membrane surrounds the cytoplasmic cell surface. It has been proposed that this semipermeable membrane protects the cellular machinery from destructive matter in the environment, but at the same time allows entry of vitamins and nutrients needed by the organism [1]. Such a membrane is unique in nature and thus is made up of many unusual components. The hydrophobic constituents are mainly phosphatidylethanolamine, located primarily on the inner lipid leaflet, and lipopolysaccharide (LPS), a very unusual molecule, located on the outer surface. The membrane is made semipermeable by a group of proteins which have been named porins. These proteins form aqueous channels which allow molecules of a particular size and charge to penetrate this membrane freely [1]. This seems to be the basic format of a gram-negative outer membrane: the LPS and phospholipids to make it impermeable and protect against lipid destructive agents, and the porin to make it semipermeable. These components are modified or others added as dictated by the particular niche exploited by the gram-negative organism.

Because *Neisseria gonorrhoeae* is constantly exposed to the selective pressures of the human immune response, it has evolved some rather surprising mechanisms to evade these and exploit its environment. Some of these involving pili are discussed by Schoolnik and Rothbard in this volume. We would like to understand the structure and the molecular interactions of the other proteins found in the gonococcal outer membrane. This information might further our knowledge of how these proteins function within the human host.

Nomenclature

The development of the simple and very powerful technique of separating proteins by SDS-PAGE has allowed us to compare easily the outer membrane proteins from numerous strains of gonococci. In such a comparison, one can observe that the electrophoretic behavior of these proteins falls into three major families. Members of each family demonstrate several common attributes. The proteins I are the most abundant protein present in the gonococcal outer membrane, have a molecular weight between 38 000 and 32 000, and are not affected either by heat or treatment with mercaptoethanol. Proteins II have varying molecular weights, depending on the temperature of the SDS extraction buffer, i.e., when these proteins are solubilized at 37°C, they have lower molecular weights than when solubilized at higher temperatures. These proteins are the so-called heat-modifiable proteins. Analogous proteins have been seen in other gram-negative bacteria. Protein III is defined by its shift to a higher molecular weight when treated with mercaptoethanol, but is unaffected by extraction temperature. All gonococci analyzed by this method so far have contained at least one member of the protein I group and one of the protein III class (lane B, Fig. 1). The presence of one or several of the protein II group may be observed, and thus appear optional (compare lanes B and G, Fig. 1).

Structure

Our knowledge of the structure of the proteins in the various families is very limited. It was derived by adding proteolytic enzymes to isolated gonococcal outer membranes and allowing the enzymes to cleave surface-exposed areas of the proteins. The bacterial membranes were then reisolated by centrifugation and the proteins analyzed by SDS-PAGE. Several different strains were used and comparisons in SDS-PAGE protein patterns were made [2].

Protein I

Each particular strain of gonococcus expressed only one member of the protein I group. The proteins I varied in molecular weight, ranging from 38 000 to 32 000, depending on the strain. In comparing numerous strains of gonococci and the ability of the enzymes to cleave protein I, it was found that proteins I of higher molecular weight were degraded by the enzymes while those of lower molecular weight were unaffected. The SDS-PAGE protein profiles of the cleaved, higher molecular weight proteins I showed that two portions of these molecules remained attached to the membrane. When chymotrypsin was used it appeared to cleave protein I at one site, and the molecular weights

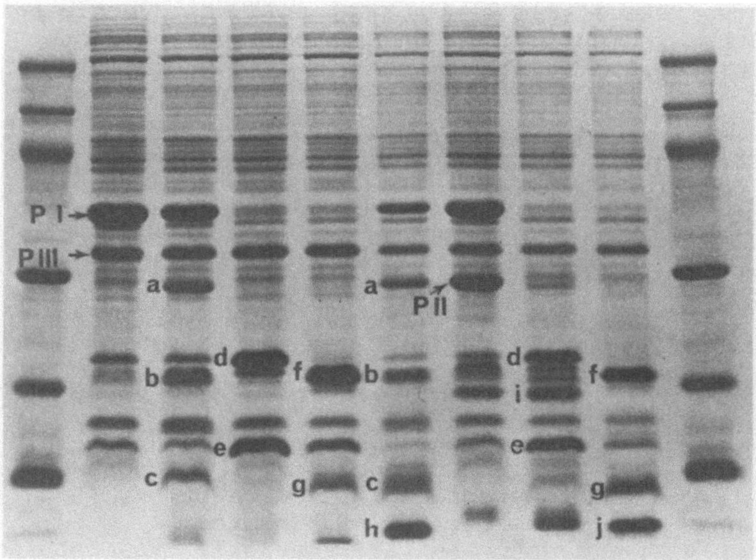

Fig. 1. SDS-PAGE analysis of purified outer membranes from Op- (*lanes B-E*) and Op+ (*lanes F-I*) variants of gonococci to which trypsin (*lanes C, F*), chymotrypsin (*lanes D, H*), and pronase (*lanes E, I*) was added. After 30 min, the membranes were reisolated by ultracentrifugation and subjected to SDS-PAGE. *Lanes B, G* contain membranes not subjected to proteolysis. The markers in lanes *A, J* are from top to bottom: human transferrin (80K), catalase (60K), ovalbumin (45K), carbonic anhydrase (30K), soybean trypsin inhibitor (21K), and cytochrome *c* (12K). The protein I (P I) species of the Op+ and Op- variants migrated identically and the Op+ control contained the opacity-associated protein II (P II). All samples contained protein III (P III). The peptide fragments of protein I are identified on the figure by *lowercase letters* as follows: *a, b, c* are trypsin fragments of protein I; *d, e* are chymotrypsin fragments of protein I; *f, g* are pronase fragments of protein I; and *h, i, j* are trypsin, chymotrypsin, and pronase fragments of protein II, respectively

of the two remaining segments equaled that of the intact protein (lane D, Fig. 1). Trypsin appeared to cleave protein I in two areas and release a portion of the molecule from the membrane. This resulted in two lower molecular weight peptides being recovered with the membrane (lane C, Fig. 1). Treatment with exopeptidases appeared to have no effect on the proteins I.

From these data, we constructed a simple representation of how protein I may be arranged in the membrane of the gonococcus. The data would suggest that protein I is associated with the membrane in at least two regions of the molecule with both the carboxy and amino terminus protected within the membrane. The middle portion of the molecule extends out of the membrane as a loop, and it is in this exposed region where the cleavage by the enzymes occurs. Because all of the protein I was hydrolyzed by the enzymes, this indicated that the molecule has only one orientation, with the loop portion exposed on the surface.

Protein II

Using the same techniques, we found that proteins II were cleaved, releasing large portions of the molecule from the membrane. After treatment with chymotrypsin, approximately two-thirds of the molecule remained with the membrane as one peptide (lane H, Fig. 1). Trypsin cleaved protein II, leaving a very small membrane-bound fragment (lane F, Fig. 1). We thus envision proteins II as extending out from the membrane surface and having only one membrane-associated segment.

Protein III

Of all the proteins of the gonococcal outer membrane, protein III remains the most enigmatic. It has been shown by cross-linking studies [3, 4] and immunoprecipitation reactions [5] that this protein is closely associated with protein I. This arrangement, although far from definite, is usually two or three proteins I to every protein III. Furthermore, when it is in a purified form, this protein can be easily cleaved by proteolytic enzymes; however, associated with the bacterial membrane (as can be seen in Fig. 1) it is completely resistant to degradation. One can hypothesize that very little of this protein is exposed on the surface and thus the sites of potential enzyme cleavage are protected by the outer membrane. However, experiments using both monoclonal [5] and polyclonal antibodies to this molecule would suggest that at least some portions of protein III are readily available to interact with antibody molecules. How this paradox is resolved in the structure of protein III remains unanswered.

Purification and Chemical Analysis

We have developed in our laboratory a very rapid method of extracting outer membrane proteins. This method has been used successfully not only with gonococci [6], but also with meningococci, *Legionella pneumophila*, and some *Yersinia* species. We have found that the outer membrane proteins from gonococci and these other gram-negative bacteria could be quantitatively solubilized in the presence of high concentrations of calcium and a zwitterionic detergent. This extraction procedure seemed to be dependent on the pH. Proteins I and proteins II were extracted at a pH of 4.0, which left protein III still associated with the bacterial membrane. By reextracting the bacteria at a pH of 10.2, protein III could then be solubilized. Further purification of the proteins was accomplished by ion exchange and molecular sieve column chromatography. The yield for each of the individual proteins varied from approximately 70% to 90%.

Protein I

The first outer membrane proteins to be isolated using this method were the various proteins I. The isoelectric points of these proteins ranged from 5.0 to 8.0, depending on the strain. By GLC analysis, no carbohydrate moieties could be detected, and no phosphates were measured by phosphorus analysis. The amino acid composition of one protein I is shown in Table 1 and is representative of all those so far examined. The purified proteins I are trimers of a single peptide somewhat analogous to the porins of other gram-negative bacteria. These trimers retained their strain-specific enzymatic susceptibility, antigenicity, and channel-forming capability. The amino terminus of many of these proteins has been sequenced and is shown in Fig. 2. As can be seen, this portion is highly conserved among the various strains of gonococci as well as in one strain of meningococcus.

Protein II

Depending on the strain and the state of colony morphology within that strain, any number of proteins II can be isolated from the gonococcus. These can be classified into two types: those associated with the phenomenon of opacity variation (pIIop) and those lacking this correlation (pIInop). Colonial opacity variation was first described by James and Swanson [7, 8]. When gonococci are grown on agar and the colonies observed with a dissecting microscope by direct lighting, the colonies appear transparent blue (Op-), granular opaque (Op+), or somewhat in between. Any one colony type can be propagated by single colony passages to obtain a uniform population. Gonococci of the Op+ colony phenotype were shown to express one or two additional proteins not present in the isogenic transparent colony-forming gonococci. These proteins have been called the opacity-associated proteins. By electron microscopy, it was also observed that organisms of

	5 10
R10 (pI 34)	ASP-VAL-THR-LEU-TYR-GLY-ALA-ILE-LYS-ALA
33 (pI 33)	VAL-THR-LEU-TYR-GLY-ALA-ILE-LYS-ALA
120176-2 (pI 32)	ASP-VAL-THR-LEU-TYR-GLY-THR-ILE-LYS-ALA
BNCV (pI 41)	ASP-VAL-SER-LEU-GLY-GLU-ILE-LYS-ALA-GLY
R10 (pIIop)	ALA-GLY-GLU-ASP-GLU-GLY-GLY-ARG-GLY-PRO
MS11 (pIIop)	ALA-SER-GLU-GLU-GLY-GLY-ARG-GLY-PRO-TYR
R10 (pIInop)	ALA-SER-GLU-ASP-GLY-GLY-ARG-GLY-PRO-TYR
R10 (pIII)	GLY-GLU-ALA-SER-VAL-GLU-GLY-TYR-XXX-VAL

Fig. 2. Amino terminal amino acid sequences of gonococcal outer membrane proteins

Table 1. Composition of proteins I, II, and III

Amino acids	Protein I	Protein II	Protein III
Neutral	206[a] (0.67)[b]	163 (0.62)	175 (0.63)
Aliphatic	162 (0.53)	147 (0.56)	138 (0.49)
Glycine	42	32	20
Alanine	27	26	34
Valine	27	29	29
Leucine	18	15	17
Isoleucine	6	11	9
Serine	27	21	18
Threonine	15	13	11
Aromatic	27 (0.09)	10 (0.04)	15 (0.05)
Phenylalanine	12	5	7
Tyrosine	15	5	8
Tryptophan			
Sulfur-containing	5 (0.02)	5 (0.02)	6 (0.02)
Half cystine	1		2
Methionine	4	5	4
Imino acids/proline	12 (0.04)	1 (0.003)	16 (0.06)
Dicarboxylic amino acids	69 (0.23)	58 (0.22)	63 (0.22)
Aspartic/asparagine	33	42	26
Glutamic/glutamine	36	16	37
Basic amino acids	30 (0.10)	41 (0.16)	41 (0.15)
Histidine	6	4	4
Arginine	6	22	20
Lysine	18	15	17
Total	305	262	279

[a]Number of moles residue per mole protein.
[b]Fraction of total number of residues represented in each class.

the opaque phenotype have numerous intracellular adhesions. These adhesions disappear when the bacteria are treated with either chymotrypsin or trypsin. The pIIop proteins have very alkaline isoelectric points, ranging from 9.5 to 10.0. The amino acid analysis of these proteins (Table 1) reflects their basic nature and their susceptibility to trypsin, as they contain several residues of lysine and arginine. These proteins migrated as monomers in contrast to the trimers of protein I. The amino terminal sequence of several pIIop (Fig. 2) shows homologous regions among these proteins and indicates their relationship to each other.

Other proteins II, pIInop, lack any correlation with the opacity phenotype. One of these proteins was first described by Swanson and co-workers [9] and later was more fully characterized by King and Swanson [10]. They called this protein the "leukocyte association factor". They examined isogenic pairs of gonococci, one expressing this protein and the other not. They found that those expressing leukocyte association factor were more adherent to human leukocytes than their isogenic counterpart lacking this protein. These pIInop proteins have a much lower isoelectric point as compared with the opacity-associated proteins II, ranging from 7.5 to 8.0. Their relationship to other proteins II is reflected in their heat modifiability, accessibility to enzyme degradation, and in their amino terminal sequence.

Protein III

As compared with proteins I which have strain-dependent variations and proteins II which have both strain and intrastrain variability, protein III seems to be the exception. This protein has been observed in all gonococcal strains and appears structurally and antigenically identical. Wong and Johnston [11] showed that the peptide maps of this protein from several strains appeared the same. The cross-reactivity of antiserum made to protein III seemed to confirm this observation. The close association of protein I with protein III has been shown with cross-linking reagents [4, 3] and by immunoprecipitation of either protein I or protein III [5]. In the purification of protein I, we found that it is important to separate protein III from protein I in the initial extraction. Once extracted, it was difficult, if not impossible, to separate the two proteins. This gave us further evidence for the interaction between the two proteins. By extracting the bacteria at pH 4.0, we found that protein I was released from protein III which remained insoluble. Protein III was then recovered by reextracting the bacteria at a higher pH. The isoelectric point of this protein is 8.6, and it is a monomer in solution. The amino acid composition is shown in Table 1. As shown in Fig. 2, its separate class distinction is seen in its amino terminal sequence being quite different from the proteins I and II.

Functional Aspects

The study of the functional contributions of surface-exposed gonococcal proteins in gonorrhea has been initiated only recently. Besides the work describing the function of gonococcal pili, very little is known about how the other gonococcal outer membrane proteins might aid in the invasion process. Some of our preliminary data will be given on the molecular interactions of pIIop and gonococcal LPS and the possible role this may play in the pathogenicity of this organism. We will further describe some of the evidence we have for the multiple functions of the proteins I.

Opacity-Associated Proteins II (pIIop)

Swanson [8], in his original description of gonococcal opacity variants, demonstrated by electron microscopy that gonococci expressing pIIop had numerous intercellular adhesions. These attachments between gonococci disappeared upon trypsin or chymotrypsin treatment. This would suggest that pIIop mediates the binding of one cell to another in a receptor-ligand fashion. Chymotrypsin, as we have shown, cleaved this protein, releasing the distal third of the molecule from the membrane. This would suggest that the active site on pIIop is located within this region. Furthermore, during the isolation of this protein, we found pIIop to migrate as a monomer with no other proteins copurifying with it. Thus, it would appear that the pIIop ligand is not protein, but another gonococcal surface component.

Using purified pIIop bound to a microtiter plate, we found in an ELISA assay that these proteins were able to bind purified gonococcal LPS. The LPS was purified from the homologous strain as the proteins II and detected either by a monoclonal antibody to the LPS or by wheat germ agglutinin. In contrast, when pIInop isolated from the same strain was used in the assay, no binding activity for LPS was found (Fig. 3). Furthermore, the purified LPS could inhibit the binding of a pIIop monoclonal antibody.

We also found the reverse to be true. LPS was bound to the microtiter plates and pIIop added thereafter. The presence of pIIop was detected by the pIIop monoclonal antibody (Fig. 4). The pIIop protein could also inhibit the binding of a monoclonal antibody to the bound LPS, but not as effectively as the acid-cleaved polysaccharide. To demonstrate that pIIop in its native membrane environment was also active, we added purified gonococcal outer membranes to LPS-sensitized ELISA plates. The membranes were detected using a monoclonal antibody to protein I of these organisms. The membranes from Op+ organisms bound to the LPS, while those from Op- organisms or chymotrypsin-treated Op+ membranes did not.

These experiments would suggest that the receptor site of pIIop is located somewhere in the distal third of the molecule. The ligand for pIIop is most likely a portion of the carbohydrate moiety of LPS. We are presently trying to define more clearly both the area on pIIop responsible for this activity and the carbohydrate to which it binds. Once this ligand is known, we will explore the possibility as to whether similar carbohydrates may exist on eukaryotic cells. Thus, the expression of pIIop by gonococci would serve two functions: (a) to hold clumps of organisms together in a microcolony which is attached to the

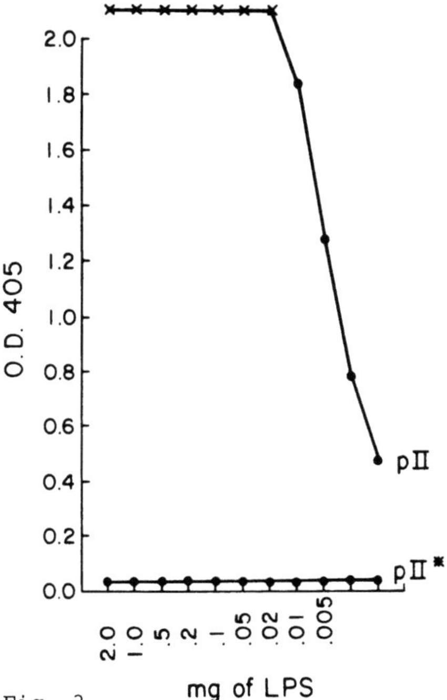

Fig. 3

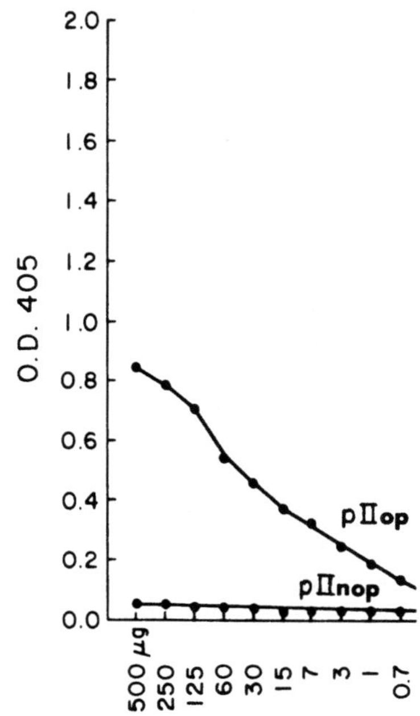

Fig. 4

Fig. 3. Microtiter plates were sensitized with an opacity-associated protein II (pII) and a non-opacity-associated protein II (pII*) at 4 µg/ml. Purified gonococcal LPS was then added and diluted as shown. After incubation and washing, the LPS bound by the proteins II was detected by sequential addition of 1.0 µg/ml wheat germ agglutinin, rabbit anti-wheat germ agglutinin, goat anti-rabbit alkaline phosphates conjugated antibody, and finally *p*-nitrophenyl phosphate

Fig. 4. Microtiter plates were sensitized with gonococcal LPS at 2.5 µg/ml. Purified proteins II were then added and diluted as shown. After incubation and washing, the proteins II bound by the LPS were detected by sequential addition of a protein II monoclonal antibody (4B12/C11), goat anti-mouse alkaline phosphatase conjugated antibody, and finally *p*-nitrophenyl phosphate

epithelium by relatively few pili; and (b) to increase the association between the bacterial membrane and the membrane of the epithelial cell.

Proteins I

Channel-forming proteins have now been documented in many gram-negative bacteria [1]. In most cases, these porins make up the majority of the proteins located in the outer membrane of these organisms. It is through these aqueous channels, it is thought, that nutrients and other small molecules are allowed to penetrate to the cytoplasmic membrane. The size and ionic preference varies between species and also within a species. Once having purified proteins I from several gonococcal strains, we began examining them for their specific channel characteristics.

Channel Characteristics

The characterization of the gonococcal channel-forming proteins I was performed in collaboration with The Rockefeller University's Biophysics Laboratory headed by Dr. Alex Mauro. Originally, protein I was inserted into Montal [12] planar lipid bilayers by mixing protein I with the lipids which made up one of the lipid leaflets [13]. In later experiments, proteins I were incorporated into liposomes of asolectin or phosphatidylethanolamine and then fused with a preformed lipid bilayer [14, 15]. The purified protein I from each of the gonococcal strains exhibited channel-forming activity, producing rapid step-like changes in conductance across the membrane [13-15]. The smallest observed step depended on the purified protein I used, with a range between 0.15 and 0.4 nS. The macroscopic conductance of all the proteins showed strain-specific voltage dependence and an asymmetric polarity dependence [14, 15]. Both the single channel fluctuations and continuous voltage ramp experiments suggested that the proteins I preferentially self-associate into functional triplets [14]. Because some of the proteins I were sensitive to proteolytic enzyme digestion, we were able to confirm that this protein is asymmetrically arranged in the artificial membrane. Chymotrypsin modified the macroscopic conductance observed, depending upon to which side of the planar lipid bilayer it was added [13]. All proteins I were anion-specific channels, each preferring chloride over sodium somewhat differently, with a range from 6 to 1 down to 3 to 1 [15].

Transfer of Protein I

Using preformed planar lipid bilayers as described and suspending viable bacteria in one of the buffer chambers, we have observed rapid changes in membrane conductance almost identical to that seen with the purified proteins I. Although the minimal channel conduction was identical to the homologous protein I, the polarity dependence is reversed [13]. Using our loop-like model of protein I, this suggested that the loop structure of protein I exposed on the gonococcus was able to penetrate the lipid bilayer and appear on the opposite side of the planar lipid bilayer. This ability to induce channels into the planar lipid bilayers seemed to be strain and protein I dependent [15]. Thus, channels from strains expressing low molecular weight, enzyme-resistant proteins I were transferred from the bacteria to the lipid bilayers more frequently than from strains expressing higher molecular weight, enzyme-susceptible proteins I. Two other neisserial species were used to compare their channel-inserting activities: one strain of *Neisseria sicca* showed no activity even at very high concentrations of bacteria, whereas the one group B *Neisseria meningitidis* strain was extremely efficient in transferring its porin into the bilayers. In these experiments, there seemed to be an interesting correlation between the frequency of channel induction and the diagnosis of the patient from whom the particular strain was isolated. With one exception, each strain producing a low molecular weight, enzyme-resistant protein I was isolated from a systemic gonococcal infection. The one exception has since been protein I serotyped by Dr. Joan Knapp at the Neisseria Reference Laboratory and found to be serologically identical to one of the other blood isolates. Each of these strains induced higher channel-forming activity than those strains isolated from patients with a local urethral infection.

The induction of channels by bacteria with reverse polarity dependence indicated to us that this transfer was not a fusion event. A fusion of outer membranes with the bilayer would orient the porin in the same way as that seen using the purified proteins. This would suggest that if gonococci with an enzyme-susceptible loop were mixed with an intact eukaryotic cell and transfer of protein I occurred, the protein would no longer be susceptible to enzyme degradation in the usual way. Using human red blood cells or HeLa cells and chymotrypsin as the enzyme, we were able to observe significant amounts of uncleaved protein I associated with the eukaryotic cells. Upon lysis of the cells and addition of the enzyme, the protein I was then degraded in a typical fashion.

The transfer of proteins between two membranes, as we have seen with the gonococcal protein I, is not without precedent. Other studies have shown that intrinsic membrane proteins can be transferred to lipid vesicles upon intimate contact [16-21]. These reports demonstrate that the transfer of proteins between membranes is facilitated when the recipient membrane is more fluid than the donor [18]. In collaboration with Dr. F.R. Landsberger, we have examined by electron spin resonance (ESR) the fluidity of both Op+ and Op- gonococcal membranes. Isolated gonococcal membranes from both phenotypes were labeled with either a C5 or C16 spin label. The ESR spectra of these membranes were compared with each other and with labeled membranes treated with proteolytic enzymes (Table 2). It was noticed in the ESR spectra of C16 spin-labeled gonococcal outer membranes (Fig. 5) that there appeared to be a superposition of two types of spectra. One is represented by the three relatively sharp line shapes (low field marked by *F* in Fig. 5) which reflected the comparatively fluid environment of the center region of the lipid bilayer. The shoulder region (marked by *B* in Fig. 5) suggested the presence of another superimposed second spectrum in which the spin label is immobilized. An arbitrary ratio of the free lipid (marked *F*) to bound can be made to semiquantitate the amount of this bound lipid. This ratio *R* would decrease as more lipid is aggregated into a bound form. Table 3 shows that, upon addition of increasing amounts of calcium, *R* decreases. The decrease in *R* would reflect an increasing amount of immobilized lipid. In summary, the ESR data indicated: (a) the membranes from Op+ organisms were less fluid than membranes from Op- organisms and this difference was unaffected by the addition of proteolytic enzymes; (b) there are lipid regions within gonococcal membranes which are relatively immobilized and these areas can be increased with calcium; and (c) in comparison with eukaryotic membranes, the gonococcal outer membrane is much less fluid. Thus, the transfer of protein I from the less fluid gonococcal outer membrane to the more fluid eukaryotic membrane

Table 2. Effect on the lipid bilayer of enzymatic treatment of gonococcal outer membranes as determined with the C5 spin label

Strains	Variant[a]	$2A'_{zz}$ (G)			
		Control	Trypsin	Chymo-trypsin	Pronase
2686	-	57.6	57.2	57.4	57.2
	+	58.2	57.9	57.9	57.9
R10	-	55.6	55.6	55.6	55.6
	+	56.0	55.8	55.9	55.8
MS11	-	55.7	55.8	55.8	55.5
	+	55.8	55.8	55.6	55.9
SR006	-	58.4	58.4	58.3	58.4
	+	58.9	58.8	58.8	58.6
120776-2	-	56.0	56.0	56.1	56.3
	+	58.4	58.2	58.4	58.4

[a]Transparent phenotype (-) and opaque phenotype (+).

Table 3. The effect of calcium on the immobilized lipid component of gonococcal outer membranes

Strain	Variant[a]	R[b]		
		Control	25 mM	100 mM
2686	-	23	11	6
	+	24	14	13

[a]Transparent phenotype (-) and opaque phenotype (+).
[b]R = ratio of C16 fluid lipid C5 divided by immobilized lipid.

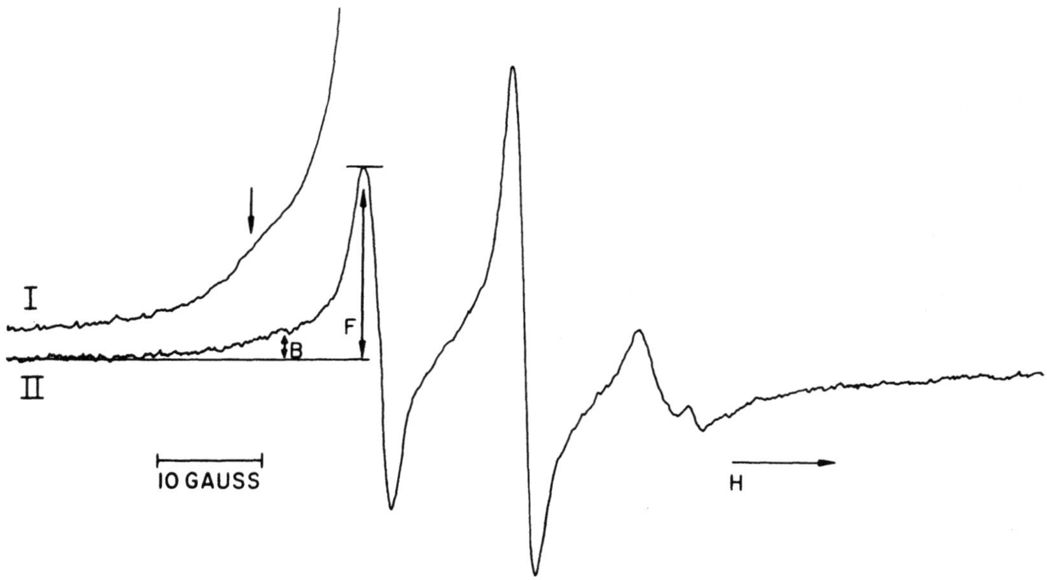

Fig. 5. The C16 ESR spectrum of an Op- variant of *Neisseria gonorrhoeae*. In spectrum II, the peak height *F* due to the C16 spin label in the bulk lipid bilayer is defined. The amplitude *B* associated with the bound lipid is arbitrarily measured 7.5 G downfield from the peak defined by *F*. The ratio *R* is defined by *F/B*. A portion (I) of spectrum II is shown recorded at higher modulation amplitude. The region of the C16 ESR spectrum indicated with the *single-headed arrow* indicates the low field peak area associated with the boundary layer

or planar bilayer would be consistent with these other observations.

The implications of this protein I transfer on the pathogenic mechanisms of gonococci are not yet clear. It has been well documented that the initiation event in professional phagocytic cells is the hyperpolarization of the plasma membrane [22-25]. It has been shown by Young et al. [26] that the macrophage Fc receptor, when aggregated by immunoglobulin, produces a channel through the membrane. Whether or not protein I activates phagocytosis of gonococci by epithelial cells in a similar manner is not known.

Two pieces of preliminary data further implicate protein I as an active participant in the infectious process. One is the interaction of protein I with the intracellular regulator, calmodulin. Schleicher et al. [27] have shown, using purified gonococcal outer membranes, the isolated protein I, or peptides derived from protein I, that calmodulin binds to this protein in a calcium-independent fashion. Most of the calmodulin binding ability was mediated by the 22 000-dalton peptide derived by a chymotrypsin digest of protein I. How attachment to calmodulin may affect this protein and its role in cellular regulation is an area of active interest.

In collaboration with Dr. A. Haines and Dr. M. Rich, we have investigated the effects of purified protein I on polymorphonuclear leukocytes (PMNs). They have observed that protein I added to human PMNs caused no damage to these cells as measured by lactate dehydrogenase release and had no stimulatory effects, except that the cells seemed to change shape, becoming rounded and less ruffled. PMNs pretreated with purified protein I and subsequently stimulated with either the chemotactic peptide FMLP or the calcium ionophore A23187 responded with a normal oxidative burst. However, when the amount of granule enzymes released from PMNs treated with protein I and stimulated with FMLP, LTB4, or A23187 was measured, the protein I-treated cells released 70% less β-glucuronidase and approximately 45% less lysozyme than the control cells. To improve our understanding of the site of inhibition of granule enzyme release, Quin 2 was used as a fluorescent probe for measuring cytoplasmic calcium. It was observed that PMNs, after treatment with protein I, equilibrated at slightly elevated cytosolic calcium levels. Upon addition of FMLP, the cytoplasmic calcium levels increased in the same proportions as leukocytes that had not been treated with protein I. This suggests that the step affected by protein I, which inhibits degranulation and enzyme release from leukocytes, must occur at some point after the mobilization of calcium. The effects of protein I do not seem to interfere with either the respiratory burst or the ability to phagocytose zymosan-coated particles. These data further add to the long-standing controversy of whether leukocytes are able to kill gonococci after phagocytosis. We are presently reexamining these issues.

As we continue to examine the properties of these outer membrane proteins, it is astounding to note the multitude of interactions they have. We have centered our observations around only two of these proteins. It will be indeed exciting to understand how the gonococcus uses its full complement of outer membrane proteins to interact with the human host and to turn the host responses to its advantage.

Acknowledgments. This work was supported in part by Public Health Service grants AI 10615 and AI 18637 from the National Institutes of Health.

References

1. Nikaido H (1979) Nonspecific transport through the outer membrane. In: Inouye M (ed) Bacterial outer membranes. Wiley, New York, pp 361-407
2. Blake MS, Gotschlich EC, Swanson JL (1981) The effect of proteolytic enzymes on the outer membrane proteins of *Neisseria gonorrhoeae*. Infect Immun 33:212-222
3. Newhall WJ, Sawyer WD, Haak RA (1980) Cross-linking analysis of the outer membrane proteins of *Neisseria gonorrhoeae*. Infect Immun 28:785-791
4. McDade RL Jr, Johnston KH (1980) Characterization of serologically dominant outer membrane proteins of *Neisseria gonorrhoeae*. J Bacteriol 141:1183-1191
5. Swanson J (1981) Surface-exposed protein antigens of the gonococcal outer membrane. Infect Immun 34:804-816

6. Blake MS, Gotschlich EC (1984) Purification and partial characterization of the opacity-associated proteins of *Neisseria gonorrhoeae*. J Exp Med 159:452-462
7. James JF, Swanson J (1978) Studies on gonococcus infection: XIII. Occurrence of color/opacity colonial variants in clinical cultures. Infect Immun 19:332-340
8. Swanson J (1978) Studies on gonococcus infection: XIV. Cell wall protein differences among color/opacity colony variants of *N. gonorrhoeae*. Infect Immun 21:292-302
9. Swanson J, Sparks E, Young D, King G (1975) Studies on gonococcus infection: X. Pili and leukocyte association factor as mediators of interactions between gonococci and eukaryotic cells in vitro. Infect Immun 11: 1352-1361
10. King GJ, Swanson J (1978) Studies on gonococcus infection: XV. Identification of surface proteins of *Neisseria gonorrhoeae* correlated with leukocyte association. Infect Immun 21:575-584
11. Wong TP, Johnston KH (1981) One-dimensional peptide mapping of the major outer membrane protein of *Neisseria gonorrhoeae*. Infect Immun 34:739-745
12. Montal M, Darszon A, Trisel HW (1977) Transmembrane channel formation in rhodopsin-containing bilayer membranes. Nature 267:221-225
13. Greco F (1981) Thesis. Rockefeller University, New York
14. Young JD-E, Blake M, Mauro A, Cohn ZA (1983) Properties of the major outer membrane protein from *Neisseria gonorrhoeae* incorporated into model lipid membranes. Proc Natl Acad Sci USA 80:3831-3835
15. Lynch EC, Blake MS, Gotschlich EC, Mauro A (1983) Studies of porins: Spontaneously transferred from whole cells and reconstituted from purified proteins of *Neisseria gonorrhoeae* and *Neisseria meningitidis*. Biophys J 45:104-107
16. Bouma SR, Drislane FW, Huestis WH (1977) Selective extraction of membrane-bound proteins by phospholipid vesicles. J Biol Chem 252:6759-6763
17. Cook SL, Bouma SR, Huestis WH (1980) Cell to vesicle transfer of intrinsic membrane proteins: effect of membrane fluidity. Biochemistry 19: 4601-4607
18. Enoch HG, Fleming PJ, Strittmatter P (1979) The binding of cytochrome b_5 to phospholipid vesicles and biological membranes. J Biol Chem 254: 6483-6488
19. Huestis WH (1977) A sodium-specific membrane permeability defect induced by phospholipid vesicle treatment of erythrocytes. J Biol Chem 252: 6764-6768
20. Roseman MA, Holloway PW, Calabro MA, Thompson TE (1977) Exchange of cytochrome b_5 between phospholipid vesicles. J Biol Chem 252: 4842-4849
21. Newton AC, Cook SL, Huestis WH (1983) Transfer of band 3, the erythrocyte anion transporter, between phospholipid vesicles. Biochemistry 22: 6110-6117
22. Gallin EK, Gallin JI (1977) Interaction of chemotactic factors with human macrophages induction of transmembrane potential changes. J Cell Biol 75:277-289
23. Korchak HM, Weissmann G (1978) Changes in membrane potential of human granulocytes antecede the metabolic responses to surface stimulation. Proc Natl Acad Sci USA 75:3818-3822
24. Seligman BE, Gallin JI (1980) Use of lipophilic probes of membrane potential to assess human neutrophil activation. J Clin Invest 66:493-503
25. Whitin JC, Chapman CE, Simons ER, Chovaniec ME, Cohen HJ (1980) Correlation between membrane potential changes and superoxide production in human granulocytes stimulated by phorbal myristate acetate. J Biol Chem 255:1874-1878

26. Young JD-E, Unkeless JC, Kaback HR, Cohn ZA (1983) Macrophage membrane potential changes associated with Fc receptor ligand binding. Proc Natl Acad Sci USA 80:1357-1361
27. Schleicher M, Noegel A, Watterson DM, Gotschlich EC (1983) Calmodulin, a eukaryotic regulator protein, binds in vitro to outer membrane proteins from neisseria species. Fed Proc 42:861

Discussion

(pp. 41-66)

Dr. Sparling noted the similarity of three sets of findings: (a) those of Dr. Anderson, indicating a factor in serum resulted in phenotypic modulation of *H. influenzae* of possible pathologic import; (b) those of Dr. Blake indicating that protein I of gonococci might enter and compromise the function of PMN leukocytes; and (c) those of Dr. Michael Cohen indicating that gonococci exposed to serum bind to PMN leukocytes less well and seem to compromise PMN function. He felt the possible change in membrane fluidity of the organisms might explain the difference in interaction with leukocytes.

Dr. Braun asked if the generally conserved nature of the binding domaine on gonococcal pili implied that the receptor was always the same. Dr. Schoolnik indicated that Dr. Heckels had shown that the same gonococcal strain could produce pili with different physical characteristics and different binding specificity. The amino acid sequence of those binding domains is unknown, but functionally, the ability of the gonococcus display more than one type of ligand so that it can bind to different receptors which may enhance its adaptability to different ecological niches in the body.

Dr. Wadström asked if the finding that gonococcal outer membrane protein II may play a role in attachment meant that there is more than one attachment factor. Dr. Blake indicated that there are probably a number of factors, pili and protein II probably being the major ones.

Dr. Bhakdi asked what is known about the immune response to various parts of the pilin subunits in naturally occurring gonococcal infection. Dr. Schoolnik indicated that he was using Western blots of various pilus fragments and serum or secretions from infected individuals to try to determine which parts were immunogenic.

Bayer-Symposium VIII
The Pathogenesis of Bacterial Infections, 68-84 (1985)

Regulation of Lipopolysaccharide Biologic Activity by Polysaccharide

D. C. Morrison, S. W. Vukajlovich, S. A. Goodman, and H.-W. Wollenweber

Summary

Bacterial lipopolysaccharides (LPS) have been implicated as a major contributing factor in the pathogenesis of gram-negative bacterial infections. Biochemical investigations have defined in detail the chemical structure of both the polysaccharide and the lipid A components. In this respect, there is now overwhelming evidence to suggest that the presence of lipid A is essential for the expression of most the multiple pathophysiologic and immunoregulatory properties of LPS. There is, in contrast, significantly less information on the role of the polysaccharide in regulating the biologic expression of the active lipid A component present in native LPS preparations. We have, therefore, performed experiments to examine this question by creating LPS macromolecules which vary significantly in their relative content of lipid A and polysaccharide. One protocol has employed the generation of LPS macromolecular hybrids in which lipid A-rich LPS molecules have been incorporated into native polysaccharide-containing LPS preparations. A second procedure has employed molecular sieve chromatography of detergent-dissociated LPS to generate LPS macromolecules with reduced subunit heterogeneity. The results of these combined studies indicate that the presence of polysaccharide can negatively regulate lipid A activity by two distinct mechanisms. They further support the concept that polysaccharide composition may be as critical a factor in the manifestation of LPS endotoxin activity as is the actual content of lipid A.

Introduction

Experiments carried out by R. Pfeiffer [1] almost a centruy ago first demonstrated the existence of a unique bacterial product present in late growth culture supernatants of *Vibrio* species, which was toxic to experimental animals. Pfeiffer termed this bacterial toxin endotoxin, to distinguish it from the more potent toxin secreted by actively growing organisms. Extensive studies by a number of investigators over the next 60 years firmly established endotoxin as a constituent of a variety of bacteria and we now recognize these toxins as characteristic products of all gram-negative bacteria, by virtue of their intimate association with the bacterial outer cell membrane.

In general, these toxic bacterial constituents are not found as distinct macromolecular species in cultures of growing bacteria, but rather are released from the outer leaflet of outer cell membrane following the loss of structural integrity of this bacterial organelle. A number of chemical procedures have been employed to promote the release of endotoxic constituents from suspensions of bacteria in vitro in order to examine their chemical composition and pathogenic responses. Such studies very early established bacterial endotoxins to be biochemically unique macromolecular structures as discussed in the following section consisting of complex mixtures of lipopolysaccharides (LPS) often in association with protein [2]. Of importance was the demonstration that these bacterial products possessed an almost limitless capacity to evoke pathologic, pharmacologic, and immunologic responses both in vitro and in vivo [3]. As a consequence, endotoxins have for many years been considered as a major contributing factor to the pathogenesis of gram-negative bacteremia and sepsis. The recent elegant experiments by Ziegler and her colleagues [4], demonstrating that antibody directed against common structural determinants of the endotoxin macromolecule will significantly increase survival of patients with gram-negative septicaemia, dramatically illustrates the importance of endotoxin-initiated host responses in the pathogenesis of human bacterial disease.

The Structure of Bacterial Endotoxin

The classic experiments of André Boivin and Lydia Mesrobeanu [2] provided some of the first detailed chemical analyses of bacterial endotoxins. Using an extraction procedure with trichloroacetic acid, these investigators documented that endotoxins contain protein, lipid, and polysaccharide. Extensive experiments by Goebel et al. [5] extended these studies and established the first concept of a toxic principle for bacterial endotoxin. In 1952, Westphal, Lüderitz, and Bister [6] published a procedure for the extraction and purification of highly purified LPS from gram-negative bacteria. The demonstration that such purified LPS preparations embodied virtually all of the endotoxin properties known at that time was a keystone to structure-function relationships in endotoxin biology. Nevertheless, more recent studies have provided convincing evidence that the protein component of endotoxin (to be discussed later) is not completely without biologic activity as manifest by its immunostimulatory properties.

Chemical Characterization of the Lipopolysaccharide Component of Endotoxin

The LPS component of bacterial endotoxins from various genera of gram-negative bacteria has been extensively purified and its unique chemical features characterized. Generally, LPS are built up of three distinct regions: the lipid part, called lipid A, which anchors the LPS to the bacterial membrane and the polysaccharide part, which in turn is subdivided into the outer O-antigen, and the inner core region.

The O-antigen of LPS represents a polysaccharide, which is made up of repeating units of one type of an oligosaccharide molecule. This generally consists of a di-, tri-, or higher oligosaccharide. The constituent components of the repeating units have been investigated in great detail and reveal an extensive diversity within different gram-negative bacteria (reviewed in [7]). Besides neutral sugars (hexoses, pentoses, and deoxy and O-methyl derivatives) and charged sugars (aminohexoses, aminopentoses, hexuronic acids, and aminohexuronic acids) a large diversity of substituents such as amino acids, phosphoryl, glyceryl, lactyl, and acetyl groups have been detected. In addition, the number of repeating units can vary considerably from zero to about 40, thus creating a high heterogeneity even within a given LPS preparation (see later discussion). As a consequence of this immense variability of the chemical compounds, sequence, type of linkage, and substitution within the repeating unit molecules, the structure of the O-polysaccharide chain is unique to each LPS and its parental bacterial strain. Therefore, the O-polysaccharide is responsible for the O-antigenicity of LPS which is determined by different O-factors, each representing a distinct immunodeterminant group. It has been shown that O-antigens may serve as pathogenicity factors of the respective bacterial strain in that they protect gram-negative bacteria from phagocytosis and killing. Moreover, antibodies against the O-antigen may protect against infection and endotoxic effects such as fever and lethality.

The isolation of rough (R)-mutants greatly enhanced the structural, biologic, and genetic studies of LPS. R-lipopolysaccharides are devoid of O-antigen and may lack part of the core region. Analysis of all *Salmonella* species (Ra to Re and S forms) revealed an identical, or closely related core structure (reviewed in [8]): an undecasaccharide, which in its outer region (proximal to the O-antigen) consists of a hexose pentasaccharide, whereas the inner core (proximal to the lipid A) contains branched trisaccharides of l-glycero-d-mannoheptose and 3-deoxy-d-mannooctulosonic acid (dOclA), formally termed KDO (2-keto-3-deoxyoctonate). Up to five different core structures have been analyzed in *E. coli* strains (R1 to R4 and K12). The innermost core region of enterobacterial LPS was found to be similar in that charged groups, such as carboxyl (dOclA), phosphoryl, and amino groups (ethanolamine) are accumulated. Thus, the core region of enterobacterial LPS expresses much less diversity than the O-polysaccharide. Because core structures represent antigens and induce core-specific antibodies, it is tempting to prepare vaccines with a broad cross-reactivity among different bacterial species.

In nonenterobacterial LPS (e.g., *Pseudomonas*, *Bacteroides*, and *Xanthomonas*) structurally distinct core types are present which may lack either heptose, dOclA, or both of these sugar components present in enterobacterial LPS. However, in contrast to the extreme variability of O-specificities, the core region seems to be of only limited diversity.

The lipid component of bacterial LPS has been analyzed in great detail because many of the pathophysiologic effects elicted by

LPS have been shown to be dependent upon the lipid A moiety (reviewed in [9]). A general structure has been proposed and proven to be present in many samples of lipid A from both closely related and taxonomically remote groups of bacteria. Long-chain fatty acids are bound to a phosphorylated backbone which, in general, consists of a 1, 6-linked d-glucosaminyldisaccharide. Characteristically, 3-hydroxylated fatty acids are linked to amino and hydroxyl groups of the glucosamine backbone. The 3-hydroxylated fatty acids may be 3-*O*-acylated by 3-hydroxy, 2-hydroxy, and nonhydroxylated fatty acids, thus forming 3-acyloxyacyl residues. The phosphate group at the reducing end of the molecule and phosphate ester linked to the 4' position may be substituted by positively charged amino compounds (e.g., phosphorylethanolamine and 4-amino-l-arabinose).

Despite the characteristics outlined, individual lipid A may vary in regard to: (a) the type (normal, branched), chain length (C-10 to C-18), and the amount of fatty acids (3-7 mol per glucosamine disaccharide) and 3-acyloxyacyl groups; (b) the presence and nature of residues attached to the backbone phosphate groups; and (c) other substituents of the glucosaminyldisaccharide. Therefore, even within one LPS preparation, a large number of related, but not identical, chemical structures, i.e., lipid A structures, may be present.

The comparable endotoxic activities of S and R form LPS and lipid A preparation pointed to the lipid A moiety as the endotoxic principle of bacterial LPS. The isolation of a lipid A precursor molecule from a dOclA synthetase-defective *Salmonella typhimurium* mutant [10] suggested that part of the ester-bound fatty acids are critical for the expression of several endotoxic activities, whereas, total removal of ester-bound fatty acid by alkaline hydrolysis resulted in a strong decrease.

Chemical Characteristics of the Protein Component of Endotoxin

Although recognized as a detectable constituent of bacterial endotoxins prepared by a number of extraction methods, the protein component of endotoxin has been significantly less well studied. This has primarily been a consequence of the fact that a vast majority of the biologic activities of endotoxin are attributable, in large measure, to the lipid A component of the LPS molecule (see later discussion). However, the discovery and extensive genetic and immunologic characterization of a mouse strain (C3H/HeJ) which is refractive to virtually all of the biologic effects of lipid A has allowed investigators to detect a number of immunologic activities characteristic of the protein component of endotoxin (reviewed in [11]). This protein component has been termed endotoxin protein (EP) or lipid A-associated protein (LAP).

Biochemical investigations have established that EP consist of a number of proteins, many of which are usually localized to the outer membrane of gram-negative bacteria. In part, the actual composition of these proteins appears to vary somewhat, depending upon the method used to extract and purify the endotoxin [12, 13]. In general, however, both porins and protein II appear to be present, as well as low but detectable amounts of lipoprotein [14]. There is good experimental evidence that the protein exists in close association with the lipid A part of the LPS molecule. In this respect, Morrison et al. [12] have shown that isolated LAP will recombine with lipid A and the LPS from *S. minnesota* R595. There is also some data to suggest that the presence of protein, in addition to manifesting immunologic activities of its own, will modify the expression of the immunologic and pathophysiologic activities of the LPS component [11]. Nevertheless, most investigators have concluded that LPS is the dominant component of endotoxin responsible for endotoxin activity.

Relationship of Lipopolysaccharide Structure to Biologic Activity

As indicated, it has been recognized for a number of years that the presence of lipid A is essential for the expression of the vast majority of the biologic activities of endotoxin. Evidence in support of this concept has derived from numerous sources, including: (a) isolation of lipid A free of contaminating polysaccharide by mild acid hydrolysis; (b) abrogation of activity by mild alkaline hydrolysis to remove selectively the ester-linked fatty acids from lipid A; and (c) the neutralization of LPS responses with agents such as polymyxin B, which bind selectively to lipid A (reviewed in [15]). These combined studies have been complemented by experiments using LPS derived from rough mutant strains of bacteria which lack the capacity to synthesize a complete LPS molecule. More recently, the demonstration that lipid A prepared by total organic synthesis manifests many of the endotoxic activities of LPS has provided unequivocal proof that activity can be expressed by lipid A independent of other endotoxic constituents [16].

In contrast to these studies with lipid A, most investigators have not ascribed a dominant biologic role to the polysaccharide component of LPS other than as an immunodominant antigenic determinant in the humoral antibody response to endotoxin. Rather, the polysaccharide has usually been viewed as a "water-soluble carrier" for the toxic lipid A component. Support for this concept is readily apparent from the notable insolubility of isolated lipid A, particularly that prepared by organic synthesis.

Some evidence to indicate that the polysaccharide component of LPS could express biologic activity has been recently provided by Morrison and Kline [28]. In these studies, it was shown that, although lipid A was required for activation of the classical pathway of serum complement, the presence of polysaccharide was essential for the lipid A-independent activation of the alternative complement pathway. Further studies have documented that polysaccharide can serve an essential role in the regulation of this complement pathway by restricting the activities of the regulator proteins H and I. More recent studies in our own laboratory have shown that the polysaccharide component of LPS may, in fact, serve a more prominent function in the expression of lipid A activity by negatively regulating the expression of lipid A activity. In this respect, it is now recognized [17, 18] that LPS macromolecules consist of a micellar aggregate of relatively heterogeneous LPS subunits which vary considerably in the numbers of O-polysaccharide repeating oligosaccharide units.

Our recent data, to be summarized in the following sections, indicate that regulation of expression of lipid A activity by polysaccharide can be manifest by at least two distinct mechanisms. With respect to the former mechanism, we demonstrate that the presence of polysaccharide-containing subunits can inhibit the normal expression of lipid A-rich subunits noncovalently contained within the same micellar aggregate. We have termed this mode of regulation extrinsic modulation. We have also shown that LPS micellar aggregates with restricted subunit heterogeneity also vary in their capacity to elicit lipid A-dependent responses in a manner not directly proportional to lipid A content. Since the LPS subunits in such preparations are relatively uniform and each consists of lipid A covalently attached to polysaccharide, we have termed this mode of polysaccharide effect intrinsic modulation. Finally, we have shown suggestive evidence for an important role for lipid A-rich subunits contained within heterogeneous micellar aggregates in their interaction with LPS-responsive cells.

In summary, therefore, our combined data presented here suggest that the tertiary configuration of the LPS aggregate macromolecular structure and the negative regulatory influences (both extrinsic and intrinsic) of polysaccharide may be of equal importance to the manifestation of LPS pathophysiologic activity as is the actual chemical structure of the lipid A component.

Regulation of Lipid A Responses by Polysaccharide

As we have stated, there is overwhelming evidence to support the concept that the majority of the endotoxin and immunostimulatory properties of LPS are associated with the lipid A region of the molecule. The best evidence in support of this concept has been the expression of biologic activity by isolated, highly purified polysaccharide-free lipid A and more recently, by lipid A prepared by total organic synthesis. It is, however, equally clear that in the vast majority of circumstances, lipid A is encountered by host cells and tissues in a molecular environment consisting primarily of polysaccharide. It is, therefore, both relevant and necessary to consider the expression of lipid A-dependent activities within the framework of core polysaccharide and/or O-antigen determinants.

Immunostimulatory Activity of LPS Hybrid Macromolecules

As one approach to assess the effect of polysaccharide on the expression of lipid A activity, we have taken advantage of the observation of Rudbach et al. [19] that LPS micellar aggregates may be reversibly dissociated in the presence of sodium deoxycholate (DOC) to form monomer LPS units. Removal of DOC by extensive dialysis results in the reformation of high molecular weight micellar aggregates.

Using this technique, we have created hybrid LPS macromolecules containing various amounts of lipid A. For these experiments, various ratios of the polysaccharide-rich *E. coli* 055/B5 LPS, prepared by extraction with aqueous phenol [20] were admixed with deep rough *S. minnesota* Re 595 LPS, prepared by the phenol-chloroform-petroleum ether procedure [21], in the presence of 0.6% DOC. For experiments in which the extent of hybrid formation was assessed, the LPS preparations were radiolabled with ^{125}I by the procedure of Ulevitch [22]. Following incubation at 37°C for 30 min, the LPS samples were dialyzed extensively against distilled water. Control experiments using ^{14}C-labeled DOC have documented that these procedures remove greater than 99.9% of the DOC.

To assess the degree of hybrid formation between these two parent molecules, we have determined their isopyknic density following equilibrium ultracentrifugation in CsCl. Owing to significant differences in the chemical composition of the two parent LPS species, they manifest considerable differences in their partial specific volumes. As shown in the top portion of Fig. 1, when centrifuged separately, the *E. coli* LPS bands at a density of approximately 1.5 g/cm^3 whereas the more lipid A-rich *S. minnesota* R595 LPS bands at about 1.40 g/cm^3. Significantly, there is little detectable association of the two parent LPS species if they are admixed in the absence of DOC prior to centrifugation and the two characteristic density peaks are again observed (Fig. 1, bottom). In contrast, if the parent LPS molecules are admixed in the presence of DOC and the detergent subsequently removed by dialysis prior to ultracentrifugation, a single LPS species results with an isopyknic density intermediate to the two parent LPS. In experiments not shown here, we have demonstrated that the average density of the various hybrid LPS macromolecules approximates the value calculated from the percentages of the two parent LPS species used to generate the hybrids. These data indicate that lipid A-rich *S. minnesota* R595 LPS subunits can be integrated into the polysaccharide-containing *E. coli* LPS parent, thus altering in a controlled way both the percentage by weight of lipid A and the net subunit composition of the LPS micellar aggregate.

We have employed these LPS macromolecular hybrids to examine the relationship between lipid A content and the expression of a lipid A-dependent biologic activity. For these studies, we have employed the in vitro proliferative response of murine B lymphocytes to LPS, now recognized as one of the prototype in vitro lipid A-dependent biologic activities of LPS. We believe this assay to be a sensitive, highly reproducible, and at least semiquantitative measure of the expression of lipid A activity. The details of this assay system, which determines incorporation of thymidine ^3H into LPS-stimulated B lymphocytes have been published elsewhere [23].

The results of one such experiment, in which the proliferative response of C3HeB/FeJ splenocytes to various concentrations of the two parent LPS preparations, as well as hybrids, containing 25%, 50%, and 75% by weight of the lipid A-rich R595 LPS, is

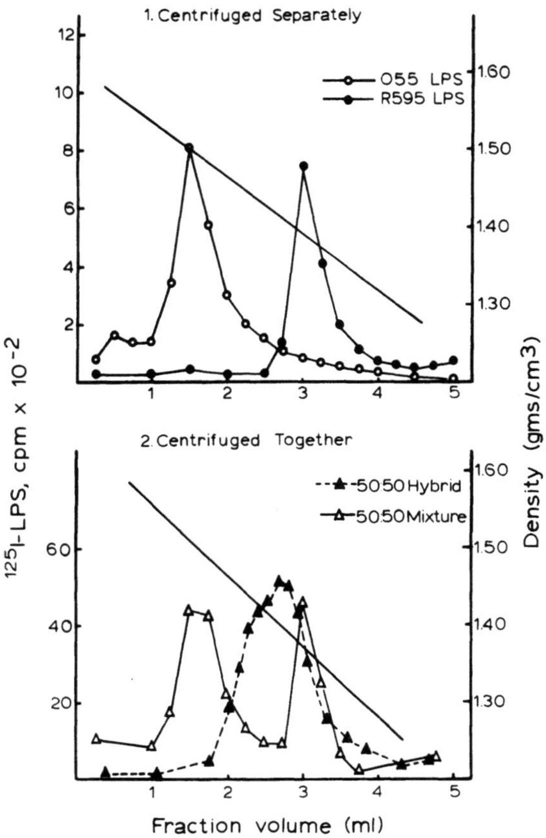

Fig. 1. Isopyknic density profiles of O55 LPS, R595 LPS, and 50-50 hybrid LPS. Samples of ^{125}I-labeled LPS plus 1 mg/ml cold carrier were diluted in 0.1 Tris pH 8.0 (0.5 mg LPS total). 2.8 g CsCl was added to the LPS samples and volume adjusted to 5.0 ml with 0.1 *M* Tris buffer. Equilibrium gradients were formed by ultracentrifugation at 42 000 rpm for 48 h in a Beckman SW50.1 rotor. 0.2-ml Fractions were collected from the tube bottom, ^{125}I was measured with a gamma radiation counter, and refractive index was used to determine fraction densities. *Top*: Density profiles of two separate gradients, R595 LPS (*full circles*) and O55 LPS, (*open circles*), *bottom*: density profiles of two separate gradients, one containing a 50-50 mixture of R595 LPS and O55 LPS (*open triangles*). Both LPS species were incubated together for 1 h at 37°C prior to additon of CsCl and ultracentrifugation. The second gradient contained a 50-50 hybrid of R595 LPS and O55 LPS (*full triangles*)

shown in Fig. 2. Several points are worthy of note. As might be anticipated, the immunostimulatory activity of the lipid A-rich R595 LPS preparation is significantly greater than that of the polysaccharide-rich *E. coli* LPS, and the hybrid LPS preparations, in general, manifest activity intermediate to the two parents. However, it is readily apparent that the immunostimulatory activity does not increase in direct proportion to the content of lipid A of the hybrid LPS. In this respect, hybrid LPS preparations containing 25% by weight R595 LPS are virtually indistinguishable from the polysaccharide-rich parent. Similar reduced responses are manifest by the other LPS hybrids.

In order to address this question more directly, experiments have been performed in which the immunostimulatory activity of a 50-50 hybrid LPS macromolecule was compared with that of an equal mixture of the two parents. In this situation, the total concentration of lipid A in the two preparations is identical. Any differences observed may therefore be attributable to the macromolecular environment of the biologically active lipid A. The results of this experiment are shown in Fig. 3. As was shown

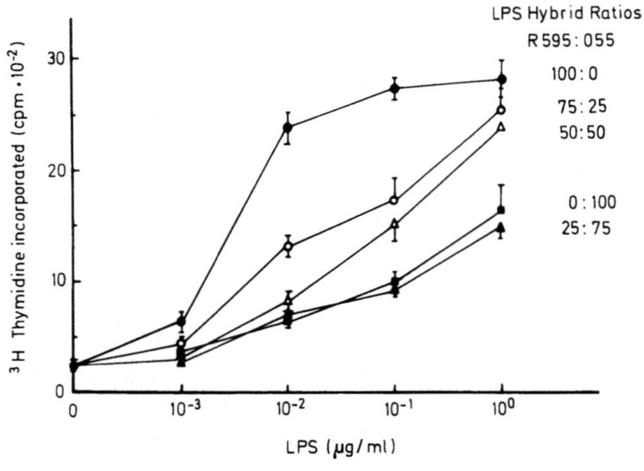

Fig. 2. Proliferative responses of murine splenocytes to R595:O55 LPS hybrids. 5×10^5 C3HeB/FeJ spleen cells in 200 µl RPMI-1640 medium supplemented with penicillin, streptomycin, and glutamine were cultured at $37^{\circ}C$ in a humidified 95% CO_2, 5% air atmosphere for 24 h with the indicated concentrations of LPS preparations, after which 0.5 µCi thymidine ^3H was added. Cells were then incubated 18 h. Background ± standard error of triplicate samples was 2231 cpm

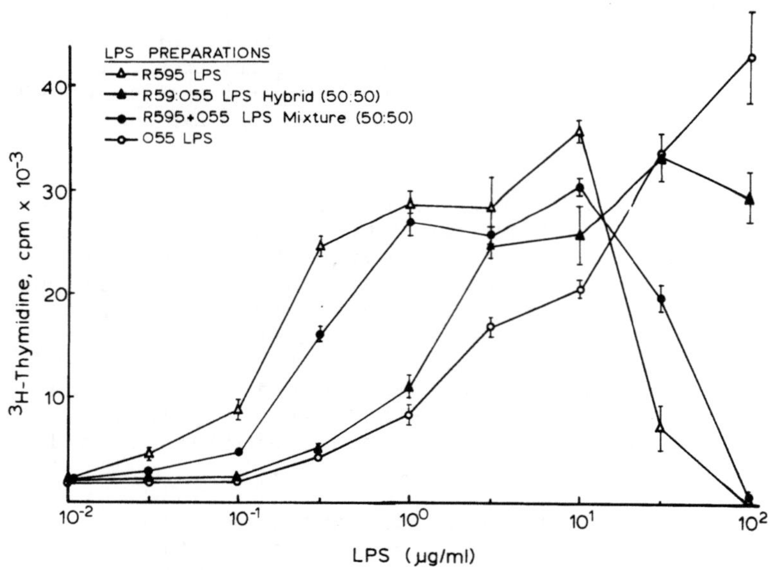

Fig. 3. Mitogenic responses of murine splenocytes to R595 + O55 LPS mixtures and R595:O55 LPS hybrids. Assay conditions were as described in Fig. 1. Dose-response curves shown for R595 LPS (*open triangles*), O55 LPS (*open circles*), R595:O55 hybrid LPS (*full triangles*), and a R595 + O55 LPS mixture (*full circles*). Background ± standard error was 1852 cpm for triplicate samples

earlier, the response to R595 LPS is considerably greater than to the polysaccharide-rich *E. coli* LPS. Of importance, however, is the fact that the activity of the hybrid LPS is significantly less than that of the mixture of the two parents, even though both contain equal amounts of lipid A. These combined data therefore indicate that the presence of polysaccharide can markedly reduce the activity of lipid A present in LPS macromolecular aggregates.

Immunostimulatory Activity of LPS Macromolecules of Reduced Subunit Heterogeneity

Although it is clear that lipid A is essential for expression of activity, and that the presence of extraneous polysaccharide-rich LPS subunits will inhibit the activity of lipid A subunits noncovalently contained within the same macromolecular aggregate, the regulatory effect of covalently associated polysaccharide on the expression of lipid A activity is not addressed by these experiments. To assess this factor, therefore, we have established procedures to prepare LPS macromolecules in which the polysaccharide/lipid A heterogeneity has been markedly reduced [23]. The evaluation of the relative immunostimulatory activity of such LPS preparations should therefore provide information which addresses directly this question.

Our approach has been to dissociate heterogeneous LPS macromolecular aggregates from *E. coli* 055:B5 using DOC as described and then to fractionate the LPS monomers on the basis of size by molecular sieve chromatography. Since the major determinant of LPS subunit heterogeneity is in the number of repeating units attached to the core polysaccharide-lipid A backbone, such procedures should fractionate LPS subunits with varying ratios of lipid A to polysaccharide. The LPS from *E. coli* 055:B5 was dissociated in 0.6% DOC and chromatographed at 37°C on an LKB AcA 44 column in Tris-buffered saline containing 0.6% DOC. Column fractions were assayed for the O-antigen-specific saccharide, abequose and the core polysaccharide-specific saccharide, 2-keto-3-deoxyoctulosonate (KDO) using a modification of published procedures [23].

The elution profiles for one such experiment are shown in Fig. 4 and indicate that the LPS monomers may be resolved into three major size fractions containing very different relative amounts of abequose/KDO. As expected, the highest molecular weight species contain the greatest amounts of abequose/KDO and the lowest molecular weight species are virtually devoid of detectable O-antigen.

Selected fractions of the column eluates were then dialyzed extensively against distilled water and lyophylized. Following resolubilization in saline, graded doses of the various LPS fractions were assayed for their relative capacity to initiate proliferation in in vitro cultures of C3HeB/FeJ splenocytes. The concentration of LPS required to stimulate thymidine incorporation 20-fold greater than background (stimulation index) was then determined and this value compared with the relative amount of lipid A by weight in the various LPS preparations.

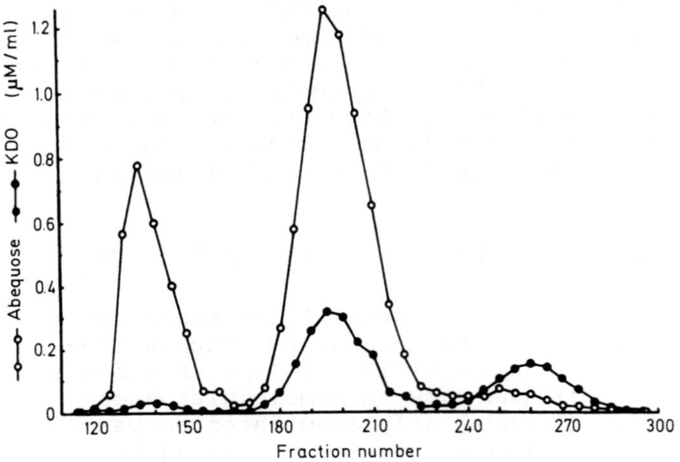

Fig. 4. Gel filtration chromatography of monomeric O55 LPS subunits. A 2-ml sample of a 50 mg/ml solution of O55:B5 LPS (100 mg) was dissociated in 2.0 ml 0.1 *M* Tris buffer, pH 7.8, 0.6% deoxycholate at 37°C for 1 h. The dissociated O55 LPS was chromatographed at 37°C on a 2.7 × 55 cm column of Ultragel AcA44 equilibrated with the same buffer. Column fractions of approximately 0.8 ml were collected and assayed for abequose (*open circles*) and KDO (*full circles*) using the thiobarbituric acid colorimetric assay as described in [23]

The results of this analysis are shown in Table 1. It is readily apparent that, although a correlation does exist between the presence of lipid A and the immunostimulatory activity of the LPS preparation, this relationship is clearly not linear. Thus, a decrease in the amount of lipid A relative to polysaccharide of approximately 10-fold is accompanied by a decrease in activity of almost 3000-fold. In addition, even minor changes in lipid A percentages by weight are accompanied by orders of magnitude changes in immunostimulatory activity. This critical dependence of activity upon polysaccharide is most pronounced with the LPS preparations containing the most extensive O-antigen polysaccharides. These results, therefore, confirm and extend those obtained with LPS macromolecular hybrids and provide convincing evidence for a dominant regulatory role of polysaccharide in modulation of the expression of lipid A activity.

Role of Defined LPS Subunits in Cellular Activation Mechanisms

The data presented, although not conclusive, suggest that much of the immunostimulatory activity (perhaps other biologic activities as well) in heterogeneous LPS micellar aggregates may be due almost exclusively to lipid A-rich subunits contained within the LPS micelle. In this respect, therefore, the regulatory role of polysaccharide- (particularly O-antigen polysaccharide)-containing LPS subunits would be to restrict the accessibility of lipid A-rich subunits to appropriate target sites on LPS/lipid A-responsive mammalian cells such as B lymphocytes.

Table 1. Immunostimulatory activity of LPS preparations with reduced subunit heterogeneity

Fraction[a]	Abequose/KDO[6 b]	Lipid A[c] (%)	Immunostimulatory activity[d]
130	58	5- 7	13
147	26	8-10	150
185	3	20-24	1370
265	0.25	50	4500

[a]Individual column fractions (see Fig. 3).
[b]Relative absorbance units (see legend to Fig. 3).
[c]Calculated from an approximate molecular weight for lipid A of 2500 and an estimate of the average number of repeating O-antigen polysaccharide units.
[d]Reciprocal of the concentration of LPS in mg/ml required to elicit 20-fold proliferation response in in vitro cultures of murine splenocytes.

We have, therefore, initiated experiments to assess directly the relative subunit specificity of the interaction of macromolecular LPS with lymphoid cells [24]. For these studies, we have employed LPS from *E. coli* O55:B5 iodinated with ^{125}I as described by Ulevitch [23]. The available evidence has suggested that LPS radioiodinated by this procedure labels selectively the substituted phosphorylethanolamine groups associated with the core polysaccharide and lipid A and thus should label with equal efficiency all of the LPS subunits contained within the macromolecular aggregate. The subsequent analysis of binding of radioiodinated LPS should thus allow a determination of selectivity in the binding of distinct LPS subunits.

For the majority of these experiments, single-cell suspensions of murine splenocytes were incubated with ^{125}I-labeled LPS RPMI-1640 culture medium containing glutamine, penicillin, and streptomycin. Following incubation, splenocytes were centrifuged and washed with medium three times. Cells were then lysed with 1% Triton X-100 and both lysates and original culture supernatants as well as the starting LPS were subsequently analyzed by polyacrylamide slab gel electrophoresis in sodium dodecylsulfate. Following electrophoresis, gels were dried onto chromatography paper (Whatman 3MM) using a gel slab dryer (BioRad Laboratories, Richmond, California) and subjected to autoradiography using Dupont Cronex Lighting Plus intensifying screens (X-Ray of Georgia, Norcross, Georgia). Autoradiographs were then scanned using a Cary 219 spectrophotometer at 66 nm.

Typical results of such an experiment are shown in Fig. 5 and illustrate several relevant points. As suggested earlier, and

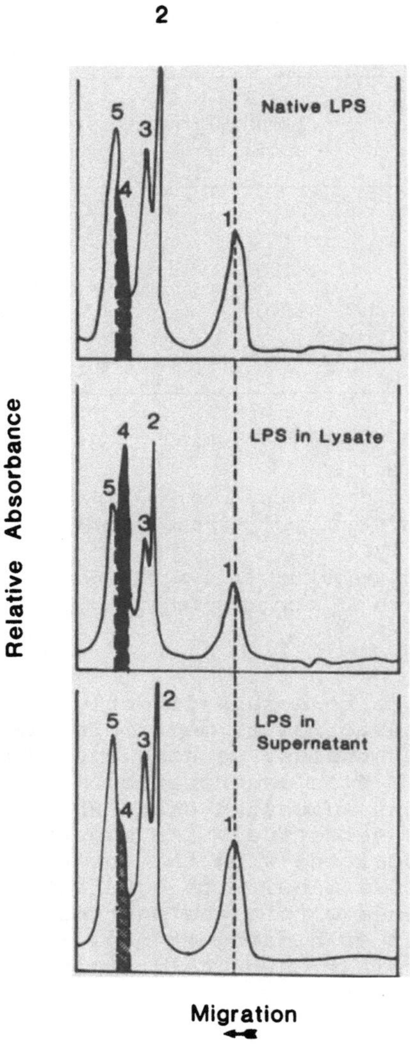

Fig. 5. Densitometric scans of autoradiographs of polyacralamide gels of LPS preparations. Washed spleen cells (10^8/ml), previously submitted to hypotonic lysis, were incubated at 37°C for 2 h in the presence of 100 µg/ml ^{125}I-labeled LPS from *E. coli* O55:B5. Cells were removed from the supernatants by centrifugation and washed further to remove unbound LPS. Cell pellets were lysed in 1% Triton X-100 for 15 min at 4°C and the debris removed by centrifugation. Samples of native LPS, LPS in cell lysates and LPS in cell supernatants were electrophoresed on SDS-10% polyacrylamide gels. After the gels were dried and submitted to autoradiography, densitometric scans were performed on the autoradiographs. Major bands are designated 1-5 in order of increasing electrophoretic mobility. *Shaded areas* show R-like subunits. The *vertical line* is for the purpose of orientation

has been shown by the gel permeation studies summarized in Fig. 4, the LPS from *E. coli* 055:B5 consists of a heterogeneous population of subunits which are also resolved on polyacrylamide gels. It is probable that LPS peaks 2 and 3 in Fig. 5 (top panel) correspond to the second peak obtained by chromatography; similarly, peaks 4 and 5 in Fig. 5 correspond to the third peak in Fig. 4. Although the results are not shown here, we have demonstrated that the peak 4 LPS migrates at a rate similar to rough LPS devoid of O-antigenic polysaccharide [24]. The precise identification of the radiolabel in peak 5, which migrates faster than the rough LPS subunits is not clear, but we believe this to be contaminating phospholipid since these may be present even in highly purified LPS preparations (M.J. Osborn, personal communication).

Also shown in Fig. 5 are the electrophoretic profiles of the LPS associated with splenocyte lysates as well as unbound LPS. Of particular interest is the observation that spleen cells have bound selectively the most lipid A-rich fraction 4 LPS component relative to the other components. Since only a relatively small fraction of the LPS (5%-10%) is bound to the splenocytes under the conditions of the experiment, this selective binding is not readily detectable in unbound LPS supernatants. Integration of the areas under the peaks of the various LPS components and normalization to control LPS indicates that the lipid A-rich component 4 is increased approximately threefold. In contrast, there is no detectable selective change in the more polysaccharide-rich LPS subunits associated with splenocyte lysates. These data thus indicate that, in addition to a selective increase in biologic immunostimulatory activity of lipid A-rich LPS components (Table 1), there is also a selective association of these subunits contained within heterogeneous LPS macromolecular aggregates to splenocytes.

We have queried whether this apparent selective association of LPS subunits is a generalized property of the interaction of LPS with mammalian cell membranes or whether such interactions are restricted to cells which can manifest a cellular response to LPS. We have therefore compared in detail the subunit association profiles of LPS bound to splenocytes from normal mice (C3HeB/FeJ) as well as from mice which are genetically refractory to the immunostimulatory and endotoxic properties of LPS (C3H/HeJ). Of importance, no significant differences were observed between these two strains in the binding profiles of their splenocytes to LPS [24]. Thus, while such selective binding may be necessary for appropriate triggering signals, such interactions would also appear not to be sufficient. On the other hand, we have demonstrated that partially purified preparations of murine hepatocytes do not manifest a selective association of lipid A-rich LPS subunits coincident with LPS binding [25]. These latter results would suggest that this phenomenon is not a generalized property attributable to the cell membranes of all mammalian cells.

Discussion and Conclusions

We have demonstrated that the presence of polysaccharide in heterogeneous macromolecular aggregates of LPS can markedly influence the expression of lipid A activity as assessed by its immunostimulatory properties in in vitro cultures of murine splenocytes. Our data suggest that regulation of lipid A expression by polysaccharide can occur by two mechanisms, an extrinsic regulation in which the molecular environments of lipid A-rich LPS subunits are inhibited from expression of activity by their (noncovalent) proximity to polysaccharide-rich LPS subunits, and an intrinsic regulation in which the extent of the O-antigen polysaccharide repeating units influences the expression of the corresponding covalently bound lipid A. We propose from these results that the presence of polysaccharide and the precise nature of the lipid A/polysaccharide relationship may be as important for the expression of lipid A activity as is the presence of lipid A itself.

Our data have shown that lipid A-rich LPS subunits are markedly more active than are polysaccharide-rich LPS subunits. This conclusion is based upon an analysis of the relative activity of LPS macromolecules in which subunit heterogeneity has been markedly reduced. It is noteworthy that an approximate 3000-fold difference can be demonstrated between LPS preparations which vary only about 10-fold in lipid A content. These large differences are not observed when native polysaccharide-containing LPS preparations such as that from *E. coli* 055:B5, are compared with the lipid A-rich LPS preparations from *S. minnesota* R595 when only 10-fold differences are noted (see Fig. 1). These data would suggest that most, if not in fact all, of the activity manifest by heterogeneous LPS preparations may be due to the presence within the macromolecular aggregate of these biologically potent lipid A-rich subunits. Consistent with this concept is our recent demonstration that these subunits appear to associate selectively with splenocytes.

It is tempting to speculate that the negative, regulatory role of polysaccharide in the expression of lipid A activity may be to limit the insertion of this phospholipid-like component into mammalian cell membrane bilayers. In this respect, the free energy of a lipid A-rich LPS subunit within a micellar LPS aggregate compared with its free energy in a biologic membrane may well be dependent upon the intrinsic hydrophobicity of the micelle, a variable which would be critically dependent upon lipid A:polysaccharide ratios. Recent evidence from our laboratory has suggested that lipid A-rich preparations from LPS interact with erythrocyte membranes in a dynamic time- and temperature-dependent manner [26], suggestive of a molecular rearrangement of LPS subsequent to a critical binding event. Additional experiments will, however, be required to confirm similar lipid A-dependent events in lymphocytes and other cells which respond to LPS/lipid A.

In addition to the role of polysaccharide as a relevant factor in the modulation of lipid A activity, there is growing evidence that, in preparations of endotoxin from at least some species, the polysaccharide itself may serve as a triggering signal. In this respect, Haeffner-Cavaillon et al. [27] have shown that rabbit peritoneal macrophages will recognize specifically the LPS from *Bordetella pertussis* and that such recognition is due to determinants on the polysaccharide component. In addition, recent experiments by McGhee and Robinson (this volume) have provided data for specific recognition of the polysaccharide of *Bacteroides* LPS by murine lymphoid cells. Thus, polysaccharide determinants on LPS can have direct as well as indirect effects on host cells.

Our combined data provide convincing support for the concept that critical attention should be paid to subunit composition of LPS preparations in the analysis of endotoxic and immunostimulatory activities of LPS. There is evidence that the distribution of subunits may vary, depending upon a number of factors, including the conditions of growth as well as phase of growth of the bacteria, strain of organism, and method of extraction and purification. These factors may vary considerably during the in vivo growth of an organism in infected tissue as compared with in vitro culture. Therefore, an appreciation for, and consideration of, the tertiary structure of LPS with respect to polysaccharide content and subunit composition will allow a more complete evaluation of the contribution of endotoxin to the pathogenesis of gram-negative infectious disease.

Acknowledgments. The authors acknowledge with appreciation the excellent secretarial assistance of Mrs. Grace Vrell. This research was supported by grants from the National Institute of Allergy and Infectious Disease AI-17225 and AI-17304.

References

1. Pfeiffer R (1892) Untersuchungen über das Choleragift. Z Hyg Infektionskran 11:393-412
2. Boivin A, Mesrobeanu L (1935) Recherches sur les antigenes somatiques et sur les endotoxines des bacteries: I. Considerations generales et expose des Techniques utilisees. Rev Immunol (Paris) 1:553-569
3. Westphal O (1975) Bacterial endotoxins. Int Arch Allergy Appl Immunol 49: 1-43
4. Ziegler EJ, McCutchen JA, Fierer J, Glauser MP, Sadoff JC, Douglas H, Braude AI (1982) N Engl J Med 307:1225-1230
5. Goebel WF, Binkley F, Perlman E (1945) Studies on the Flexner group of dysentery Bacilli: I. The specific antigens of *S. paradysenteriae*. J Med 81:315-330
6. Westphal O, Luderitz O, Bister F (1952) Über die Extraktion von Bakterien mit Phenol-Wasser. Z Naturforsch 7B:148-155
7. Luderitz O, Freundenberg MA, Galanos C, Lehmann V, Rietschel ET, Shaw DW (1982) In: Razin S, Rottem S (eds) Microbial membrane lipids. Academic, New York, pp 79-151
8. Rietschel ET, Galanos C, Luderitz O, Westphal O (1982) In: Webb DR (ed) Immunopharmacology and the regulation of leukocyte function. Dekker, New York, pp 183-229
9. Morrison DC, Alving CA (eds) (1984) Symposium Molecular Concepts of Lipid A. Rev Infect Dis 4:427-587

10. Rick PD, Osborn MJ (1977) Lipid A mutants of *Salmonella typhimurium*. Characterization of a conditional lethal mutant in 3-deoxy-D-mannooctulosonate-8-phosphate synthetase. J Biol Chem 252:4895-4903
11. Hitchcock PJ, Morrison DC (1984) The protein component of bacterial endotoxins. In: Rietschel ET (ed) Chemistry of endotoxin. Elsevier North Holland, Amsterdam
12. Morrison DC, Oades ZG, Betz SJ (1980) The role of lipid A and lipid A-associated protein in cell degranulation mechanisms. In: Eaker D, Wadstrom T (eds) Natural toxins. Pergammon, New York, pp 287-294
13. Sultzer BM, Goodman GW, Eisenstein TK (1980) Endotoxin protein as an immunostimulant. In: Schlessinger D (ed) Microbiology-80. American Society for Microbiology, Washington, pp 61-65
14. Goldman RC, White C, Leive L (1981) Identification of outer membrane proteins, including known lymphocyte mitogens as the endotoxin protein of *E. coli* 0111. J Immunol 127:1290-1294
15. Morrison DC, Ulevitch RJ (1978) A review – The interaction of bacterial endotoxins with cellular and humoral mediation systems. Am J Pathol 93: 527-618
16. Tanamoto K-I, Zahringer U, McKenzie GR, Galanos C, Rietschel ET, Luderitz O, Kusumoto S, Shiba T (1984) Biological activities of synthetic lipid A analogs: Pyrogenicity, lethal toxicity, anticomplement activity, and induction of gelation of *Limulus* amoebocyte lysate. Infect Immun 44:421-426
17. Palva ET, Makela PH (1980) Lipopolysaccharide heterogeneity in *Salmonella typhimurium* analyzed by sodium dodecyl sulfate/polyacrylamide gel electrophoresis. Eur J Biochem 107:137
18. Goldman RC, Leive L (1980) Heterogeneity of antigenic-side-chain length in lipopolysaccharide from *Escherichia coli* 0111 and *Salmonella typhimurium* LT2. Eur J Biochem 107:145
19. Rudbach JA, Milner KC, Ribi E (1967) Hybrid formation between bacterial endotoxins. J Exp Med 126:62-79
20. Westphal O, Lüderitz O, Bister F (1952) Über die Extraktion von Bakterien mit Phenol-Wasser. Z Naturforsch [C] 7B:148-155
21. Galanos C, Luderitz O, Westphal O (1969) A new method for the extraction of R lipopolysaccharides. Eur J Biochem 9:945
22. Ulevitch RJ (1978) The preparation and characterization of a radioiodinated bacterial lipopolysaccharide. Immunochemistry 15:164
23. Vukajlovich SW, Morrison DC (1983) Conversion of lipopolysaccharides to molecular aggregates with reduced subunit heterogeneity: demonstration of LPS-responsiveness in "endotoxin-unresponsive" C3H/HeJ splenocytes. J Immunol 130:2804-2808
24. Goodman SA, Morrison DC (1984) Selective association of lipid rich R-like lipopolysaccharide (LPS) subunits with murine spleen cells. Mol Immunol 21:689-697
25. Morrison DC, Oades ZG, Vukajlovich SJ, Goodman SA, Duncan RL (1984) Mechanism of action of endotoxin at the cellular level. In: Keppler D (ed) Mechanisms of hepatocyte injury and death. MTP, Lancaster
26. Carr C, Morrison DC (1984) Lipopolysaccharide interaction with rabbit erythrocyte membranes. Infect Immun 43:600-606
27. Haeffner-Cavaillon N, Chaby R, Cavaillon JM, Szabo L (1982) Lipopolysaccharide receptor on rabbit peritoneal macrophages: I. Binding characteristics. J Immunol 128:1950-1954
28. Morrison DC, Kline LF (1977) Activation of the classical and properdin pathways of complement by bacterial lipopolysaccharides. J Immunol 118: 362-368

Bayer-Symposium VIII
The Pathogenesis of Bacterial Infections, 85-98 (1985)

Mucosal Immunoregulation: IgA Inductive Sites, Isotype-Specific Helper T Cells, Gut LPS Influence, and Subclass Distribution of IgA Antibodies

J. R. McGhee, S. M. Michalek, H. Kiyono, S. I. Williamson, T. A. Brown, and J. Mestecky

Summary

In this brief review, we have discussed several aspects of the common mucosal immune defense system which are important in protecting the host against infections at mucosal surfaces. GALT contains subpopulations of T cells, including isotype-specific helper cells, which act on IgA-committed B cells for support of IgA immune responses. T cell help is antigen specific and requires H-2-compatible B cells and accessory cells for maximum IgA responses. Evidence was presented that LPS from the gram-negative gut microbial flora influences IgA responses. Studies with LPS from *Bacteroides* indicate that the lipid A moiety exerts similar biologic activity to the lipid A derived from *Enterobacteriaceae*, whereas the carbohydrate component of *Bacteroides* LPS exhibits biologic activity for lymphoreticular cells from LPS-responsive and LPS-hyporesponsive mice. The results of these studies indicate that purified cell populations and LPS components must be assessed separately when the biologic activities of different LPS molecules are compared. Other studies were presented which demonstrate that human IgA responses to environmental antigens such as bacterial LPS are largely of the IgA_2 subclass, while responses to other antigens such as glucosyltransferase and influenza A virus hemagglutinin are mainly IgA_1. The significance of IgA_2 antibody responses and the role of IgA_1 protease in host infection and immunity has also been briefly considered in this review.

Introduction

Immunoglobulin A (IgA) is the principal antibody isotype found in human external secretions and is a major host defense mechanism against infections involving mucosal surfaces [18, 19, 27]. Gut-associated lymphoreticular tissue (GALT) consists mainly of Peyer's patches (PP) which are distinct lymphoid nodules located along the gastrointestinal tract of most experimental animals, and represent major IgA inductive sites for ingested antigens, including pathogens, allergens, food components, milk proteins, and environmental toxicants. Ingested antigens are selectively taken up by specialized epithelial cells, termed M cells [24] or follicular-associated epithelial (FAE) cells [2], which cover the dome regions of the PP, and subsequently reach the underlying B and T cell zones. The PP contain regulatory T cells (Lyt-1 inducer and helper cells and Lyt-2 suppressor and cytotoxic cells), B cells, including those committed to IgA, and the two principal accessory cell types, i.e., macrophages (MΦ) [15] and dendritic cells – all cell types involved in host immune responses. However, local antigenic stimulation of PP cells does not result in the final differentiation of IgA-committed B cells to plasma cells synthesizing IgA in this tissue. Instead, antigen-stimulated lymphoid cells leave PP via the efferent lymphatics and enter the mesenteric lymph nodes (Fig. 1). These migrating cells pass through the thoracic duct lymphatics, enter the blood circulation, and selectively home to the lamina propria regions of the gastrointestinal, upper respiratory, and genitourinary tracts, and to the interstitium of glands, including salivary, lacrimal, and mammary tissues (Fig. 1). Although poorly understood, it is in these tissues that the precursor IgA B cells (which originated in GALT) receive the final inductive signals for their differentiation into fully mature plasma cells synthesizing IgA antibodies with specificity to the antigen first encountered in the PP. This homing network of antigen-sensitized lymphoid cells from the PP to mucosal tissues comprises a *common mucosal immune defense system* which continually provides mucosal tissues with precursor IgA B cells, committed to the synthesis of IgA antibodies with specificity to the ingested environmental antigens. Although evidence has accumulated during the past several years which supports the existence of a common mucosal im-

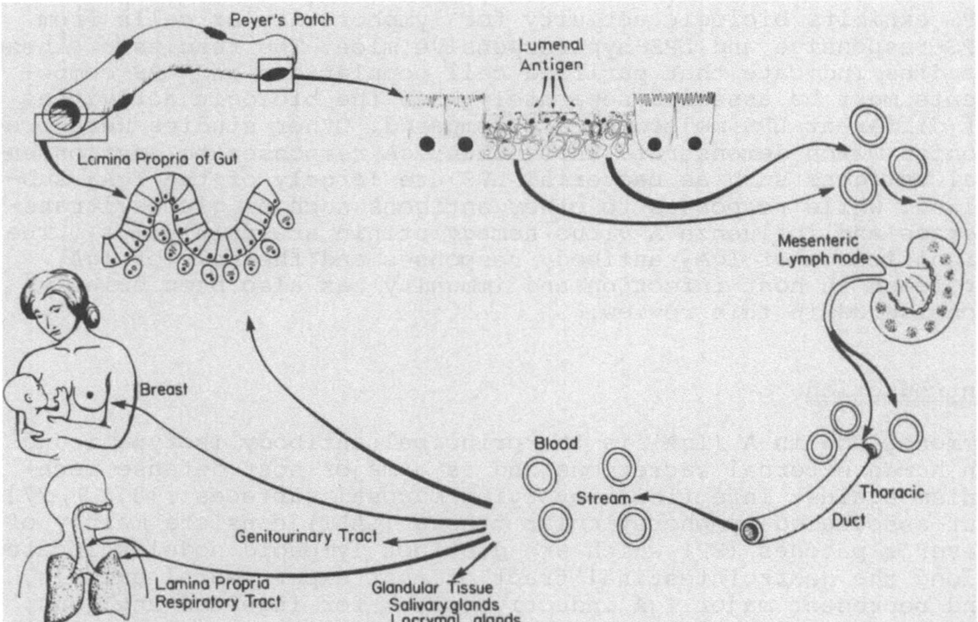

Fig. 1. The common mucosal immune system

mune system ([18, 19, 33] and numerous others), many aspects are still undefined, including: (a) isotype switching events resulting in a high frequency of IgA-committed B cells in GALT; (b) failure to induce IgA responses in the PP; (c) the mechanisms involved in the selective migration of IgA-committed B cells from the PP and the cell interactions required for their final differentiation in various mucosal tissues; (d) the effector functions and subclass distribution of IgA antibodies; and (e) environmental factors which regulate the induction of IgA responses.

In this brief review, we have summarized recent evidence on the role of T helper (Th) cells in PP for IgA B cell responses, the influence of gut microbial lipopolysaccharide (LPS) on the induction of IgA immune responses, and the human IgA_1 and IgA_2 subclass responses to various antigens first encountered at mucosal surfaces. The biologic significance of human pathogens which produce IgA_1 protease is also briefly discussed in terms of host infection and immunity.

T Cell Regulation of the IgA Response

IgA responses to antigens are thymic dependent; however, in the past, it has been difficult to study T cell regulation of IgA responses because of technical difficulties in obtaining uniform T cell populations from IgA inductive sites. We have previously shown that murine PP contain approximately equal numbers of regulatory T cells (including 40%-50% $Lyt\text{-}1^+$ and 15%-20% $Lyt\text{-}2^+$ cells) and B cells, a high proportion (12%-15%) of which express surface IgA (sIgA) [15, 20]. Furthermore, in vitro cultures of PP cells from mice orally primed with sheep erythrocytes (SRBC) give good IgA anti-SRBC plaque-forming cell (PFC) responses [15]. The availability of methods for the continuous growth of T cells [30] has allowed the isolation of regulatory T cells from murine PP, and extensive studies are currently under way to determine the precise mechanisms involved in Th-B cell collaboration for IgA isotype-specific immune responses. Recently, we have established several Th cell clones which were derived from the PP of C3H/HeJ mice orally primed with SRBC [14]. These Th cell clones support largely IgA responses (Table 1) and can be divided into two broad categories; one type of Th cells supports IgM and largely IgA anti-SRBC responses, while the second type supports low IgM, IgG_1 IgG_2, IgG_3, and high IgA responses. These T cell clones preferentially support IgA responses and have been designated PP Th A. All PP Th A cell clones are antigen (SRBC) specific and require H-2 compatible B cells for support of optimal IgA responses (Table 1); however, small IgA responses occur across the H-2 barrier. The PP Th A cells are Thy 1.2^+, $Lyt\text{-}1^+$, $Lyt\text{-}2^-$, and sIg^- and possess Fc receptors for IgA ($Fc_{\alpha}R$) (Table 1).

We have recently shown that PP Th A cells support higher IgA responses in cultures of B cells from PP than from spleen [14]. These results suggest that PP Th A cells could act directly on the postswitched $sIgA^+$ B cell subpopulation, perhaps via the

Table 1. Salient characteristics of PP Th A clones

1. PP Th A cells support largely IgA responses
2. PP Th A cells are antigen (SRBC) specific, and fail to support polyclonal or immune responses to other TD antigens
3. PP Th A cells do not support carrier-specific (SRBC) anti-hapten responses, and thus exhibit noncognate recognition
4. PP Th A cells give maximum help with fully histocompatible B cells; however, small IgA responses occur across the H-2 barrier
5. PP Th cells are Thy-1^+, Lyt-1^+, and Lyt-2^-
6. PP Th A cells bear Fc receptors for IgA ($Fc_\alpha R^+$), and are $Fc_\mu R^-$ and $Fc_\gamma R^-$

$Fc_\alpha R$ for Th-B cell collaboration for IgA responses. Alternatively, the PP Th A cells could induce isotype switching in the B cell population, and recent studies by Kawanishi and co-workers [8, 9] with mitogen-induced PP T cell clones support this possibility. Therefore, in order to distinguish between an isotype switch mechanism and preferential induction of $sIgA^+$ B cells, we have examined the nature of the B cell which collaborates with our PP Th A cell clones for IgA responses.

Purified PP B cells were separated into $sIgA^+$ and $sIgA^-$ subpopulations by flow cytometry (FACS) or by panning [13]. The addition of PP Th A cells to $sIgA^+$ B cell-enriched cultures resulted in IgA responses which were significantly higher than those obtained in cultures containing the total PP B cell population (Table 2). Interestingly, cultures containing PP B cells depleted of $sIgA^+$ B cells gave low IgA, but similar IgM, anti-SRBC PFC responses when compared with the total B cell cultures. These results indicate that the PP Th A cells collaborate with mature IgA-committed B cells and suggest that the cloned T cells help different subsets of B cells for IgM or IgA isotype responses.

In other studies, we have investigated the importance of $Fc_\alpha R$ on PP Th A cells in providing isotype-specific help to $sIgA^+$ B cells [20]. When PP Th A cells were preincubated with purified myeloma or hybridoma IgA, washed and then added to B cell cultures, the IgA anti-SRBC PFC response was reduced by approximately 90% (Fig. 2). Both 7 *S* and 11 *S* IgA produced a similar inhibitory effect on the ability of PP Th A cells to support IgA isotype-specific responses in B cell cultures. The failure of purified IgM, IgG_1, IgG_2, or IgG_3 to inhibit helper function of PP Th A cells suggests that abrogation of PP Th A cell helper activity was isotype specific. These results demonstrate that PP Th A cells collaborate with mature IgA-committed B cells and that the $Fc_\alpha R$ expressed on PP Th A cells is of central importance for T cell collaboration with B cells expressing sIgA.

A summary of possible mechanisms by which GALT T cells regulate IgA isotype responses is presented in Fig. 3. Kawanishi and coworkers [8, 9] isolated T cell clones from murine PP T cells

Table 2. PP Th A cells direct Peyer's patch sIgA$^+$ B cells toward IgA responses

Purification procedure[a]	PP B cell preparation	Anti-SRBC PFC per culture[b]	
		IgM	IgA
	Total B cells	62 ± 2	182 ± 7
FACS	sIgA$^-$	57 ± 8	28 ± 2
	sIgA$^+$	11 ± 1	308 ± 65
	Total B cells	203 ± 27	671 ± 71
Panning	sIgA$^-$	233 ± 16	131 ± 15
	sIgA$^+$	63 ± 4	1173 ± 94

[a] Peyer's patch B cells were prepared by two methods; cells were incubated with FITC-labeled anti-mouse α antibody and cells sorted by FACS into sIgA$^-$ and sIgA$^+$ populations, or cells were treated with goat IgG anti-mouse α antibody and then incubated in rabbit anti-goat IgG-coated Petri plates. The B cells were cultured with PP Th A cells and SRBC. IgM and IgA anti-SRBC PFC responses were assessed on day 5 of culture.
[b] Values are the mean anti-SRBC PFC responses per culture ± standard error.

treated with Con A. Two clones were characterized which acted on sIgM$^+$ (sIgA$^-$) B cells and induced them to switch to sIgA$^+$B cells. However, these sIgA$^+$ B cells, presumed to be committed to IgA, do not synthesize IgA following stimulation with mitogen, a finding which could explain the high frequency of sIgA$^+$ B cells in GALT. Our results with PP Th A cell clones indicate that IgA-specific T cells recognize sIgA$^+$ (committed) B cells, presumably via $Fc_{\alpha}R$ and sIgA on committed B cells, and induce these cells to final differentiation and IgA synthesis. Thus, two distinct types of T cells are present in GALT, both of which could play important roles in the regulation of IgA responses.

Influence of Gut Microbial LPS on IgA Responses

Previous results from our laboratory [1, 12, 22] have suggested that IgA responses to orally administered antigens are influenced by the *Lps* gene which is located on chromosome 4 of the mouse and regulates responsiveness to LPS [31, 32]. This conclusion was based on studies which demonstrated that the LPS-hyporesponsive C3H/HeJ mice, when compared with syngeneic LPS-responsive C3H/HeN mice, gave higher IgA splenic PFC and serum and secretory IgA antibody responses to various orally administered, T-dependent antigens. The induction of high IgA responses

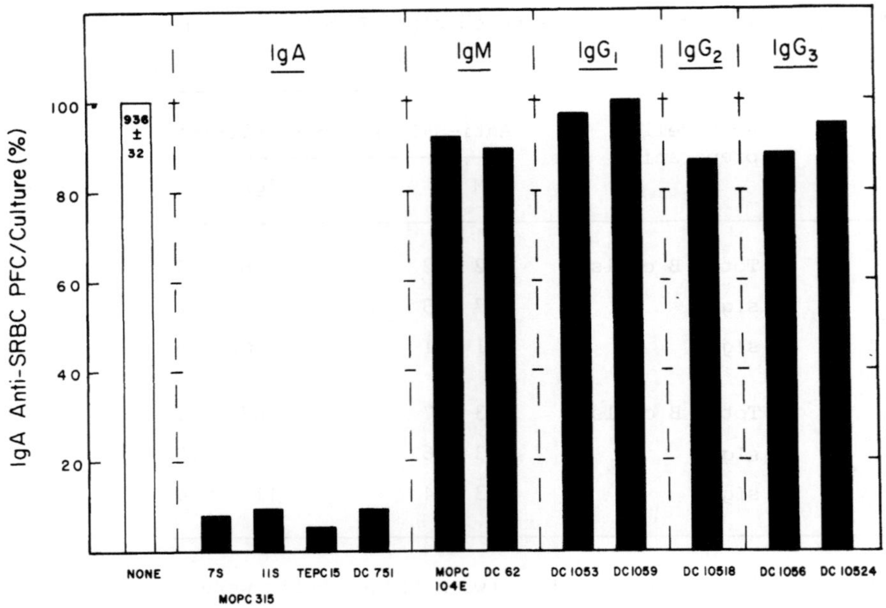

Fig. 2. Role of $Fc_{\alpha}R$ on PP Th A cells for providing isotype-specific help to B cells. PP Th A cells were incubated with purified IgA (from MOPC 315 or TEPC 15 plasmacytomas or hybridoma DC 751), IgM (from MOPC 104E plasmacytoma or hybridoma DC 62), IgG_1 (from hybridoma DC 1053 or DC 1059), IgG_2 (from hybridoma DC 10518), or IgG_3 (from hybridoma DC 1056 or DC 10524). Untreated or treated PP Th A cells were added to purified C3H/HeN splenic B cells and immunized with SRBC. IgA anti-SRBC PFC were determined on day 5 of culture. Data is expressed as the percentage of the response obtained in cultures containing Ig-treated PP Th A cells compared with the response in cultures containing untreated PP Th A cells

correlated with higher numbers of Th cells in GALT and spleen of orally immunized C3H/HeJ mice [12]. Genetic studies with offspring from crosses with C3H/HeN (Lps^n/Lps^n ; n = normal) and C3H/HeJ (Lps^d/Lps^d ; d = defective) mice confirmed the finding that elevated IgA responses are linked to expression of the Lps^d gene.

The *Lps* gene controls responses to LPS, specifically to the lipid A moiety of members of the Enterobacteriaceae, including *Escherichia coli* and *Salmonella*. However, less than 1% of the microbial flora in the gut of mammals, including humans, is comprised of members of the Enterobacteriaceae, while greater than 99% consists of the anaerobic genus, *Bacteroides*. Recent studies have shown that LPS from nonenterobacteria, including *Bacteroides*, *Brucella*, and *Pseudomonas*, stimulate lymphoid cells from C3H/HeJ mice [7, 23, 25]. Since our results clearly indicate that gut microbial LPS influences IgA immune responses to orally administered antigens, we have further investigated the biologic activity of *Bacteroides fragilis* LPS purified by phenol-water extraction.

When spleen cells (8×10^5 cells per well) from C3H mice were incubated with a phenol-water-extracted preparation of LPS from *B. fragilis* ATCC 25285 (B-LPS), significant mitogenic responses

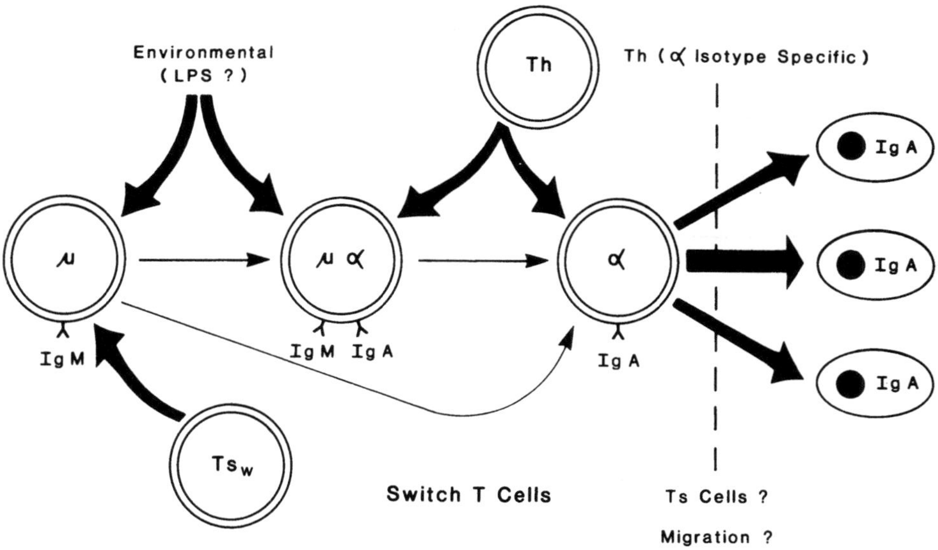

Fig. 3. Model for T cell regulation of IgA responses

were obtained; however, the responses to various doses of B-LPS of classical LPS-hyporesponsive C3H/HeJ cultures were always lower than those seen in similarly treated spleen cell cultures from C3H/HeN mice (Fig. 4A). The difference in responses to B-LPS of C3H/HeN and C3H/HeJ mice was even more apparent when limited numbers of spleen cells (8×10^4 cells per well) were tested. In fact, the response pattern resembled that observed with LPS derived from Enterobacteriaceae, in that C3H/HeN spleen cells were fully responsive, while C3H/HeJ cells gave significantly lower responses to B-LPS (Fig. 4B). These results suggested that C3H/HeJ mice are low responders to B-LPS and indicate that the *Lps* gene defect in this mouse strain is not limited to responses to LPS derived from Enterobacteriaceae.

We next examined whether B-LPS and the lipid A and carbohydrate components of B-LPS were mitogenic for splenic B cells (Table 3). B-LPS and the lipid A component induced mitogenic responses in purified splenic B cell cultures from C3H/HeN mice and essentially no responses in B cell cultures from C3H/HeJ animals. The carbohydrate component did not induce splenic B cell responses from either mouse strain. These results demonstrate that the lipid A from B-LPS is similar to that of lipid A from Enterobacteriaceae in its ability to trigger responses in C3H/HeN, but not C3H/HeJ mice. Of interest was the demonstration that the carbohydrate component of B-LPS induced mitogenic responses in whole spleen cell cultures from both C3H/HeN and C3H/HeJ mice. This observation suggests that the carbohydrate component of B-LPS is inducing B cell responses via a second cell type and could explain the earlier findings [7] which showed that B-LPS induced responses in both C3H/HeN and C3H/HeJ mice. In recent studies, we have shown that B-LPS will induce C3H/HeN B cells

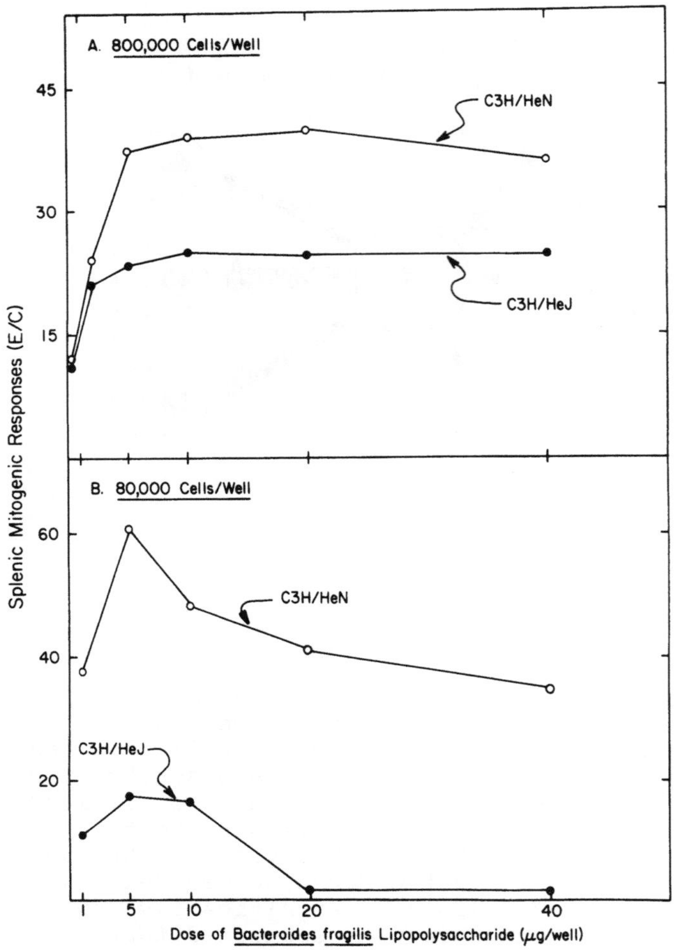

Fig. 4. Spleen cells (either 8×10^5 or 8×10^4) from C3H/HeN or C3H/HeJ mice were cultured with the amount of B-LPS indicated and incubated at 37°C in a humidified atmosphere of 5% CO_2 in air. Cultures were pulsed with ^{3}HTdR during the last 6 h of a 48-h incubation period. Values are expressed as the mean of the stimulation ratio *E/C*, defined as ^{3}HTdR uptake by cultures with LPS divided by ^{3}HTdR uptake in cultures containing medium only

to respond in the presence or absence of macrophages, while C3H/HeJ B cells will only respond when macrophages are present. These results indicate that the carbohydrate component of B-LPS stimulates macrophages, which results in B cell proliferation by a mechanism unrelated to lipid A stimulation. Therefore, in studies comparing the biologic effects of different LPS preparations, it is essential to test responses in both purified lymphoid cell cultures and whole spleen cell preparations. Furthermore, the biologic effects of the lipid A and carbohydrate components of the LPS on proliferative responses should be determined. In summary, our results indicate that the *Lps* gene regulates responses to lipid A of *Bacteroides* and these lipid A effects on GALT cells may be similar to those induced by lipid A from Enterobacteriaceae.

Table 3. Mitogenic responses of whole spleen cells or purified splenic B cells from C3H/HeN and C3H/HeJ mice to the lipid A and carbohydrate components of *Bacteroides* LPS[a]

Spleen cell culture	LPS preparation	Mitogenic response (E/C)[b]	
		C3H/HeN	C3H/HeJ
Purified B cells	B-LPS	18.0	1.0
	Lipid A	12.3	1.1
	Carbohydrate	1.4	1.3
Whole spleen cells	B-LPS	18.8	2.6
	Lipid A	8.2	1.4
	Carbohydrate	11.1	12.9

[a]Purified splenic B cells or whole spleen cells (5×10^5 cells per well) were cultured with B-LPS or the purified lipid A or carbohydrate components of B-LPS (10 μg per culture) and incubated at 37°C in 5% CO_2 in air. Cultures were pulsed with ^{3}HTdR during the last 6 h of a 48-h incubation period.
[b]Values are expressed as the mean of the stimulation ratio E/C, defined as ^{3}HTdR uptake by cultures with LPS divided by ^{3}HTdR uptake in cultures containing medium only.

Subclass Distribution of Human IgA Antibodies to Environmental Antigens

As discussed in the introduction, there is now considerable evidence to suggest that the human IgA response is under separate regulatory mechanisms from those influencing systemic IgG subclass or IgM responses. Two subclasses of IgA occur in humans: IgA_1 and IgA_2 [5, 17, 28], which exhibit a different distribution pattern in various body fluids (Table 4). Serum IgA consists of approximately 90% IgA_1 and 10% IgA_2, whereas external secretions contain equivalent amounts of the two IgA subclasses [4, 29]. Essentially all IgA found in external secretions is polymeric [27], and a recent study [3] has demonstrated a high percentage of IgA_2 plasma cells containing J chain in mucosal tissues which could help explain the relative increase of this IgA subclass in external secretions. This distribution of IgA_1 and IgA_2 in serum and external secretions and of IgA_1-, IgA_2-, and J chain-containing cells in various human tissues provides additional evidence that mucosal IgA responses are regulated by mechanisms which are separate from those that influence systemic humoral immune responses.

Table 4. Subclass distribution of IgA in human serum and external secretions and of IgA antibodies to bacterial antigens in parotid saliva

General distribution of IgA

Serum IgA	Percentage
IgA_1	~90
IgA_2	~10

90% is monomeric (7 *S*) and 10% is polymeric (pIgA)

Secretory IgA (pIgA)	Percentage		
	Colostrum	Saliva	Tears
IgA_1	50-60	~50	~50
IgA_2	40-50	~50	~50

Most pIgA is 11 *S* with lesser amounts of 15.5 *S*

Predominant subclass of IgA antibodies in parotid saliva to environmental antigens

IgA_1	IgA_2
Glucosyltransferase (*S. mutans* 6715)	Lipoteichoic acid (*S. pyogenes*)
Bacterial dextrans (B512, B1355S)	Lipopolysaccharide
Hemagglutinin (influenza A virus)	Lipid A

A major question regarding the distribution of IgA subclasses involves the specificity of IgA_1 and IgA_2 antibodies to environmental antigens. We have recently addressed this question by examining external secretions (parotid saliva and nasal washes) and serum for the presence of specific IgA_1 and IgA_2 antibodies against microbial and environmental antigens. IgA responses to a given antigen are generally similar among individuals and include antibodies in both subclasses. In parotid saliva, naturally occurring IgA antibodies to bacterial antigens such as the glucosyltransferase enzyme of *Streptococcus mutans* and dextrans preferentially occur in the IgA_1 subclass, while antibodies to lipoteichoic acid, and LPS from *Salmonella*, *E. coli*, *Bacteroides gingivalis*, and *B. fragilis* are primarily of the IgA_2 subclass (Table 4). Furthermore, it appears that the major specificity of these IgA anti-LPS antibodies is to the lipid A moiety. The parotid saliva samples used in these studies were obtained from normal, healthy subjects and should therefore represent a steady state pattern. However, it is possible that during an infection, the subclass and specificity of IgA antibodies induced may vary.

In one study (Brown et al., manuscript submitted for publication), nasal washes from human volunteers undergoing experimental intranasal infection with live influenza A virus showed a rise in the amount of IgA antibody to the hemagglutinin which was almost exclusively of the IgA_1 subclass, even though preexisting IgA_2 antibodies were also observed.

IgA_1 Protease in Host Immunity and Infection

Although the ability of IgA_1 and IgA_2 antibodies to react with the same microbial or environmental antigen and afford protection may be comparable, the presence on mucosal surfaces of bacteria which produce an enzyme capable of selectively cleaving human IgA_1 (IgA_1 protease) may considerably compromise the protective effect of antibodies of this subclass. The initial report that bacteria can produce an enzyme which specifically cleaves human IgA in the hinge region to generate intact Fab and Fc fragments [21] has led to numerous investigations to determine the spectrum of microorganisms which produce IgA_1 protease, the mode of action of this enzyme, and the possible effects of this enzyme in host immunity and infection [11, 16].

A variety of bacteria have been shown to produce IgA_1 protease (reviewed in reference [11]), and as indicated from the partial list presented in Table 5, these bacteria are associated with mucosal surfaces. Specific groups of pathogens clearly exist, e.g., the bacteria which commonly produce meningitis and upper respiratory tract infections all produce IgA_1 protease. The same is true of venereal disease bacteria and *Ureaplasma urealyticum* [10]. Finally, it is becoming clear that the two major oral diseases: dental caries and periodontal disease have contributions from IgA_1 protease-producing bacteria. *Bacteroides gingivalis* and the other major bacteria associated with destructive periodontal disease all produce IgA_1 [11]. Furthermore, the two oral streptococci involved in the initial dental plaque formation are also major IgA_1 protease producers [11].

IgA_1 proteases have a unique specificity for either prolyl-seryl or prolyl-threonyl peptide bonds which are located in the hinge region of the heavy chain of IgA_1 [11, 16]. The region is restricted to a 13-amino acid sequence which is deleted in the heavy chain of IgA_2. Although we know that IgA_1 represents approximately 90% of the IgA in serum and 50% in external secretions, we do not yet know the biologic significance of IgA_1 protease.

A number of possible consequences of IgA_1 protease on host infection and immunity have been suggested. We still do not know whether the $F(ab')_2$ fragments of IgA_1 are able to interact with antigen and retain biologic activity. It is difficult to determine whether this occurs in external secretions, since low levels of secretory IgA antibodies to IgA_1 protease have been demonstrated [6]. It is also possible that the $Fc_{\alpha 1}$ fragment which is generated could exert biologic activity, including polyclonal B cell activation and either enhancement or suppression of regu-

Table 5. Bacteria which produce IgA_1 protease and their association with disease

Species	Disease	Ecological site
Neisseria meningitidis *Hemophilus influenzae* *Streptococcus pneumoniae*	Meningitis, URT infections	Upper respiratory tract
Neisseria gonorrhoeae *Ureaplasma urealyticum*	Gonorrhea, nongonococcal urethritis	Genitourinary tract
Bacteroides gingivalis *Bacteroides loescheii* *Bacteroides melaninogenicus* Other *Bacteroides* sp. *Capnocytophaga* sp.	Periodontal disease	Dental plaque
Streptococcus sanguis *Streptococcus mitior*	Initial plaque formation	Dental plaque

latory T cells. Finally, it has recently been shown that secretory IgA can mediate bacterial killing via ADCC [25] and released $Fc_{\alpha 1}$ could have specific effects on GALT K cells and diminish ADCC activity. Additional studies are required in order to determine why pathogenic microorganisms produce IgA_1 protease and the significance of this enzyme in host infection and immunity.

Acknowledgments. We wish to thank Ms. Betty Wells for typing this manuscript. This work was supported by United States Public Health Service Grants AI 19674, AI 18958, DE 04217, AI 18745, CA 13148, DE 06068, and DE 02670. S.M.M. is the recipient of a Research Career Development Award (DE 00092).

References

1. Babb JL, McGhee JR (1980) Mice refractory to lipopolysaccharide manifest high immunoglobulin A responses to orally administered antigen. Infect Immun 29:322-328
2. Bockman DE, Cooper MD (1973) Pinocytosis by epithelium associated with lymphoid follicles in the bursa of Fabricius, appendix and Peyer's patches. An electron microscopic study. Am J Anat 136:455-478
3. Crago SS, Kutteh WH, Moro I, Allansmith MR, Radl J, Haaijman JJ, Mestecky J (1984) Distribution of IgA1-, IgA2-, and J chain-containing cells in human tissues. J Immunol 132:16-18

4. Delacroix DL, Dive C, Rambaud JC, Vaerman JP (1982) IgA subclasses in various secretions and in serum. Immunology 47:383-385
5. Feinstein D, Franklin EC (1966) Two antigenically distinguishable subclasses of human A myeloma proteins differing in their heavy chain. Nature 212:1496-1498
6. Gilbert JV, Plaut AG, Longmaid B (1983) Inhibiton of bacterial IgA proteases by human secretory IgA and serum. Ann NY Acad Sci 409:625-636
7. Joiner KA, McAdam KPWJ, Kasper DL (1982) Lipopolysaccharides from *Bacteroides fragilis* are mitogenic for spleen cells from endotoxin responder and nonresponder mice. Infect Immun 36:1139-1145
8. Kawanishi H, Saltzman LE, Strober W (1983) Mechanisms regulating IgA class-specific immunoglobulin production in murine gut-associated lymphoid tissue: I. T cells derived from Peyer's patches that switch sIgM B cells to sIgA B cells in vitro. J Exp Med 157:433-450
9. Kawanishi H, Saltzman L, Strober W (1983) Mechanisms regulating IgA class-specific immunoglobulin production in murine gut-associated lymphoid tissue: II. Terminal differention of post switch sIgA-bearing Peyer's patch B cells. J Exp Med 158:649-669
10. Kilian M, Brown MB, Brown TA, Freundt EA, Cassell GH (1984) Immunoglobulin A1 protease activity in strains of *Ureaplasma urealyticum*. Acta Path Microbiol Immunol Scand [B] 92:61-64
11. Kilian M, Thomsen B, Petersen TE, Bleeg HS (1983) Occurrence and nature of bacterial IgA proteases. Ann NY Acad Sci 409:612-624
12. Kiyono H, Babb JL, Michalek SM, McGhee JR (1980) Cellular basis for elevated IgA responses in C3H/HeJ mice. J Immunol 125:732-737
13. Kiyono H, Cooper MD, Kearney JF, Mosteller LM, Michalek SM, Koopman WJ, McGhee JR (1984) Isotype specificity of helper T cell clones. Peyer's patch Th cells preferentially collaborate with mature IgA B cells for IgA responses. J Exp Med 159:798-811
14. Kiyono H, McGhee JR, Mosteller LM, Eldridge JH, Koopman WJ, Kearney JF, Michalek SM (1982) Murine Peyer's patch T cell clones. Characterization of antigen-specific helper T cells for immunoglobulin A responses. J Exp Med 156:1115-1130
15. Kiyono H, McGhee JR, Wannemuehler MJ, Frangakis MV, Spalding DM, Michalek SM, Koopman WJ (1982) In vitro immune responses to a T cell-dependent antigen by cultures of disassociated murine Peyer's patch. Proc Natl Acad Sci USA 79:596-600
16. Kornfeld SJ, Plaut AG (1981) Secretory immunity and the bacterial IgA protease. Rev Infec Dis 3:521-534
17. Kunkel HG, Prendergast RA (1966) Subgroups of γA immune globulins. Proc Soc Exp Biol Med 122:910-913
18. McGhee JR, Mestecky J (eds) (1983) The secretory immune system. Ann NY Acad Sci 409:1-896
19. McGhee JR, Michalek SM (1981) Immunobiology of dental caries: microbial aspects and local immunity. Annu Rev Microbiol 35:595-638
20. McGhee JR, Michalek SM, Kiyono H, Eldridge JH, Colwell DE, Williamson SI, Wannemuehler MJ, Jirillo E, Mosteller LM, Spalding DM, Hamada S, Gollahon KA, Morisaki I, Gregory RL, Koopman JW (1984) Mucosal immunoregulation: environment lipopolysaccharide and GALT T lymphocytes regulate the IgA response. Microbiol Immunol 28:261-280
21. Metha SK, Plaut AG, Calvanico JH, Tomasi TB Jr (1973) Human immunoglobulin A: production of an Fc fragment by an enteric microbial proteolytic enzyme. J Immunol 111:1274-1276
22. Michalek SM, Kiyono H, Babb JL, McGhee JR (1980) Inheritance of LPS nonresponsiveness and elevated splenic IgA immune responses in mice orally immunized with heterologous erythrocytes. J Immunol 125:2220-2224

23. Moreno E, Berman DT (1979) *Brucella abortus* lipopolysaccharide is mitogenic for spleen cells of endotoxin-resistant C3H/HeJ mice. J Immunol 123:2915-2919
24. Owen RL, Jones AL (1974) Epithelial cell specialization within human Peyer's patches: an ultrastructural study of intestinal lymphoid follicles. Gastroenterology 66:189-203
25. Pier GB, Markham RB, Eardley D (1981) Correlation of the biological responses of C3H/HeJ mice to endotoxin with the chemical and structural properties of the lipopolysaccharides from *Pseudomonas aeruginosa* and *Escherichia coli*. J Immunol 127:184-191
26. Tagliabue A, Nencioni L, Villa L, Keren DF, Lowell GH, Boraschi D (1983) Antibody-dependent cell-mediated antibacterial activity of intestinal lymphocytes with secretory IgA. Nature 306:184-186
27. Tomasi TB (ed) (1976) The immune system of secretions. Prentice-Hall, New Jersey
28. Vaerman JP, Heremans JF (1966) Subclasses of human immunoglobulin A based on differences in the α polypeptide chain. Science 153:647-649
29. Vaerman JP, Heremans JF, Laurell CB (1968) Distribution of α chain subclasses in normal and pathological IgA-globulins. Immunology 14:425-432
30. Watson J (1979) Continuous proliferation of murine antigen-specific helper T lymphocytes in culture. J Exp Med 150:1510-1519
31. Watson J, Kelly K, Largen M, Taylor BA (1978) The genetic mapping of defective LPS response gene. J Immunol 120:422-424
32. Watson J, Riblet R, Taylor BA (1977) The response of inbred strains of mice to bacterial lipopolysaccharide. J Immunol 118:2088-2093
33. Weisz-Carrington P, Roux ME, McWilliams M, Phillips-Quagliata JM, Lamm ME (1979) Organ and isotype distribution of plasma cells producing specific antibody after oral immunization: evidence for a generalized secretory system. J Immunol 123:1705-1708

Discussion

(pp. 68-98)

Dr. Patterson inquired of Dr. Morrison why he relied on the B-cell proliferative assay as a means for assessing the biological activity of lipopolysaccharide (LPS). Dr. Morrison indicated that there are a number of biological activities which are elicited by LPS, both in vitro and in vivo. There is a reasonable correlation between the ability of LPS to act as a B-cell mitogen, the ability of LPS to elicit a lethal response in mice, and the ability of LPS to stimulate procoagulant activity in mononuclear cells. He postulated from these results that the measure of proliferative activity of an LPS preparation will approximate its ability to interact with cells of bone-marrow origin. There is good data suggesting that cells of bone-marrow origin are critical for the manifestations of endotoxin lethality in mice.

Dr. Morrison asked two questions: 1. Is there evidence that aggregated or monomeric Fc-alpha will initiate a polyclonal B-cell response? 2. Is there evidence that the concept of isotype-specific T-helper cells extend to the subclass level? Dr. McGhee replied that at his institution they are using IgA_1 protease to cleave the Fc, so that they can pursue this point. They plan to study peridontal disease and determine whether they can induce a polyclonal activation with peripheral blood cells. With regard to isotype-specific T-helper cells, others have been able to cell sort using fluoresceinated IgA_1 to bind to peripheral blood cells, cell sort those out, and put them back into a pokeweed mitogen culture. Under those conditions a very nice IgA response is seen. Examination of whether the response is A_1 or A_2 has not been done but is underway.

Dr. Joiner asked what Dr. Morrison thought the state of aggregation of the LPS would contribute to the biological activity measured. Dr. Morrison indicated that one must think about LPS macromolecules as high molecular weight mycellar aggregates. They are not homogeneous materials, but rather extremely heterogeneous and of extremely high molecular weight. Equally as important as the presence of lipid A is the molecular environment in which the lipid A finds itself – the relative hydrophobicity or hydrophilicity. There is good evidence now that at least some LPS will in fact bind with relatively high affinity to lipoproteins. There is some species dependence for these interactions and the precise role of divalent cations as a negative regulatory influence for these interactions has yet to be determined.

Session 2

Extension of Infection Beyond the Surface Cells - Circumvention of the Host Defense System

Chairman: W. Opferkuch

Bayer-Symposium VIII
The Pathogenesis of Bacterial Infections, 102-120 (1985)

Molecular Interaction Between the Third Complement Protein and Bacterial Cell-Surface Macromolecules

R. P. Levine

Summary

When C3, the third complement protein, is activated it can bind covalently to bacterial cell-surface macromolecules where its presence can lead to cell death by either phagocytosis or cytolysis. *Haemophilus influenzae* type B, O18:K1 *Escherichia coli*, and group A streptococci are three examples of complement resistant pathogens and this paper describes certain features of the chemistry of C3 activities and binding that relate to the resistance of these organisms to be bactericidal effects of complement.

Introduction

The deposition of the third complement protein (C3) on a bacterial cell marks the cell for death because the activation of the classical and the alternative complement pathways can lead to either phagocytosis or cytolysis. Phagocytosis can take place because of the presence on the cell surface of one of several different molecular forms of C3 that are able to initiate phagocytosis through the attachment of the cell-bound form of C3 to complement receptors on phagocytic cells. Cytolysis can occur because the cell-bound C3 can initiate the formation of the membrane attack complex (MAC) composed of the fifth through the ninth complement proteins (C5-C9), which, acting as an ion channel, disrupts the ionic integrity of the bacterial cell. Figure 1 is a highly abbreviated view of the complement system that intentionally emphasizes the central role of C3 (see [1-4] for reviews of the complement system).

One is not surprised by the occurrence of complement-resistant bacteria, particularly among those that cause systemic infections. Nor is one surprised that normal human serum can serve as an excellent growth medium for certain of these organisms. Several examples of complement resistance have been described to date, and the properties of a few of the resistant organisms are summarized in Table 1. In general, these organisms are "resistant" to either the binding and/or action of C3 [5-11] or to the binding and/or action of the MAC [12-18]. This paper is concerned with C3 and its interaction with bacterial cell-surface macromolecules. It will focus first on the chemistry of C3 activation and binding and then on three bacterial pathogens that have evol-

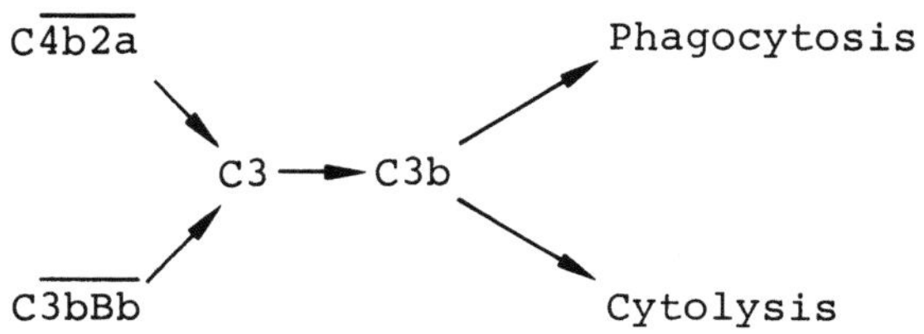

Fig. 1. The activation of C3 by either the classical pathway enzyme ($\overline{C4b2a}$) or the alternative pathway enzyme ($\overline{C3bBb}$) can lead to either phagocytosis or cytolysis. Phagocytosis is induced by the presence of one of several different molecular forms of C3 that can bind to receptors on phagocytic cells, and cytolysis can occur when cell-bound C3 initates the formation of the membrane attack complex composed of complement proteins C5-C9

Table 1. Resistance to complement-mediated killing

	Resistance "factor"	Resistance "mechanism"	References
A. *Examples of C3b resistance*			
K1 *E. coli*	Sialic acid	Inhibits activation of the alternative pathway	[5,6]
Group B streptococci	Sialic acid	Inhibits activation of the alternative pathway	[7,8]
Group A streptococci	M protein	Limits C3b binding	[9,10]
Hemophilus influenzae	Polyribose ribitol phosphate capsular polysaccharide	Inhibits activation of the alternative pathway	[11]
B. *Examples of membrane attack complex (MAC) Resistance*			
E. coli K12	traT protein (?)	Prevents MAC insertion and/or function	[12,13]
Salmonella minnesota S218	Long-chain LPS (?)	Prevents MAC insertion	[14,15]
Neisseria gonorrhoeae	(?)	Prevents MAC function	[16,17]
Acholeplasma laidlawii	Lipoglycan (?)	Prevents MAC insertion and/or function	[18]

ved resistance to C3 activation and/or binding, O18:K1 *Escherichia coli*, *Hemophilus influenzae* type b, and group A streptococci.

The Activation and Binding of C3

C3 is composed of two polypeptides, α and β, having molecular weights of approximately 120 000 and 75 000, respectively. During the course of the action of either the classical or alternative pathways, an arginyl-serine bond in the α polypeptide is cleaved to produce a 77-residue peptide (C3a) and a major component (C3b). C3b has the transient capacity to bind covalently [19] to cell-surface macromolecules, immune complexes, and a variety of molecules in solution [20-22]. The binding occurs via an acyl transfer reaction [20,21] that results in the formation of either an acyl ester or amide bond. The α chain of C3 contains an internal thioester [23-26] in the sequence -Gly-Cys-Gly-Glu-Glu-Asn-Met and, upon activation, the thioester is either hydrolyzed or the active glutamyl residue reacts with hydroxyl or amino groups to form either acyl ester or amide-linked complexes, respectively [22,27,28].

The activation of C3 can occur either enzymatically or chemically [22,28,29]. Enzymatic activation by the classical pathway is brought about by a complex composed of subunits of C2 and C4, $\overline{\mathrm{C4b2a}}$, in which C2a is a serine protease and C4b is a cofactor. Activation of C3 via the alternative pathway [3] occurs through the action of a serine protease known as Bb in a complex with C3b ($\overline{\mathrm{C3bBb}}$) in which C3b acts as a cofactor. Thus, the alternative pathway contains a feedback loop in which the generation of additional C3b amplifies the activity of the pathway. This pathway is subject to regulation by two proteins: I, a serine protease that can cleave C3 and hence inactivate it, and its cofactor, H. Certain cell surfaces are not conducive to the activation of the alternative pathway because H, in competition for binding with B, binds more efficiently than B to establish an environment in which protein I can inactivate the C3b molecules that are generated by the $\overline{\mathrm{C3bBb}}$ enzyme. It is in this manner that the feedback or amplification loop is broken, thus preventing the activation of the alternative pathway.

C3 can also be activated with trypsin which cleaves the α polypeptide between the same arginyl-serine bond that is attacked by the complement enzymes [1]. The chemical activation of C3 (Table 2) comes about through the action of chaotropic agents and certain protein denaturants [28]. In this case, however, the α polypeptide of C3 remains intact.

The mechanism of the enzymatic or chemical activation of C3 and formation of either acyl ester or amido ester bonds is poorly understood. The initiating event may be a conformational change in the protein [30-32] induced either by the cleavage of the α polypeptide or by the disruptive action of a chaotropic agent or a denaturant. The nature of the conformational change is not clear; apparently is exposes the internal thioester bond to direct nucleophillic attack by either hydroxyl or amino groups [29]. Since these groups, at least on biologically relevant molecules and at physiologic pH, are relatively weak nucleophiles, it is possible that an internal assistance mechanism accounts for their attack on the bond.

Table 2. C3 activation (after Law [28])

(In)activating reagent	Concentration	Inactivation (%)	Specific binding of glycerol ^{3}H (cpm/μl C3)
KBr	2 M	99	43.1 ± 3.4
KSCN	0.5 M	73	34.9 ± 3.6
Guanidinium chloride	1 M	97	32.2 ± 3.0
Urea	3 M	106	41.2 ± 3.7
SDS	0.015%	71	9.0 ± 3.2
Trypsin	0.5%	100	26.9 ± 3.4
Methylamine	0.1 M	94	1.5 ± 4.3

The spectrum of receptive cell surfaces and receptive molecules to which C3 can bind covalently is very broad [22,29], but the thioester is not equally accessible to all molecules. For example, the alcohols of the simple alkanes show differences in their reactivity, depending on the bulk of the alkyl groups (Table 3). This observation suggests that the structure of C3 and of the covalent binding site impose certain restrictions on the accessibility of the site to bulkier molecules [29].

Table 3. Efficiency of binding of alcohols to C3 as measured by the inhibition of glycerol ^{3}H binding (after Law et al. [29])

Alcohol	Binding efficiency
None	
Glycerol	1 (by definition)
Methanol	1.12
Ethanol	1.13
n-Propanol	1.25
Isopropanol	0.28
n-Butanol	1.26
sec-Butanol	0.22
tert-Butanol	-0.02

Recently [29], we have compared the binding of glycerol ^3H and putresine ^3H to C3 at different pH values. The results in Fig. 2 show that the binding of glycerol at pH 6 is about twice that at pH 10. In contrast, the pH dependence of putrescine binding to C3 is quite different since binding is negligible at pH values of 7.5 or less. These results support the idea that binding occurs by a nucleophilic attack on the thioester by either OH or NH_2 groups. That the efficiency of glycerol binding is relatively constant over the pH range studied reflects the fact that the nucleophilicity of OH groups is rather insensitive to pH. The binding of putrescine, on the other hand, is sensitive to pH since only the unprotonated form of the amino group is nucleophilic; indeed, the curve of putrescine binding efficiency approximates the deprotonation of its first amino group (pK_a about 9.0). This difference in potential for acyl ester versus amide bond formation may be of significance to the resistance of certain bacteria to the binding of C3 (see the section on group A streptococci).

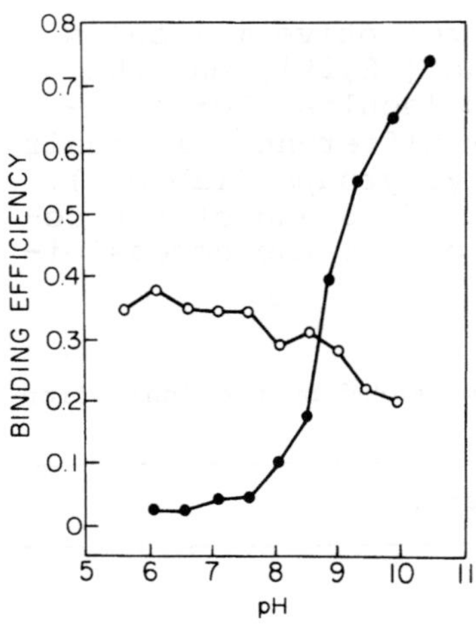

Fig. 2. The fluid phase activation and binding [22] of glycerol ^3H (*open circles*) and putrescine ^3H (*full circles*) to C3 at different pH values. Trypsin was used to activate C3. The concentration of glycerol was 24 mM and that of putrescine was 14 mM. From Law et al. [29]

The Resistance of Bacteria to the Action of C3

Several bacterial pathogens are resistant to complement-mediated killing at the stages of complement action at which C3 is either activated or becomes bound to the bacterial cell surface [5-11]. Since C3 binds to cell surfaces by either acyl ester or amide bonds and since bacterial cell surfaces are presumably rich in the hydroxyl and amino groups to which C3 can bind, the ways by which pathogens have evolved resistance are of considerable biologic and chemical interest.

K1 *E. coli*

E. coli strains that possess the K1 capsular polysaccharide are a common cause of neonatal meningitis and bacteremia [33]. Thus, in host organisms whose immature immune systems are not yet fully capable of producing antibodies, the antibody-independent alter-

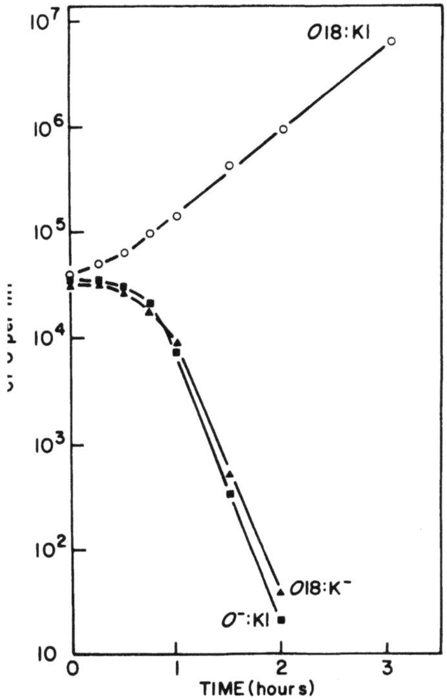

Fig. 3

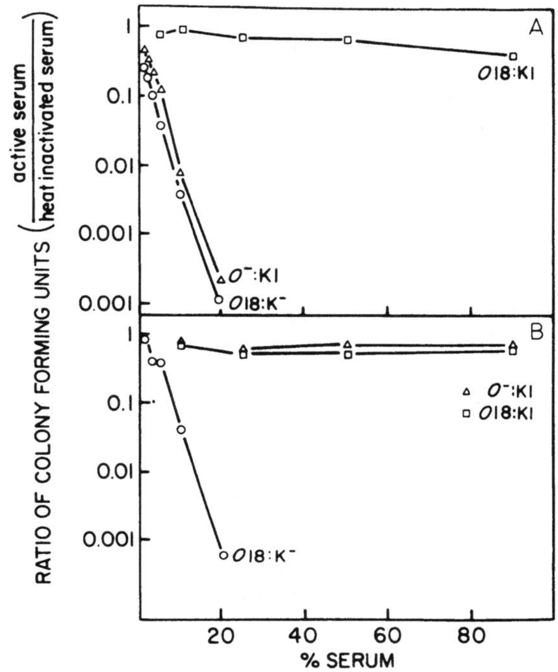

Fig. 4

Fig. 3. The bactericidal effects of 90% normal guinea pig serum on O18:K1, O18:K⁻, and O⁻:K1 strains of *E. coli*. After Pluschke et al. [5]

Fig. 4. The bactericidal effects of normal guinea pig serum (A) and C4-deficient guinea pig serum (B) on O18:K1, O18K⁻, and O⁻:K1 strains of *E. coli*. After Pluschke et al. [5]

native pathway rather than the antibody-dependent classical pathway would seem to be a pirmary line of defense.

Studies [56] of the bactericidal effects of complement on an O18:K1 strain (RS228) of *E. coli* and mutant strains derived from it that lack either the K1 capsule (strain A691) or the O antigen (strain A691) are summarized in Fig. 3-6 and Table 4. The bactericidal effects of 90% normal guinea pig serum are shown in Fig. 3 where it will be noted that the O18:K1 strain is totally resistant whereas both of the mutant strains are sensitive. Figure 4a shows the effect of serum concentration on the viability of the three strains. Since one or both of the complement pathways could be responsible for the killing of the O18:K1 and O18:K⁻strains, the identical experiment was carried out using C4-deficient guinea pig serum (Fig. 4b) in which only the alternative pathway is operative. In this instance, it is seen that only the O18:K⁻strain is sensitive, suggesting that the presence of the K1 capsular polysaccharide is responsible for the resistance of the cells to the bactericidal effects of the alternative pathway. Several different sera were then tested for both their

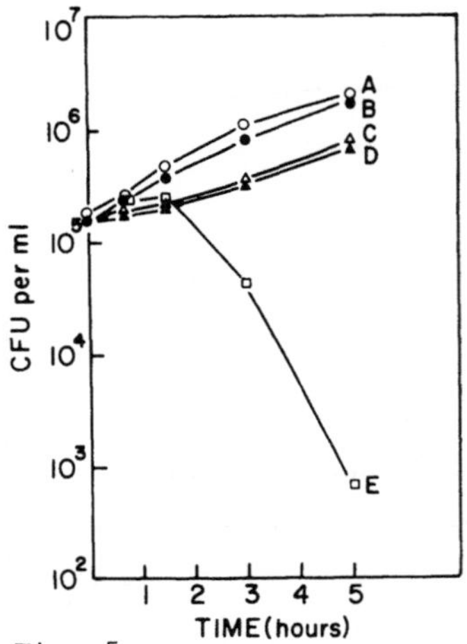

Fig. 5

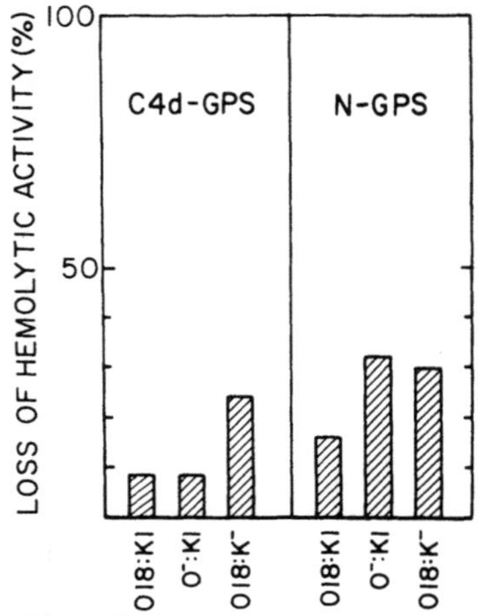

Fig. 6

Fig. 5. The effect of antibody on the bactericidal activity of complement from normal rat serum on O18:K1 *E. coli*. Curve *A* rat anti-O7:K1, in normal rat serum; curve *B* normal rat serum; curve *C* normal rat serum in Mg-EGTA; curve *D* rat anti-O18:K1 in normal rat serum containing Mg-EGTA; curve *E* rat anti-O18:K1 in normal rat serum. After Pluschke and Achtmann [6]

Fig. 6. Complement-consuming activities in normal guinea pig serum (N-GPS) and C4-deficient guinea pig serum (C4D-GPS) of O18:K1, O^-:K1, and O18:K^- strains of *E. coli*. Residual hemolytic activity was measured in serum samples after they had been incubated with bacteria for 30 min at 37°C. The percentage activity lost relative to control samples incubated without bacteria is shown. The control values were 19 600 hemolytic units per milliliter and 19 000 hemolytic units per milliliter for N-GPS and C4d-GPS, respectively. The values are the averages from four experiments. From Pluschke et al. [5]

classical and alternative pathway bactericidal effects, and the results are summarized in Table 4, where it can be seen that the O18:K1 strain is resistant to the bactericidal effects of human serum and sera that possess alternative and/or classical pathway activity. O^-:K1 cells, on the other hand, are resistant to sera that have only alternative pathway activity, but sensitive to sera that have only classical pathway activity. The O18:K^- cells are sensitive to all of the sera tested. It appears, therefore, that the presence of the K1 capsular polysaccharide alone is sufficient to prevent the bactericidal action of the alternative pathway. The loss of the O antigen (strain A454) results in a rough derivative of the O18:K1 strain that remains resistant to the alternative pathway, but becomes sensitive to the classical pathway in the absence of added antibody. This is seen most particularly in guinea pig classical pathway reagent that lacks alternative pathway activity. Since, however, the O^-:K1 cells are also sensitive in antibody-free colustrum-derived calf serum and in the germ-freee rat serum, it appears that antibody is not entirely essential for the classical pathway-mediated effects of these sera. This independence of antibody for classical pathway killing has been demonstrated to occur by the so-called C1

Table 4. Bactericidal effects of different sera on *E. coli* strains[a] (after Pluschke et al. [5])

	Serum					
	C2d-HS	C4d-GPS	N-GPS	CPR-GPS	CD-CS	GF-RS
Classical pathway	-	-	+	+	+	+
Alternative pathway	+	+	+	-	+	+
Bacterial strains						
Rs228 (o18:K1)	R	R	R	R	R	R
A464 (O^-:K1)	R	R	S	S	S	S
A691 (O18:$K1^-$)	S	S	S	S	S	S

[a] 2×10^3 bacteria were incubated in 0.1 ml containing 90% serum and the change in viable count was determined after 3 h at 37°C. R indicates that these bacteria had multiplied at least fivefold. S indicates that less than 1% of the original inoculum survived the incubation. C2d-HS C2-deficient human serum; C4d-GPS C4-deficient guinea pig serum; N-GPS normal guinea pig serum; CPR-GPS classical pathway reagent guinea pig serum; CD-CS colostum-deprived calf serum; and GF-RS germ-free rat serum. CPR is prepared by inactivating the alternative pathway by treating serum with a combination of bentonite and diisopropylfluorophosphate

bypass, [34,35] a classical pathway route that has been observed to occur in the presence of certain organisms. This route is apparently blocked in O18:K1 cells, perhaps because the O18 antigen blocks deeper structures on the cell surface from activating the C1. Addition of antibody directed specifically against the O18 antigen, however, renders O18 cells sensitive to the bactericidal effects of killing by the antibody dependent classical pathway (see Fig. 5), demonstrating that the antibody-mediated classical pathway can be effective on these cells.

The observations made with these strains of *E. coli* demonstrate: (a) that the K1 capsular polysaccharide is related to resistance to the alternative pathway; (b) that the presence of the O antigen renders the cells resistant to antibody-independent activation of the classical pathway, presumably by the C1 bypass; and (c) that in the presence of added anti-O18 antibody, the cells are sensitive to the classical pathway killing. Thus, in neonatal hosts, the virulence of O18:K1 *E. coli* can be explained, at least in part, on the basis of resistance to complement-mediated killing via the alternative pathway, and if the antibody-independent activation of the C1 bypass is of significance as a host defense mechanism, the presence of the O18 antigen appears to prevent its operation as well.

In view of the results summarized here, it is of interest to examine the capacity of the cells of the three strains to consume complement in the absence of added antibody. Figure 6 shows the results of complement fixation assays using C4-deficient and normal guinea pig serum as sources of complement. When C4-deficient serum is incubated with cells of the O18:K$^-$type, it loses 20%-30% of its hemolytic activity whereas incubation of this serum with cells that possess the K1 capsular polysaccharide leads to less than a 10% loss of hemolytic activity. There is a considerable loss of hemolytic activity in normal guinea pig serum after it is incubated with O18:K1, and O18:K$^-$cells. The loss of activity after incubation with O18:K1 and O$^-$:K1 cells is presumably due to classical pathway activation of the complement in normal guinea pig serum. It is of interest in this regard to note that O18 cells are resistant to classical pathway-mediated killing, even though complement is activated via the classical pathway and hence consumed. It is not known, however, which if any of the complement proteins have become bound to the cells. In contrast to the classical pathway activation of complement by O18 cells, the activation of the alternative pathway in the presence of K1 cells is minimal, suggesting that the K1 capsular polysaccharide inhibits alternative pathway activation.

The K1 capsular polysaccharide is a homopolymer of sialic acid, and the presence of sialic acid has been correlated with the invasiveness of certain bacterial pathogens [33,34-39]. It is known that sialic acid plays a role in preventing the activation of the alternative pathway on mammalian cell surfaces where its presence on these cell surfaces enhances the efficiency of the regulatory proteins, I and H, that bring about the proteolysis of the alternative pathway C3 activating enzyme [40-42]. Hence, under normal circumstances, the alternative pathway is not activated on mammalian cell surfaces. Thus, by apparently mimicking their host cell surfaces, K1 *E. coli* and other invasive pathogens, such as type III, group B streptococci, that also possess sialic acid in the capsule [7,8] can inhibit a major, nonspecific defense mechanism of the preimmune hosts to bacterial invasion.

Hemophilus influenzae b

H. influenzae b causes meningitis and bacteremic infections in children in whom susceptibility is correlated with either undetectable or low concentrations of antibody directed against the type b polyribose ribitol phosphate (PRP), capsular polysaccharide [43], and noncapsular antigens. Both anti-capsular and anti-noncapsular antibodies may provide a mechanism for host defense by activating the classical pathway of complement action [44,45].

We have investigated both the classical and alternative pathway bactericidal activity of human complement and of human antibody directed against specific *H. influenzae* type b strain Eagan cell-surface antigens [11]. Figure 7 shows the effects of different antibody-free complement sources on the survival of *H. influenzae* b. It can be seen that cells grow in agammaglobulinemic serum (AGS) that provides both classical and alternative pathway activities and in C2-deficient serum and AGS containing Mg and EGTA, both of which provide alternative pathway activity only. Figure 8 shows that AGS is bactericidal in the presence of either a total IgG fraction containing both anti-capsular and anti-noncapsular antibodies or IgG-absorbed PRP, and IgG fraction absorbed with PRP-Sepharose. Since both pathways operate under the conditions

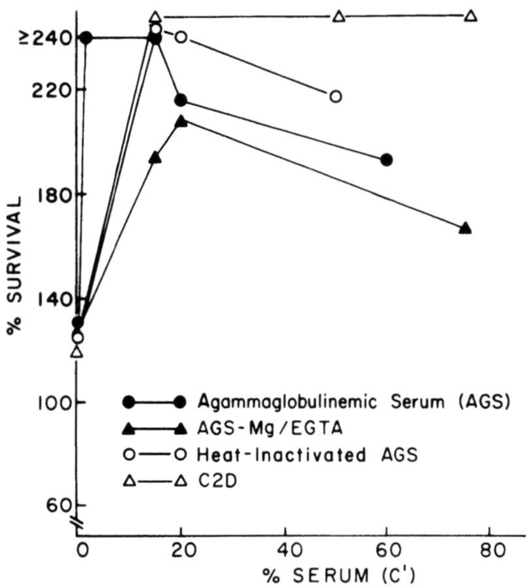

Fig. 7. Bactericidal effects on *H. influenzae* type b strain Eagan of different complement sources without added antibody. From Steele et al. [11]

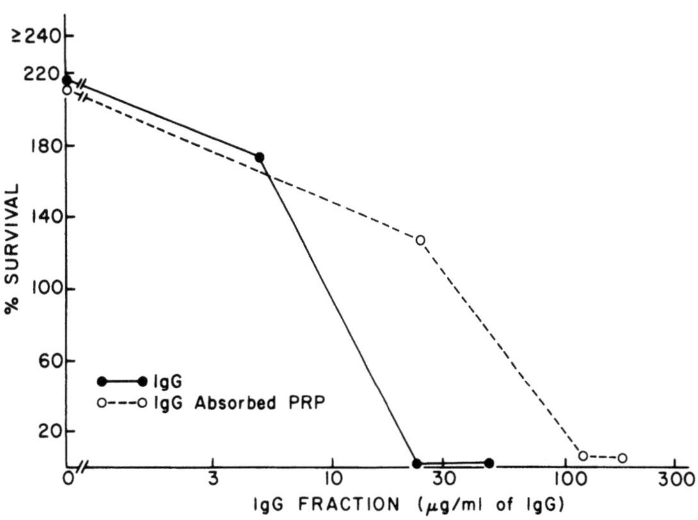

Fig. 8. Bactericidal effects of 15% AGS with added IgG or IgG-absorbed PRP on *H. influenzae* type b. Both sources of antibodies elicited bactericidal activity. However, a greater concentration of IgG-absorbed PRP (noncapsular antibody) was required to achieve killing comparable to unabsorbed IgG. From Steele et al. [11]

of this experiment, we examined the alternative pathway activity of AGS containing Mg and EGTA in the presence of either the total IgG fraction or IgG-absorbed PRP. Figure 9 shows that the unabsorbed antibody is effective in bringing about the alternative pathway killing of *H. influenzae* b whereas the antibody lacking anti-PRP has only a marginal effect and that this is seen only at antibody concentrations above 190 μg/ml. Thus, it appears that the alternative pathway resistance of *H. influenzae* b can be overcome in the presence of an IgG fraction containing antibodies directed against the PRP capsular polysaccharide. This observation is in agreement with that of Tarr et al. [46] who noted that alternative pathway activity against *H. influenzae* b could be

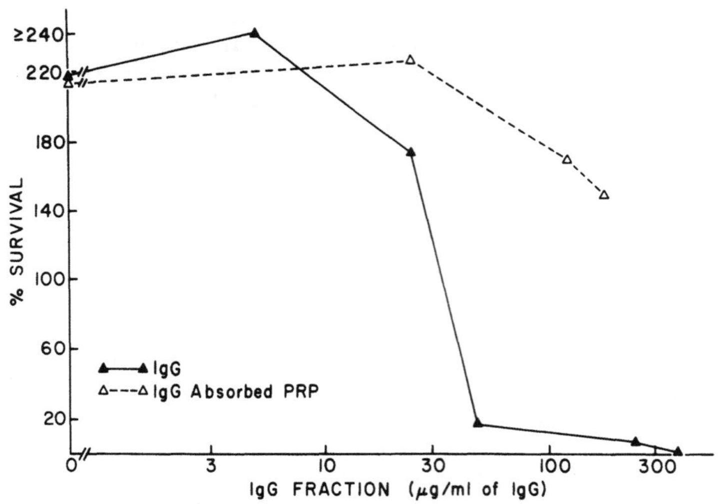

Fig. 9. Bactericidal effects on *H. influenzae* type b of 15% AGS-Mg/EGTA with added IgG or IgG-absorbed PRP. The IgG fraction elicited alternative pathway killing of this organism. However, at the concentrations tested, IgG-absorbed PRP did not. From Steele et al. [11]

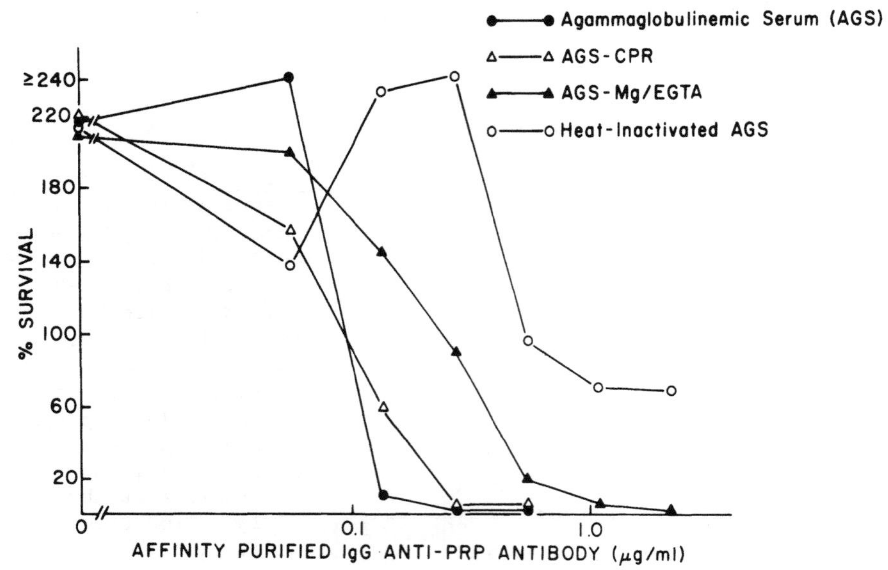

Fig. 10. Bactericidal effects on *H. influenzae* type b of 15% AGS, 15% AGS-Mg/EGTA, and 20% AGS-CPR with added affinity-purified anticapsular antibody. A higher concentration of AGS-CPR was used to compensate for loss of complement activity during preparation of this reagent. In the presence of AGS or AGS-CPR, killing was observed at comparable concentrations of antibody. In contrast, in AGS-Mg/EGTA, a more than three-fold increase in anti-PRP antibody was required for comparable killing. From Steele et al. [11]

initiated in C4-deficient guinea pig serum upon the addition of human IgG containing anti-PRP antibody. Figure 10 shows both the classical and alternative pathway activity of AGS in the presence of added affinity-purified anti-capsular antibody. Also shown

Table 5. Alternative pathway complement consumption[a] by *H. influenzae* type b (Steele et al. [11])

% Total consumed			% C3 consumed	
Complement source	No added antibody	IgG anti-PRP	No added antibody	IgG anti-PRP
10% AGS-Mg/EGTA (human)	0	52	N.T.[b]	N.T.
10% C2-deficient (human)	0	25	0	41
10% C4-deficient (guinea-pig)	29	N.T.	N.T.	N.T.

[a]Consumption of total hemolytic complement or C3 by *H. influenzae* b (2.8×10^7 CFU/ml), or by *H. influenzae* b plus affinity-purified anti-capsular (anti-PRP) antibody (1.0 µg/ml). Complement activity was measured by hemolytic assays using rabbit erythrocytes (1.25×10^7 µl) for total complement or sheep EAC142 for C3 consumption. Results are reported as percentage consumption compared with controls (10% AGS-Mg/EGTA or 10% C2-deficient serum with added antibody, but not incubated with *H. influenzae* b cells). C4-deficient guinea pig serum contained 0.08 µg/ml anti-PRP antibody.

[b]N.T. not tested

is the activity of a classical pathway reagent prepared from AGS (AGS-CPR), and the alternative pathway activity of AGS containing Mg and EGTA.

The findings described here confirm previous observations that suggest that cells of *H. influenzae* b are resistant to the bactericidal effects of the alternative pathway in the absence of added antibody. Complement is either not activated or, if activation occurs, one or more of the complement proteins that are essential to bring about cytolysis either fail to bind or they bind in a fashion that is not effective in allowing cytolysis to occur. Complement consumption should be detected in the latter case, and indeed it has been reported [46-47] that complement consumption of C4-deficient guinea pig serum does occur in the absence of cytolysis. We have also investigated total complement consumption using C4-deficient guinea pig serum and have confirmed these earlier reports (Table 5). Our results with C2-deficient human serum, and with AGS containing Mg and EGTA, however, show that there is only insignificant alternative pathway consumption unless IgG anti-PRP antibody is present. We have, at present no explanation for the differences in the results obtained for guinea pig serum and human serum, but they show the need to consider differences between animal species with regard to differences in complement activation. We also measured C3 consumption in C2-deficient human serum in both the presence and absence of added anti-PRP antibody and found that C3 was not consumed in the absence of the added antibody.

The results of the complement fixation assays reveal that the resistance of *H. influenzae* b to alternative pathway-mediated killing lies at the level of C3 activation rather than to a step in the pathway that lies beyond C3. They also are in accord with the results obtained in the bactericidal assays in that total complement as well as C3 consumption occur in the presence of added anti-PRP antibody.

Next, we turned to the question of the nature of the resistance of *H. influenzae* b to the bactericidal action of the alternative pathway and to the role of antibody in bypassing the resistance. Antibody-*stimulated* alternative pathway has been reported [48-52] and antibody-*dependent* alternative pathway has been described for the opsonization of type III, group B streptococci [7,8].

In contrast to the specific role played by antibody in initiating the classical pathway, the precise role of antibody in activating the alternative pathway is obscure. Antibody may either mask groups, such as sialic acid residues, that are known to inhibit alternative pathway activation, or, on the other hand, the presence of an antibody on an inhospitable cell surface may merely provide new sites for alternative pathway activation. In the case of type III, group B streptococci, whose capsular polysaccharide chains terminate with sialic acid residues, removal of the sialic acid residues, renders these organisms sensitive to opsonization by C3b generated via the alternative pathway, and the role of antibody in the opsonization of group B streptococci via the alternative pathway may be to mask sialic acid residues or to provide sites removed from the sialic acid where the C3 cleaving enzyme is protected from degradation by the proteins H and I that regulate the alternative pathway. Except for the fact that the cell surface of *H. influenzae* b lacks sialic acid residues, its resistance to the alternative pathway appears to be analogous to that of type III, group B streptococci.

As described in the section on its activation and binding, C3 has the capacity to form covalent bonds with cell-surface macromolecules and, at neutral pH, covalent attachment is most likely to be by acyl ester rather than by amido ester bonds. It is conceivable that OH groups on the cell surface of *H. influenzae* b are oriented in a fashion that makes them inaccessible to the covalent binding site of C3 so that too little C3b becomes bound to establish sufficient $\overline{C3bBb}$ to convert additional C3 into C3b. It is also conceivable that the polyanionic nature of the capsular polysaccharide somehow excludes C3b from binding to the cell surfaces. Additionally, it is possible that the components of the polysaccharide, either the ribose or the ribitol phosphate, act to inhibit the activation of the alternative pathway in a manner similar to that of sialic acid. At this juncture, we know only that trypsin-activated C3 does not bind to PRP in the fluid phase [22]. Clearly, the chemical nature of *H. influenzae* b resistance to the bactericidal effects of the alternative pathway is intriguing, and a knowledge of its nature may be important for better understanding of the virulence of this organism in non-immune hosts.

Group A Streptococci

The virulence of group A streptococci is associated with the rigid, α-helical coiled-coil M protein, a component of the cell surface [53,54]. In immune hosts, M+ cells can be opsonized with C3b produced via the classical pathway; in nonimmune hosts, in which presumably only the alternative pathway is operative, however, the cells are resistant to phagocytosis [8-9]. M- cells on the other hand, are sensitive to phagocytosis follwing opsonization with C3b generated by the alternative pathway. M+ cells, in contrast to M- cells, activate the alternative pathway less efficiently and bind about 50% less C3, but even though they bind less C3, the amount deposited per cell is sufficient for the promotion of phagocytosis of an M- cell [10]. Hence, a deficiency of cell-bound C3b cannot be solely responsible for resistance of the M- cells to phagocytosis.

Recently, Dr. Janis J. Weis [62] has carried out a series of experiments concerned with C3 and the alternative pathway resistance of M+, group A streptococci, and some of her results are summarized here. Since the C3b bound to M+ cells does not promote adherance between group A streptococci and PMNs, it is conceivable that the C3 detected on M+ cells is either in a molecular form that is not recognized by complement receptors on PMNs or that it is inaccessible to these receptors. Possibly the M protein blocks the receptor binding site on the C3b or alternatively its rigid helical structure might impose constraints on the capacity of C3b to interact with these receptors.

The attachment of M- cells to PMNs is facilitated by the presence on the bacterial cell surface of C3b that can bind to the CR1 receptor and of iC3b and C3d,g that can bind to the CR3 receptor on PMNs [4,55,56]. The observation that opsonized M+ cells do not promote phagocytosis under conditions in which opsonized M- cells adhere readily suggests that the C3 detected on the surface M+ bacteria is either inaccessible to CR1 and CR3 or that it is in a molecular form that is not recognized by these receptors. In order to determine the molecular form of the C3 bound to M+ and M- cells, ^{125}I-labeled C3 was added to serum during opsonization after which the cell-bound C3 was released by various treatments that disrupt hydrophobic and/or covalent interactions between C3 and the bacterial surface [18,19]. SDS-polyacrylamide gel electrophoresis of C3 extracted by 25 m*M* methylamine and 1% SDS revealed that greater than 90% of the C3 deposited on both M+ and M- cells was in the opsonic form of either C3b or iC3b.

Further analysis revealed that 90% of the C3 bound to M+ cells was released by three extractions with 1% SDS at neutral pH whereas less than 50% of that associated with M- cells was released under these conditions. Electrophoretic analysis of the detergent-released C3 demonstrated that 74% and 66% of the C3 associated with M+ and M- cells, respectively, migrated with polypeptides of molecular weight greater than the α chain of native C3. These polypeptides are presumed to represent the α chains of C3 covalently attached to detergent-releasable bacterial membrane components. The quantitative difference in susceptibility to detergent release of C3 bound to M+ and M- cells may reflect different topographical sites of C3 deposition on those surfaces, and it is likely that remaining C3 bound to M- surfaces after SDS extraction is covalently attached to a component of the cell wall, possibly peptidoglycan which is an efficient activator of the alternative pathway [57]. In contrast, no more than 10% of the C3 bound to M+ surfaces appears to be covalently attached to detergent-insoluble structures, and this may reflect the greater complexity of the M protein-bearing surface upon which cell-surface components other than the cell wall provide an efficient site for covalent bond formation. Alternatively, the M protein may mask the cell wall and hence inhibit its complement-activating properties. No obvious differences appear in the profile of the C3 membrane polypeptide complexes of the SDS-soluble material of the two strains that might reflect unique sites for covalent bond formation on the M protein-bearing surface. The fraction of covalently bound C3 that bound to both SDS-soluble and SDS-insoluble membrane components was approximately 80% for both cell types. Therefore, not only do M+ cells bear opsonic forms of C3, but most of the bound C3b has formed a covalent bond with the cell surface and should be recognized by receptors on PMNS. It is possible that the C3 covalently bound to the M+ surface is attached to a structure that, because of its loose association with the rest of the cell, cannot mediate adherence of the entire cell to receptor-positive cells, on the other hand, the receptor binding site on M+ cell-associated C3 may be blocked or buried so that it cannot interact with membrane receptors.

Other serum and plasma proteins have been found to influence susceptibility of group A streptococci to phagocytosis. Plasma fibrinogen has been reported to act as a cofactor in resistance to phagocytosis of an M24 organism [58], however, unlike the strains used here and in previous studies [8,9,59], this M+ culture was susceptible to phagocytosis upon opsonization with nonimmune serum. Fibronectin in decomplemented human plasma appears to promote adherence of several M- strains to PMNs, although at only 2% of the level of complement-containing plasma [60]. This is of interest since fibronectin has recently been shown to enhance C3b- and iC3b-dependent phagocytosis by human monocytes and macrophages [61] and may therefore have an enhancing effect on ingestion of bacteria.

The observations set forth here can be summarized in the following way. First, M+ cells bind 50% less C3 than do M- cells. Nevertheless, the C3 is covalently bound. The absolute difference between the amount of C3 that is bound to M+ and M- cells may be the consequence of a difference in the availability of OH compared with NH_2 groups on the two cell surfaces. It will be recalled (see the section on activation and binding) that, upon activation, C3 forms acyl ester, but not amide bonds in the pH range 6-9. Accordingly, the decreased C3 binding to M+ cells could be explained by the fact that these cells possess a greater abundance of NH_2 groups relative to OH groups. Second, the fact that the number of opsonic forms of C3 bound to M+ cells is deemed to be sufficient to enhance phagocytosis suggests that the binding sites on these forms of C3 are either masked or somehow constrained from binding to complement receptors in PMNs.

Third, this masking or constraint may result from the covalent binding of C3 to SDS-soluble membrane proteins rather than to SDS-insoluble cell wall components.

Acknowledgments. Research in the author's laboratory is supported by a research grant (AI-16543) from the National Institute of Allergy and Infectious Diseases of the N.I.H.

References

1. Reid KBM, Porter RR (1981) The proteolytic activation systems of complement. Annu Rev Biochem 50:433
2. Brown EJ, Frank MM (1981) Complement activation. Immunol Today 2:129
3. Müller-Eberhard HJ, Schreiber RD (1980) Molecular biology and chemistry of the alternative pathway of complement. Adv Immunol 29:1-53
4. Fearon DT, Wong WW (1983) Complement ligand-receptor interactions that mediate biological responses. Ann Rev Immunol 1:243-272
5. Pluschke G, Mayden J, Achtman M, Levine RP (1983) Role of the capsule and the O antigen in resistance of O18:K1 *Escherichia coli* to complement-mediated killing. Infect Immun 42:907-913
6. Pluschke G, Achtmann M (1984) Degree of antibody-independent activation of the classical complement pathway ba K1 *Escherichia coli* differs with O antigen type and correlates with virulence of meningitis in newborns. Infect Immun 43:684-692
7. Edwards MS, Kasper DL, Jennings HJ, Baker CJ, Nicholson-Weller A (1982) Capsular sialic acid prevents activation of the alternative complement pathway by type III, group B streptococci. J Immunol 128:1278-1283
8. Edwards MS, Nicholson-Weller A, Baker CJ, Kasper DL (1980) The role of specific antibody in alternative complement pathway-mediated opsonophagocytosis of type III, group B *Streptococcus*. J Exp Med 151:1275-1287
9. Peterson PK, Schmeling D, Clearly PP, Wilkinson BJ, Kim Y, Quie PG (1977) Inhibition of alternative complement pathway opsonization by group A streptococcal M protein. J Infect Dis 139:575-585
10. Jacks-Weis J, Kim Y, Cleary PP (1981) Restricted deposition of C3 on M+ group A streptococci: Correlation with resistance to phagocytosis. J Immunol 128:1897-1902
11. Steel NP, Munson RS, Granoff DM, Cummins JR, Levine RP (1984) Antibody independent alternative pathway killing of *Haenophilus influenzae* Type b. Infect Immun 44:452-458
12. Ogata RT, Levine RP (1980) Characterization of complement resistance in *Escherichia coli* conferred by the antibiotic resistance plasmid R100. J Immunol 125:1494-1498
13. Binns MM, Mayden J, Levine RP (1982) Further characterization of complement resistance conferred in *Escherichia coli* by the plasmid genes *traT* of R100 and *iss* of ColV, I-94. Infect Immun 35:654-659
14. Joiner KA, Hammer CH, Brown EJ, Cole RJ, Frank MM (1982) Studies on the mechanism of bacterial resistance to complement-mediated killing: I. Terminal complex components are deposited and released from *Salmonella minnesota* S218 without causing bacterial death. J Exp Med 155:797-808
15. Joiner KA, Hammer CH, Brown EJ, Frank MM (1982) Studies on the mechanism of bacterial resistance to complement-mediated killing: II. C8 and C9 release C5b67 from the surface of *Salmonella minnesota* S218 because the terminal complex does not insert into the bacterial outer membrane. J Exp Med 155:809-819

16. Harriman GR, Podack ER, Braude AI, Corbeil LD, Esser AF, Curd JG (1982) Activation of complement by serum-resistant *Neisseria gonorrhoeae:* Assembly of the membrane attack complex without subsequent cell death. J Exp Med 156:1235-1249
17. Joiner KA, Warren KA, Brown EJ, Swanson J, Frank MM (1983) Studies on the mechanism of bacterial resistance to complement-mediated killing: IV. C5b-9 forms high molecular weight complexes with bacterial outer membrane constituents on serum-resistant but not on serum-sensitive *Neisseria gonorrhoeae.* J Immunol 131:1443-1451
18. Dahl JS, Hellewell SB, Levine RP (1977) A mycoplasma mutant resistant to lysis by C: Variation in membrane composition and altered response to the terminal C complex. J Immunol 119:1419-1426
19. Law Sk, Levine RP (1977) Interaction between the third complement protein and cell surface macromolecules. Proc Natl Acad Sci USA 74:2701
20. Law SK, Lichtenberg NA, Levine RP (1979) Evidence for an ester linkage between the labile binding site of C3b and receptive surfaces. J Immunol 123:1388
21. Gadd KJ, Reid KBM (1981) The binding of complement component C3 to antibody-antigen aggregates after activation of the alternative pathway in human serum. Biochem J 195:471
22. Law SK, Minich TM, Levine RP (1981) Binding reaction between the third human complement protein and small molecules. Biochemistry 20:7457
23. Howard JB (1980) Methylamine reaction and denaturation-dependent fragmentation of complement component 3: Comparison with α_2-macroglobulin. J Biol Chem 255:7082
24. Tack BF, Harrison RA, Janatova J, Thomas ML, Prahl JW (1980) Evidence for presence of an internal thiolester bond in third component of human complement. Proc Natl Acad Sci USA 77:5764
25. Pangburn MK, Müller-Eberhard HJ (1980) Relation of a putative thioester bond in C3 to activation of the alternative pathway and the binding of C3b to biological targets of complement. J Exp Med 152:1102
26. Thomas ML, Janatova J, Gray WR, Tack BF (1982) Third component of human complement: Localization of the internal thiolester bond. Proc Natl Acad Sci USA 79:1054
27. Hostetter MK, Thomas ML, Rosen FS, Tack BF (1982) Binding of C3b proceeds by a tranesterification reaction at the thiolester site. Nature 298:72
28. Law SK (1983) Non-enzymic activation of the covalent binding reaction of the complement protein C3. Biochem J 211:381
29. Law SK, Minich TM, Levine RP (1984) The covalent binding efficiency of the third and fourth complement proteins in relation to pH, nucleophilicity, and availability of hydroxyl groups. Biochemistry 23:3267-3272
30. Isenman DE, Cooper NR (1981) The structure and function of the third component of human complement: I. The nature and extent of conformational changes accompanying C3 activation. Mol Immunol 18:331-339
31. Isenman DE, Kells DIC, Cooper NR, Müller-Eberhard HJ, Pangburn MK (1981) Nucleophilic modification of human complement protein C3: Correlation of conformational changes with acquisition of C3b-like functional properties. Biochemistry 20:4458-4467
32. Isenman DE (1983) Conformational changes accompanying proteolytic cleavage of human complement protein C3b by the regulatory enzyme factor I and its cofactor H: Spectroscopic and enzymological studies. J Biol Chem 258: 4238-4244
33. Robbins JB, McCracken GH, Gotschlich EC, Ørskov F, Ørskov I, Hanson LA (1974) *Escherichia coli* K1 capsular polysaccharide associated with neonatal meningitis. N Engl J Med 290:1216-1220

34. Leist-Welsh P, Bjornson AB (1982) Immunoglobulin-independent utilization of the classical complement pathway in opsonophagocytosis of *Escherichia coli* by human peripheral leukocytes. J Immunol 128:2643-2651
35. Loos M, Wellek B, Thesen R, Opferkuch W (1978) Antibody-independent interaction of the first component of complement with gram-negative bacteria. Infect Immun 22:5-9
36. Glode MP, Sutton A, Moxon ER, Robbins JB (1977) Pathogenesis of neonatal *Escherichia coli* meningitis: Induction of bacteremia and meningitis in infant rats fed *E. coli* K1. Infect Immun 16:75-80
37. Pluschke G, Mercer A, Kusečék B, Pohl A, Achtman M (1983) Induction of bacteremia in newborn rats by *Escherichia coli* K1 is correlated with only certain O (lipopolysaccharide) antigens. Infect Immun 39: 599-608
38. Siegel JD, McCracken GH (1981) Sepsis neonatrum. N Engl J Med 304:642-647
39. Smith HW, Huggins MB (1980) The association of the O18, K1 and H7 antigens and the Col V plasmid of a strain of *Escherichia coli* with its virulence and immunogenicity. J Gen Microbiol 121:387-400
40. Kazatchkine MD, Fearon DT, Austen KF (1979) Human alternative complement pathway: Membrane-associated sialic acid regulates the competition between B and β1H for cell bound C3b. J Immunol 122:75-81
41. Okada N, Yasuda T, Okada H (1982) Restriction of alternative complement pathway activation by sialosyl-glycolipids. Nature 299:261-263
42. Pangburn MK, Müller-Eberhard HJ (1978) Complement C3 convertase: Cell surface restriction of β1H control and generation of restriction on neuraminidase-treated cells. Proc Natl Acad Sci USA 75:2416-2420
43. Peltola H, Kayhty H, Sivonen A, Mäkelä PH (1977) *Haemophilus influenzae* type b capsular polysaccharide vaccine in children: A double-blind field study of 100,000 vaccinees three months to five years of age in Finland. Pediatrics 60:730-737
44. Anderson P, Johnston Jr RB, Smith DH (1972) Human serum activities against *Haemophilus influenzae*, type b. J Clin Invest 51:31-38
45. Fothergill LD, Wright J (1933) Influenzal meningitis. The relation of age incidence to the bactericidal power of blood against the causal organism. J Immunol 24:273-284
46. Tarr PI, Hosea SW, Brown EJ, Schneerson R, Sutton A, Frank MM (1982) The requirement of specific anticapsular IgG for killing of *Haemophilus influenzae* by the alternative pathway of complement activation. J Immunol 128:1772-1775
47. Quinn PH, Crossen Jr FJ, Winkelstein JA, Moxon ER (1977) Activation of the alternative complement pathway by *Haemophilus influenzae* type B. Infect Immun 16:400-402
48. Boackle RJ, Pruitt KM, Mestecky J (1974) The interaction of human complement with interfacially aggregated preparations of human secretory IgA. Immunochemistry 11:543
49. Joseph BS, Cooper NR, Oldstone MBA (1975) Immunologic injury of cultivated cells infected with measles virus: I. Role of IgG antibody and the alternative pathway. J Exp Med 141:761
50. Nelson B, Ruddy S (1979) Enhancing role of IgG in lysis of rabbit erythrocytes by the alternative pathway of human complement. J Immunol 122:1994
51. Polhill RB, Newman SL, Pruitt KM, Johnston RB (1978) Kinetic assessment of alternative complement pathway activity in a hemolytic system: II. Influence of antibody on alternative pathway activation. J Immunol 121: 371
52. Winkelstein JA, Shin HS (1974) The role of immunoglobulin in the interaction of pneumococci and the properdin pathway: Evidence for its specificity and lack of requirement for the Fc portion of the molecule. J Immunol 112:1635

53. Lancefield RC (1962) Current knowledge of type-specific M antigens of group A streptococci. J Exp Med 89:307-313
54. Fox EN (1974) M proteins of group A streptococci. Bacteriol Rev 38:57-86
55. Lachmann PJ, Pangburn MK, Oldroyd RG (1982) Breakdown of C3 after complement activation. Identification of a new fragment. C3g, using monoclonal antibodies. J Exp Med 156:205-216
56. Beller DI, Springer TA, Schreiber RD (1982) Anti-Mac-1 selectively inhibits the mouse and human type three complement receptor. J Exp Med 156:1000-1009
57. Greenblatt JR, Baackle J, Schwab JH (1978) Activation of the alternative complement pathway by peptidoglycan from streptococcal cell wall. Infect Immun 19:296-303
58. Whithack E, Beachey EH (1982) Antiopsonic activity of fibrinogen bound to M protein on the surface of group A streptococci. J Clin Invest 69: 1042-1045
59. Bisno AL (1979) Alternative complement pathway activation by group A streptococci: Role of M protein. Infect Immun 26:1172-1176
60. Simpson WA, Hasty DL, Mason JM, Beachey EH (1982) Fibronectin-mediated binding of group A streptococci to human polymorphonuclear leukocytes. Infect Immun 37:805-810
61. Wright SD, Craigmyle LS, Silverstein SC (1983) Fibronectin and serum amyloid P component stimulate C3b and C3bi mediated phagocytosis in cluture human monocytes. J Exp Med 158:1338-1343
62. Weis JJ, Law SK, Levine RP, Cleary PP (1985) Resistance to phagocytosis by group A streptococci: Failure of deposited complement opsonins to interact with cellular receptors. J. Immunol 134:500-505

Discussion

(pp.102-120)

The question came up as to where the energy for the esterification comes from. The answer was that the attack upon the internal thioester bond of C3 and C4 by weak nucleotides follows upon the induction of a conformational change in these proteins; but the mechanism of the reaction between the nucleotides and C3 or C4 is poorly understood. It may be that the conformational change alters the reactivity of the bond and an internal assistance mechanism provides the means for the attack upon the bond by the weak nucleophiles.

Another question concerned whether bacterial proteases are known to be capable of splitting C3 and C4. Knowledge is very limited and very few examples can be found in the literature. Sunquist recently showed that C3 could be degraded in vivo in a guinea pig model by a *Bacteroides* strain.

Bayer-Symposium VIII
The Pathogenesis of Bacterial Infections, 122-136 (1985)

Mechanisms of Bacterial Resistance to Complement-Mediated Killing

K. A. Joiner and M. M. Frank

Summary

The mechanisms of bacterial resistance to complement-mediated killing were investigated. Initial studies showed that the C5b-9 complex of complement was formed rapidly on smooth, serum resistant (ser-R) Salmonella and *E. coli* strains incubated in serum. However, the complex did not insert into hydrophobic domains of the outer membrane, was shed from the bacterial surface and was not bactericidal. Recent work shows that complement is being deposited on only the longest lipopolysaccharide molecules in these strains, suggesting that C5b-9 is sterically blocked from access to complement susceptible sites on the outer membrane. Ser-R *Neisseria gonorrhoeae* (GC) also activate complement efficiently, but the non-bactericidal C5b-9 complex which forms on and remains stably bound to the outer membrane of ser-R GC is in a different molecular configuration than the bactericidal C5b-9 formed on serum-sensitive GC or ser-R GC rendered sensitive with antibody. Additional studies with polyclonal and monoclonal antibodies suggest that bactericidal antibody may function by increasing the bactericidal efficiency of C5b-9 in the bacterial surface.

Introduction

The capacity of fresh blood to cause killing of certain types of bacteria was the first recognized function of the complement system. Although much of the initial research on the interaction of the complement system with bacteria involved gram-negative organisms which were susceptible to direct complement attack (so-called serum sensitive (Ser-S) organisms), it is now apparent that those gram-negative bacteria that can resist direct complement-mediated killing are more virulent and pathogenic than their serum-susceptible counterparts. Thus, in animal models of infection involving gram-negative bacteria, serum-resistant (Ser-R) bacteria cause more sustained bacteremia [24,34], are better able to cause infective endocarditis [4,8], and survive better in implanted tissue chambers [24] than do susceptible strains. More importantly, a large number of clinical circumstances have been defined in which the ability to evade complement lysis is a distinct virulence factor. This was first appreciated in the studies of Roantree and Rantz [35], who found that bloodstream isolates of gram-negative organisms were generally Ser-R whereas isolates from the stool and urine of the same individuals were more susceptible to serum killing. This finding has been documented repeatedly [39,44,45]. There is also a suggestion that bacteremia caused by Ser-R organisms is associated with a higher incidence of shock and death than is bacteremia caused by serum-sensitive strains [22,29]. Localized deep tissue infections within the urinary tract (pyelonephritis) are more commonly caused by Ser-R isolates than are cystitis or assymptomatic bacteriuria, again implying a selective advantage in invasive potential for those strains capable of evading lytic attack by complement.

Serum resistance appears to be a particularly important virulence determinant for *Neisseria* species. Schoolnik et al. [37] demonstrated that gonococci causing localized genital infections are frequently Ser-S, whereas those isolates causing disseminated infection are almost invariably Ser-R, and other workers have confirmed and extended this observation [33]. Similarly, disseminated infection with *N. meningitidis* is typically caused by strains which evade direct complement killing, whereas meningococcal isolates from pharyngeal carriers are more susceptible to human serum. The most convincing evidence for the importance of complement-mediated bacteriolysis in host defense is provided by those patients with a congential deficiency of one the terminal complement components. These individuals have a particular propensity for disseminated infection with *Neisseria* species.

There is a complex interplay between levels of "natural" bactericidal antibody to various organisms and susceptibility of the host to infection. The current rise in the incidence of serious infection with *Hemophilus influenzae*, and the striking age-related distribution of *H. influenzae* infections has been ascribed to the absence of bactericidal antibody in susceptible individuals. The target of natural or immune antibody (e.g., LPS, outer membrane protein, capsule, pilus) and the antibody isotype are important determinants of bactericidal activity. For example, antibodies to pili are not generally bactericidal, perhaps because complement is being activated at too great a distance from the cell wall. Antibodies to LPS and outer membrane proteins are typically, but not invariably bactericidal, especially when in vitro killing studies limit activation to the alternative complement pathway [40]. The demonstration that anti-capsular antibodies for *N. meningitidis* and *H. influenzae* are bactericidal is of both practical and theoretical interest. Practically, vaccine trials with the polysaccharide capsules from these organisms have demonstrated protective efficacy of anti-capsular antibodies. Theoretically, it would be of importance to determine the mechanism by which an antibody to a capsular structure renders the outer membrane of an organism susceptible to complement attack. Finally, the presence of blocking antibodies which are present in normal human serum and which can override or circumvent the bactericidal activity of coexisting bactericidal antibodies for *N. gonorrhoeae* and *N. meningitidis* has been clearly elucidated [6,23,32].

The characteristics of gram-negative bacteria which render them resistant to complement attack have been extensively investigated. The clearest association with Ser-R is the possession within Enterobacteriaceae of the smooth phenotype (e.g., LPS molecules bearing long *O*-polysaccharide side-chains) [3,27,36,43]. Many such isolates resist serum killing, even in the presence of high-titered antibody to the *O*-polysaccharide. There is an emerging recognition that LPS variations within bacteria possessing exclusively rough LPS, such as *Neisseria* [25,38] and *Hemophilus* [1], or organisms possessing relatively short *O*-polysaccharide side-chains within LPS, such as *Pseudomonas* [9], can also be associated with serum resistance. The mechanism of resistance in these cases apparently represents either the absence of bactericidal antibody directed against LPS from the Ser-R isolates or the presence of blocking antibody. There is a clear association in *E. coli* [42], *Yersinia enterocolitica* and *Aeromonas salmonicida* [26] between the presence of specific outer membrane proteins and Ser-R, although the mechanism mediating resistance is unclear. The presence of certain polysaccharide capsules (K1 in *E. coli*, type B in *N. meningitidis*, type b in *H. influenzae*) has a clear association with Ser-R. Finally, it should be mentioned here that all gram-positive bacteria evade direct complement killing, possibly as a consequence of the thick peptidoglycan layer. Much less is known about the actual mechanism by which organisms evade complement killing. The central question in this regard is whether complement resistance represents inefficient complement activation or instead represents subversion of the membrane attack process at some later step. There is growing evidence that the latter mechanism is operative in most circumstances. Many Ser-R strains are well opsonized in nonimmune serum, and C3b is demonstrable on these isolates by immunofluorescence following serum incubation. Fierer and Finley [5] demonstrated equivalent deposition of C3 by immunofluorescence on a Ser-R *E. coli* strain before and after conversion of the strain to a Ser-S form with diphenylamine. Reynolds et al. [31] demonstrated C3, but were unable to demonstrate C5b on a Ser-R strain of *Salmonella* following incubation in C6-deficient rabbit serum. This finding was likely due to the instability of C5b binding to target sites. Ogata and Levine [28] initially reported that equivalent amounts of C3 and C5 were consumed by two *E. coli* strains varying in complement susceptibility owing to the presence of a specific outer membrane protein (tra-t) in one isolate. Workers from the same laboratory [2] have subsequently shown that C8 and C9 consumption did not differ when the two *E. coli* isolates were compared, thus illustrating that the relative complement resistance of the tra-t-containing strain did not represent inability to activate complement through C9.

Over the last 3 1/2 years, we have systematically investigated the mechanism of Ser-R for a number of bacterial studies. We initially examined the mechanism by which smooth, Ser-R isolates of *E. coli* and *Salmonella* were able to evade serum killing, and studies are continuing on this issue. More recently, we have turned our attention to the question of Ser-R in *N. gonorrhoeae* (GC), and to the mechanism by which bactericidal antibody renders GC susceptible to complement attack.

Serum Resistance in *Salmonella* and *E. coli*

Our initial studies compared the interaction of complement with a smooth, Ser-R isolate of *Salmonella minnesota* and an isogenic, deep rough, Ser-S mutant of the parent strain [11,12]. The Ser-R organism was not killed by any concentration of pooled normal human serum (PNHS), even in the presence of high-titered agglutinating antibody. The Ser-S organism was killed in a dose-related fashion as serum concentration was raised, with over 99.9% killing of the strain in 10% PNHS. Early studies indicated that both organisms were capable of causing rapid C3 depletion from serum. Deposition of C3 on the Ser-R isolate actually exceeded C3 deposition on the Ser-S strain, clearly demonstrating that the mechanism of Ser-R for the smooth *S. minnesota* isolate was not an inability to active complement efficiently through C3. We therefore turned our attention to the interaction of the terminal complement components with both organisms. Less than 25% consumption of C5, C7, and C9 from serum occurred with the Ser-S strain, compared with rapid and complete utilization of these three representative late components by Ser-R *S. minnesota*. It was clear, therefore, that consumption of terminal components was not translatable into formation of bactericidal C5b-9. To investigate this further, direct binding studies of purified terminal components were performed. These showed that, while as many as 8×10^3 C5b-9 complexes per bacterium rapidly formed on the Ser-R bacterial surface, the complexes were shed from the bacterial surface with continued incubation (Fig. 1). This was quite unlike the situation with Ser-S *S. minnesota* in which stable binding of $5\text{-}7 \times 10^3$ C5b-9 complexes occurred. This same pattern of stable C5b-9 attachment to Ser-S strains and transient C5b-9 binding followed by release from Ser-R organisms was observed

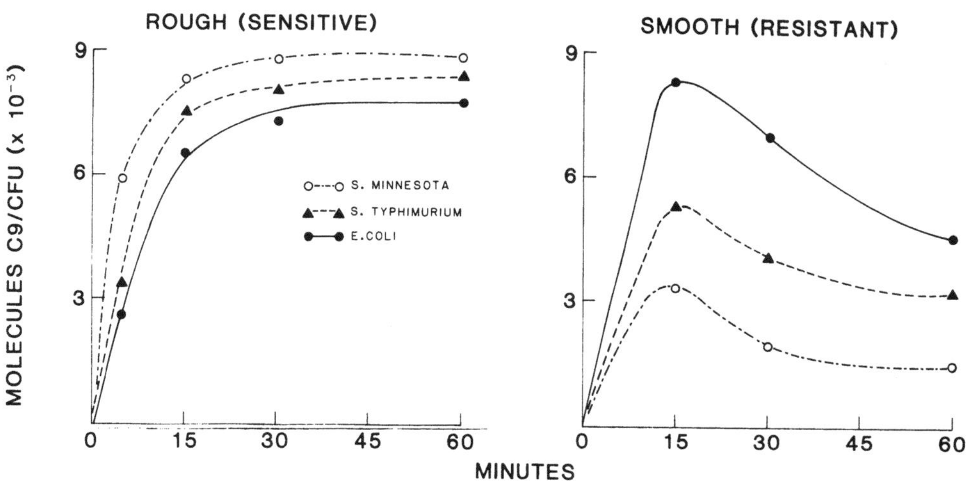

Fig. 1. Kinetics of C9 uptake on isogenic pairs of rough, Ser-S and smooth, Ser-R *Salmonella* and *E. coli*. The rough strains were *S. minnesota* Re595 (Re mutant), *E. coli* J5 (Rc mutant), and *S. typhimurium* TV119 (Ra mutant). The smooth, parent strains were *S. minnesota* S218, *E. coli* O111B4 (ATCC 29552), and *S. typhimurium*

for two additional isogenic pairs of rough and smooth *E. coli* and *Salmonella*. C5b-9 release from Ser-R organisms did not result from bacterial metabolism or cell wall shedding since the process occurred equally well with heat-killed or glutaraldehyde-fixed organisms. Also, organisms intrinsically labeled with ^{14}C glucose did not show shedding of labeled material during serum incubation.

Release of C5b-9 from the Ser-R organism required the presence of C8 and C9 since: (a) the intermediate complex C5b67 was stably attached; and (b) addition of C8 with or without C9 to the bacteria-bound C5b67 resulted in dose-dependent release of the entire C5b-8 or C5b-9 complex. These results suggested that the C5b-9 complex was attached in a different way to the Ser-R and Ser-S bacteria. This possibility was pursued by measuring the release of C5b-9 from Ser-R and Ser-S organisms under different elution conditions (Fig. 2). Less than 20% of bound C5b-(^{125}I) C9 on Ser-S was eluted by 1 *M* NaC1 or 0.1% trypsin, compared with 60%-72% release by NaC1 and 89%-95% release by 0.1% trypsin from Ser-R. This experiment suggested that the bulk of the C5b-9 on Ser-S was intimately associated with hydrophobic portions of the outer membrane, probably by actual insertion into

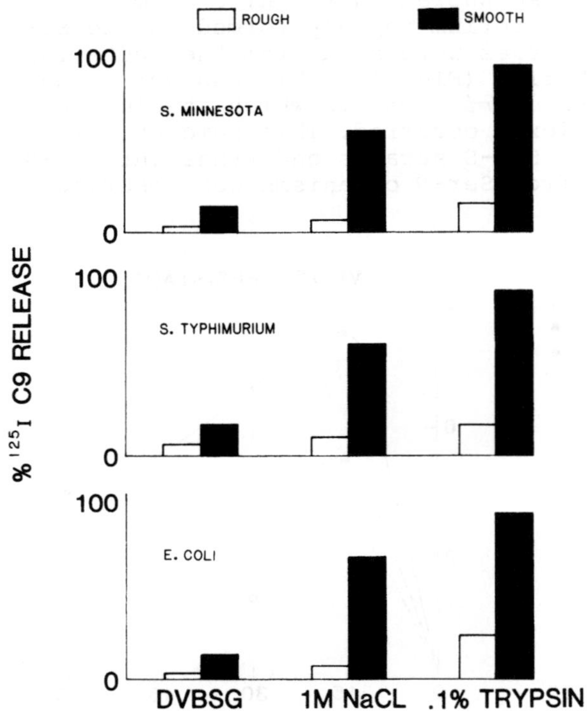

Fig. 2. Release of C5b-9 from rough, Ser-S and smooth, Ser-R *Salmonella* and *E. coli* by DVBSG, NaC1, and trypsin. Bacterial strains were as described in the legend to Fig. 1, and experimental methodology was as described in reference [12] (DVBSG: *D*extrose-*V*eronal-*b*uffered *s*aline containing *g*elatin)

the outer membrane since the complex was not released by ionic manipulations or proteolytic attack. Conversely, salt-susceptible bonds between C5b-9 and the Ser-R organism implied that the C5b-9 complex had not inserted into hydrophobic domains of the outer membrane. In fact, recent studies have evaluated the nature of C5b-9 attachment to the isolated outer membrane of three isogenic strains of *E. coli* varying in serum sensitivity [21]. Killing was associated with C5b-9 deposition on the outer membrane in a form which was resistant to elution with NaC1 and proteolytic removal by trypsin. Complement-mediated lysis of erythrocytes and phospholipid vesicles, by way of analogy, is known to be dependent upon insertion of C5b-9 into the lipid bilayer. Furthermore, complement-mediated killing of gram-negative bacteria is generally associated with partial dissolution of the outer membrane by the detergent-like action of C5b-9. Our experiments suggested that neither the insertion step nor the dissolution step was occurring with Ser-R strains of *E. coli* and *Salmonella* and thus demonstrated a mechanism for serum resistance in bacteria capable of efficiently activating complement.

We have pursued the idea that smooth LPS within *Salmonella* and *E. coli* renders organisms resistant to complement killing by acting as a physical barrier to complement attack. The acceptor site for C3 deposition on Ser-R isolates of *Salmonella* and *E. coli* was sought. Since C3b is an obligate constituent of both the classical pathway (C4b2a3b) and alternative pathway (C3bBbC3b) C5 convertase, an understanding of the molecular localization of C3b deposition provides a direct clue as to the localization of the subsequently formed C5b-9 complex. C3 binding to acceptor molecules on the bacterial surface is via a covalent interaction, as clearly outlined in the paper by Levine (this volume), and thus is unlike the situation with C5b-9 which has exclusively noncovalent interactions. The C3-acceptor bond is not broken during solubilization of organisms in denaturing detergents, permitting a biochemical and immunochemical analysis of individual acceptor molecules for C3 on the bacterial surface.

In initial studies, we found that C3b deposited predominantly on LPS when a smooth, nonencapsulated, Ser-R strain of *E. coli* was incubated in serum [18]. These studies were performed with an organism which was intrinsically labeled in either LPS or outer membrane protein. Bacteria were incubated in serum, and the bacterial molecules bearing C3 were identified by affinity purification with anti-C3. Subsequently, we have used this technique to evaluate the subset of LPS molecules bearing C3 after incubation of a Ser-R strain of *Salmonella montevideo* in serum [19]. This strain possesses a double mutation in the LPS synthetic pathway, since it lacks both UDP-4-galactose epimerase and phosphomannose isomerase. It is therefore possible to differentially label the organism with galactose ^{14}C in the core oligosaccharide (one copy per LPS molecule) and with mannose ^{3}H in the *O*-polysaccharide (0-55 copies per LPS molecule), such that the ratio of ^{3}H:^{14}C for any given molecule will reflect the length of the *O*-polysaccharide side-chain. When organisms grown in this way are incubated in serum, the LPS molecules bearing C3 are on the average eightfold longer than the LPS molecules on non-serum-incubated bacteria. Altering the LPS profile of the organism to

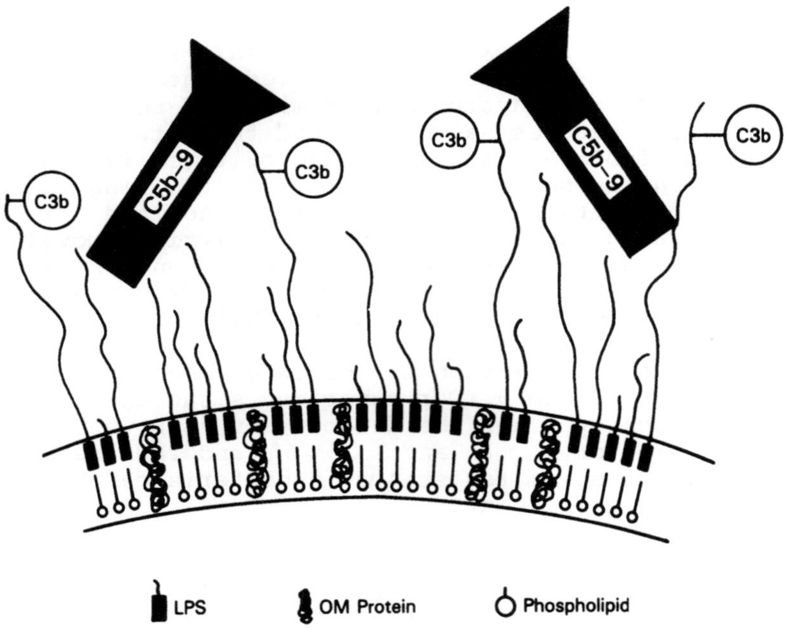

Fig. 3. Model for Ser-R in smooth *Salmonella* and *E. coli*. Complement is activated by and C3b attaches to LPS molecules bearing the longest *O*-polysaccharide side-chains. Steric hindrance by LPS prevents access of C3b and C5b-9 to the bacterial cell wall. C3b remains covalently attached, but C5b-9 is bound by weak hydrophilic interactions and is shed from the surface

render it sensitive to serum killing, which can be accomplished by growth in suboptimal concentrations of mannose, results in attachment of C3 to shorter LPS molecules. Changes in the LPS profile are associated with abrupt rather than gradual changes in serum sensitivity; furthermore, sharp cutoffs can be established for the percentage coverage of lipid A core with *O*-polysaccharide and for the *O*-polysaccharide lengths which are required to render an organism Ser-R [7].

On the basis of these findings, we have developed a model for the mechanism of serum resistance in smooth gram-negative bacteria (Fig. 3). Complement is activated by and C3 attaches to the longest LPS molecules on these organisms. Steric hindrance by LPS prevents access of C3b and C5b-9 to the bacterial cell wall. C3 remains covalently attached, but C5b-9 is shed from the surface. A high percentage of lipid A core oligosaccharide molecules must bear *O*-polysaccharide, and a substantial fraction of these must be long if the organism is to subvert attack by complement by sterically hindering access of the C5b-9 complex to the outer membrane.

Serum Resistance in *Neisseria gonorrhoeae*

We have also been interested in the mechanism of Ser-R in *N. gonorrhoeae* (GC) [14]. As pointed out earlier, serum resistance in

GC represents an important biologic problem since strains causing disseminated gonococcal infection (DGI) are almost invariably resistant to the bactericidal action of PNHS. In contrast to Enterobacteriaceae, GC have not been demonstrated to possess smooth LPS. It is also known that Ser-R GC are not absolutely refractory to serum killing, as is the case with some Enterobacteriaceae, since virtually all Ser-R GC can be killed by the addition of sufficient bactericidal antibody. For these reasons, it was of interest to examine the mechanism of Ser-R in GC.

The initial strategy was similar to that for studies with *Salmonella*. Complement consumption and terminal component binding were compared on three Ser-S strains from localized genital infections and two Ser-R strains from DGI isolates. We found equivalent terminal component consumption and binding when sensitive and resistant strains were compared, in support of recently published work [10]. The binding of C5b-9 to the bacterial surface of both Ser-S and Ser-R organisms was stable during extended incubation, implying that the mechanism of serum resistance that was operative in GC was different from that in the Enterobacteriaceae.

The addition of immune rabbit antisera or purified IgG prepared against one of the Ser-R DGI strains resulted in serum killing. It was clear from C9 binding studies that antibody was exerting its effect on bacterial killing by a mechanism other than simply increasing terminal component uptake on the bacterial surface. When incubation conditions were adjusted to permit equivalent deposition of C5b-9 in the presence and absence of antibody, only in the presence of antibody did killing occur (Fig. 4). Thus, it appeared that antibody might be altering the nature of attachment of C5b-9 to the bacteria. Although the complex was apparently attached by hydrophobic bonds to both Ser-S and Ser-R

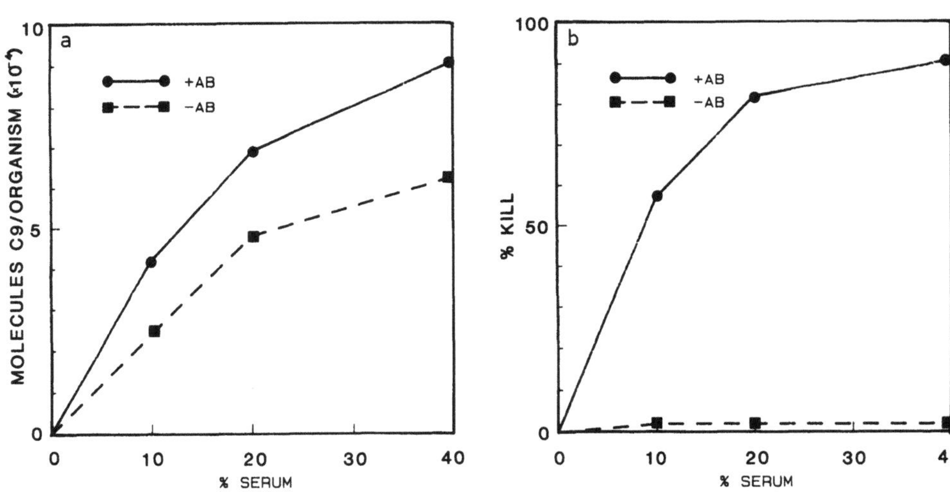

Fig. 4. Deposition of C9 (a) and killing (b) of Ser-R GC strain 6305 incubated in 10% agammaglobulinemic serum. The organism was presensitized prior to serum incubation with either bactericidal rabbit IgG *(circles)* or normal rabbit IgG *(squares)*. Reprinted with permission of the *Journal of Immunology*

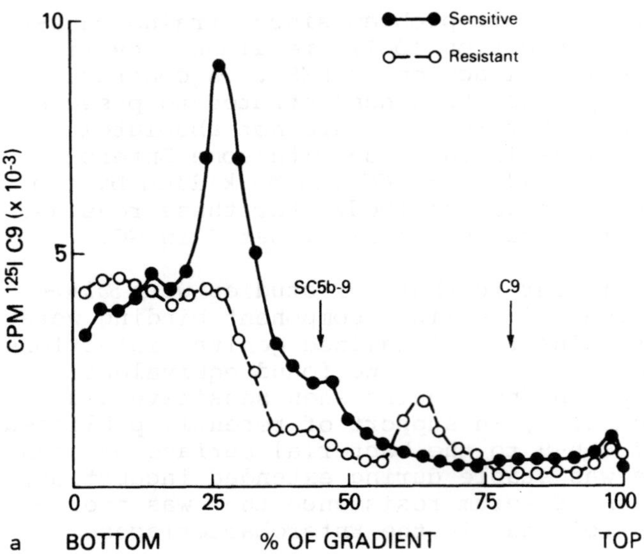

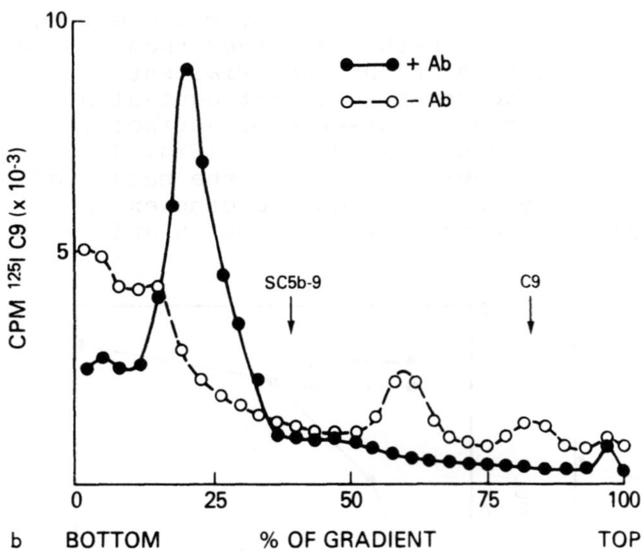

Fig. 5a-c. Sucrose density gradient profiles of C5b-9 extracted from Ser-S and Ser-R GC. Samples were prepared as described in reference [14], applied to 10%-40% sucrose gradients, and centrifuged for 16 h at 33 000 rpm. a: Ser-S 7189 (*full circles*); Ser-R 6305 (*open circles*); extraction with 1% SB_{12}, b: Ser-R 6305+Ab (*full circles*); Ser-R 6305-Ab (*open circles*); extraction with 1% SB_{12}, c: Ser-R 6305; extraction with 1% naDOC (*full circles*), extraction with 1% SB_{12} (*open circles*)

GC, trypsin released nearly 2.5 times as much C9 from the Ser-R strains as from the Ser-S organism or the Ser-R isolate that was rendered Ser-S with antibody.

We examined the form of C5b-9 on Ser-S and Ser-R GC by sucrose density gradient analysis of the detergent extracted C5-(^{125}I)C9 complex (Fig. 5). This analysis showed that: (a) the major bactericidal form of C5b-9 on the surface of Ser-S or presensitized Ser-R GC sedimented as a 33*S* complex when extracted from the organisms with either 1% sodium deoxycholate (NaDOC) or the zwit-

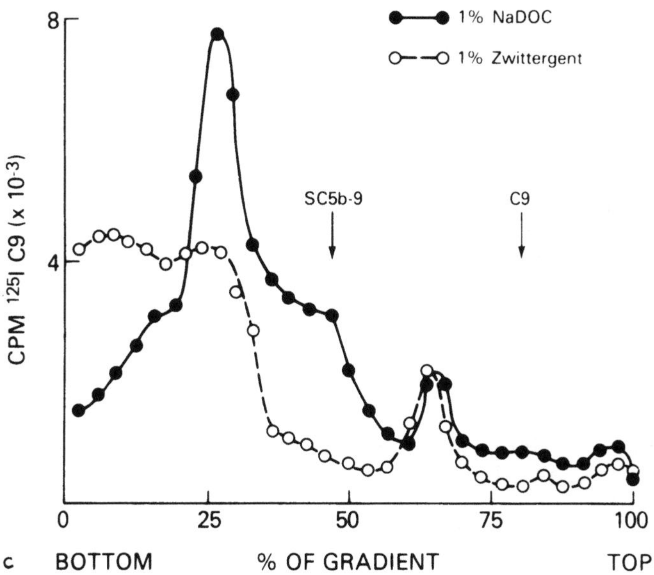

c

terionic sulfobetaine detergent, SB_{12}; (b) the nonbactericidal C5b-9 on Ser-R GC existed in larger 35 and 43 *S* aggregates when extracted with SB_{12}; but not NaDOC; and (c) a 13.5 *S* peak containing C9 was uniquely extracted with NaDOC and SB_{12} from the Ser-R DGI strain, but the peak disappeared when the organism was rendered Ser-S by presensitization with IgG.

The unusual sedimentation pattern of C5b-9 from Ser-R GC raised the possibility that complex formation was occurring between C5b-9 and GC outer membrane constituents in SB_{12} extracts, even though the C5b-9 was not covalently bound to the membrane. This possibility was confirmed by coprecipitation experiments and double diffusion analysis of SB_{12} extracts.

A series of experiments were than undertaken to investigate the specific outer membrane constituents of GC with which bactericidal and nonbactericidal C5b-9 were associated [15]. By immunoprecipitating the C5b-9 complex extracted from surface-labeled bacteria following serum incubation, we demonstrated that bactericidal, but non nonbactericidal C5b-9 was associated with distinctive surface-iodinated proteins. This observation was made for both a Ser-S organism (7189) and for a Ser-R strain (6305) which had been rendered sensitive by presensitization with bactericidal rabbit antibody (6305+Ab). Analysis of non-serum-incubated GC ^{125}I showed prominent PI, PIII, and diffuse 15-19 K bands for both 6305 and 7189. For those organisms bearing bactericidal C5b-9 (6305+Ab and 7189), but not for those lacking bactericidal C5b-9 (6305-Ab), distinctive bands coprecipitated with C5b-9. These bands were of molecular weight 93, 44, 40, and 15 K for 6305+Ab and of molecular weight 90, 50, 44, and 19K for 7189. The association of bacterial constituents with C5b-9 was also studied by transmission electron microscopy. The C5b-9 lesion on 6305+Ab was attached to only small pieces of bacteria or was free of associated material. In contrast, the C5b-9 lesion on 6305-Ab was associated with larger bacterial fragments. These results indicate that bactericidal, but not nonbactericidal C5b-9 on GC is associated with distinctive surface-iodinatable constituents and that bactericidal C5b-9 has a different association with bacterial constituents by electron microscopy than does nonbactericidal C5b-9. These studies suggest the possibility that bactericidal antibody, through an as yet undiscovered mechanism, is required for effective insertion of C5b-9 into and disruption of the outer membrane of GC. The corollary of this statement is that surface structures of GC may subvert effective insertion of C5b-9 into the outer membrane in the absence of bactericidal antibody.

Studies have continued on the mechanism by which bactericidal antibody renders GC susceptible to complement-mediated killing. In all of our initial studies done with serum resistant GC, we used polyclonal bactericidal antibody raised in rabbits and directed against PI, PIII, and LPS on intact GC. In order to pursue these studies further, we have examined the binding and bactericidal activity of a series of Mab directed against gonococcal PI [20]. Three Mab (4G5, 1D3, and 1G6) were studied which bound to the surface of Ser-R GC strain R11, as assessed by a coagglutination assay and by specific uptake of ^{125}I-labeled protein A by presensitized isolates. All three Mab activated and deposited complement on the surface of GC R11 as assessed by C9 ^{125}I binding. Approximately 30 000 molecules of C9 were bound per organism when GC R11 was presensitized with either 4G5, 1D3, or 1G6 and incubated in agammaglobulinemic serum. Surprisingly, only 4G5 and 1D3 were bactericidal. Further studies have shown that all three Mab can compete with one another for binding to intact GC R11, raising the possibility that they recognize identical or closely related epitopes. Coagglutination data with a large panel of GC strains varying in PI serotype would suggest that 1D3 and 1G6 recognize identical epitopes whereas 4G5 recognizes a different, but closely related determinant. These data demonstrate that Mab directed against identical or closely associated, surface-exposed epitopes on gonococcal PI differ markedly in bactericidal activity, despite leading to deposition of nearly equivalent numbers of C9 molecules per organism during serum incubation.

Bactericidal Antibody for *E. coli* O111

The concept that bactericidal antibody may alter the bactericidal efficiency of C5b-9 rather than simply increasing the number of bound terminal complexes applies to organisms other than GC. This was initially suggested in studies by Tarr et al. [41] on alternative pathway-mediated killing of *H. influenzae* by antibody to the type b capsule. In addition, we have recently completed a more detailed series of experiments examining the mechanism of antibody-dependent serum killing of *E. coli* O111B4 [16,17]. This strain is killed via the alternative pathway in the presence of antibody, but not in its absence. Presensitization with IgG or $F(ab')_2$, but not F(ab'), results in a dose-related killing and increase in C3 binding in 10% PNHS, but only a minimal increase in C9 binding. Additional experiments demonstrated that antibody must be present at the time of C5 convertase formation to mediate its effect. These experiments suggest that antibody must be influencing the site and/or organization of C3b deposition and C5 convertase formation in such a way as to increase the bactericidal efficiency of subsequently deposited C5b-9.

Serum Resistance in *S. pneumoniae*

Finally, we have investigated the reason for the well-known inability of antibody and complement to kill gram-positive bacteria. We have shown that a C5b-9 complex forms and is stably attached to the surface of both rough and type 7 *S. pneumoniae* when these organisms are incubated in serum [13]. Complement-mediated killing of these strains does not occur, as has been repeatedly documented with gram-positive organisms as a group. It appears that the thick peptidoglycan cell wall of the gram-positive organism serves as a physical barrier to C5b-9 disruption of the cytoplasmic membrane, a necessary requirement for serum killing. Thus, although the membrane attack complex is stably bound to the bacterial wall, the inner membrane bilayer is not disrupted.

Conclusions

These studies have demonstrated at least three different mechanisms for bacterial resistance to complement-mediated killing: (a) smooth LPS of Enterobacteriaceae may sterically hinder access of C5b-9 to complement-susceptible sites on the outer membrane; (b) noncovalent associations of C5b-9 with outer membrane constituents of GC may prevent effective insertion of the membrane attack complex, and (c) the thick peptidoglycan layer of *S. pneumoniae* shields the vulnerable inner membrane from attack by C5b-9. Our results indicate that bactericidal antibody can mediate serum killing by increasing the bactericidal efficiency of C5b-9; however, not all complement-activating antibodies can subserve this function. We believe these and future studies will aid in the development of more efficacious vaccines and in the development of other strategies designed to augment the host's natural bactericidal capacity against gram-negative bacteria.

References

1. Anderson P, Johnston RB Jr, Smith DH (1972) Human serum activities against *Hemophilus influenzae*, Type b. J Clin Invest 51:31
2. Binns MM, Mayden J, Levine RP (1982) Further characterization of complement resistance conferred on *Escherichia coli* by the plasmid genes *traT* of R100 and *iss* of ColV,I-K94. Infect Immun 35:654-659
3. Dlabac V (1968) The sensitivity of smooth and rough mutants of *Salmonella typhimurium* to bactericidal and bacteriolytic action of serum, lysozyme and to phagocytosis. Folia Microbiol (Praha) 13:439-449
4. Durack DT, Beeson PB (1977) Protective role of complement in experimental *Escherichia coli* endocarditus. Infect Immun 16:213-217

5. Fierrer J, Finley F (1979) Lethal effect of complement and lysozyme on polymyxin-treated, serum resistant gram-negative bacteria. J Infect Dis 140:581-589
6. Griffis JM, Bertram MA (1977) Immunoepidemiology of meningococcal disease in military recruits: II. Blocking of serum bactericidal activity by circulating IgA early in the course of invasive disease. J Infect Dis 136: 733-739
7. Grossman N, Schmetz M, Klima EN, Leive L, Joiner KA (1984) Changes in the distribution of lengths of lipopolysaccharide (LPS) of *Salmonella montevideo* (O-6,7) after serum sensitivity. Fed Proc 43:1447
8. Gutschik E, Norwood RS, Møller S, Olling S (1980) Experimental endocarditis in rabbits: IV. Experiments with *Serratia marcescens:* on the significance of serum susceptibility and proteolytic capacity of the strains and the influence of an indwelling catheter. Acta Pathol Microbiol Scand [B]88:269-276
9. Hancock REW, Mutharia LM, Chan L, Darveau RP, Speert DP, Pier GB (1983) *Pseudomonas aeruginosa* isolates from patients with cystic fibrosis: a class of serum-sensitive, nontypable strains deficient in lipopolysaccharide O side chains. Infect Immun 42:170-177
10. Harriman G, Podack ER, Braude AI, Corbeil LC, Esser AF, Curd JG (1982) Activation of complement by serum-resistant *Neisseria gonorrhoeae*. Assembly of the membrane attack complex without subsequent cell death. J Exp Med 156:1235
11. Joiner KA, Hammer CH, Brown EJ, Cole RJ, Frank MM (1982a) Studies on the mechanism of bacterial resistance to complement-mediated killing: I. Terminal complement components are deposited and released from *Salmonella minnesota* S218 without causing bacterial death. J Exp Med 155:797
12. Joiner KA, Hammer CH, Brown EJ, Frank MM (1982b) Studies on the mechanism of bacterial resistance to complement-mediated killing: II. C8 and C9 release C5b67 from the surface of *Salmonella minnesota* S218 because the terminal complex does not insert into the bacterial outer membrane. J Exp Med 155:809
13. Joiner KA, Brown E, Hammer C, Warren K, Frank M (1983a) Studies on the mechanism of bacterial resistance to complement-mediated killing: III. C5b-9 deposits stably on rough and type 7 *S. pneumoniae* without causing bacterial killing. J Immunol 130:345
14. Joiner KA, Wa-ren KA, Brown EJ, Swanson J, Frank MM (1983b) Studies on the mechanism of bacterial resistance to complement-mediated killing: IV. C5b-9 forms high molecular weight complexes with bacterial outer membrane constituents on serum-resistant but not serum-sensitive *Neisseria gonorrhoeae*. J Immunol 131:1443
15. Joiner K, Warren K, Frank M (1983c) Mechanism of serum resistance in *Neisseria gonorrhoeae* (GC). Interscience Conference on Antimicrobial Agents and Chemotherapy, Oct 1983, Las Vegas, Nevada
16. Joiner K, Goldman R, Hammer C, Leive L, Frank M (1983d) Studies of the mechanism of bacterial resistance to complement-mediated killing: V. IgG and $F(ab)'_2$ mediate killing of *E. coli* O111B4 by the alternative complement pathway without increasing C5b-9 deposition. J Immunol 131:2563
17. Joiner KA, Goldman R, Hammer C, Leive L, Frank MM (1983e) Studies on the mechanism of bacterial resistance to complement-mediated killing: VI. IgG increases the bactericidal efficiency of C5b-9 for *E. coli* O111B4 by acting at a step prior to C5 cleavage. J Immunol 131:2570
18. Joiner KA, Goldman R, Schmetz M, Berger M, Hammer CH, Frank MM, Leive L (1984a) A quantitative analysis of C3 binding to O-antigen capsule, lipopolysaccharide, and outer membrane protein of *E. coli* O111B4. J Immunol 132:369

19. Joiner K, Grossman N, Schmetz M, Leive L (1984b) C3 binds preferentially to long chain LPS in serum resistant *Salmonella montevideo*. Clin Res 32: 371A
20. Joiner K, Warren K, Tam M, Frank M (1984c) Bactericidal activity of monoclonal antibodies (Mab) directed against protein I of *Neisseria gonorrhoeae* (GC). Clin Res 32:371A
21. Joiner KA, Schmetz MA, Goldman RC, Leive L, Frank MM (1984d) Mechanism of bacterial resistance to complement-mediated killing: Inserted C5b-9 correlates with killing for *Escherichia coli* O111B4 varying in O-antigen capsule and O-polysaccharide coverage of lipid A core oligosaccharide. Infect Immun 45:113-117
22. McCabe WR, Kaijser B, Olling S, Uwaydah M and Hanson LA (1978) *Escherichia coli* in bacteremia: K and O antigens and serum sensitivity of strains from adults and neonates. J Infect Dis 138:33-41
23. McCutchan JA, Katzenstein D, Norquist D, Chikami G, Wunderlich A, Braude AI (1978) Role of blocking antibody in disseminated gonococcal infection. J Immunol 121:1884-1888
24. Medhurst FA, Glynn AA (1970) *In vivo* bactericidal activity of mouse complement against *Escherichia coli*. Br J Exp Pathol 51:498-506
25. Morse SA, Mintz CS, Sarafian SK, Bartenstein L, Bertram M, Apirella MA (1983) The effect of dilution rate on lipopolysaccharide and serum resistance of *Neisseria gonorrhoeae* grown in continuous culture. Infect Immun 41:74-82
26. Munn CB, Ishiguro EE, Kay WW, Trust TJ (1982) Role of surface components in serum resistance of virulent *Aeromonas salmonicida*. Infect Immun 36: 1069-1075
27. Muschel LH, Larsen LJ (1970) The sensitivity of smooth and rough gram-negative bacteria to the immune bactericidal reaction. Proc Soc Exp Biol Med 133:345-348
28. Ogata RT, Levine RP (1980) Characterization of complement resistance in *Escherichia coli* conferred by the antibiotic resistance plasmid R100. J Immunol 125:1494-1498
29. Olling S (1977) Sensitivity of gram-negative bacilli to the serum bactericidal activity: a marker of the host-parasite relationship in acute and persisting infections. Scand J Infect Dis [Suppl] 10:1-40
30. Olling S, Hanson LA, Holmgren J, Jodal U, Lincoln K, Lindberg U (1973) The bactericidal effect of normal human serum on *E. coli* strains from normals and from patients with urinary tract infections. Infection 1: 24-28
31. Reynolds BL, Rother KO (1975) Interaction of complement components with a serum-resistant strain of *Salmonella typhimurium*. Infect Immun 11:944-948
32. Rice PA, Kasper DL (1982) Characterization of serum resistance of *Neisseria gonorrhoeae* that disseminate. J Clin Invest 70:157
33. Rice PA, McCormack WM, Kasper DL (1980) Natural serum bactericidal activity against *Neisseria gonorrhoeae* isolates from disseminated, locally invasive and uncomplicated disease. J Immunol 124:2105-9
34. Roantree RJ, Pappas NC (1960) The survival of strains of enteric bacilli in the bloodstream as related to their sensitivity to the bactericidal effect of serum. J Clin Invest 39:82-88
35. Roantree RJ, Rantz LA (1960) A study of the relationship of the normal bactericidal activity of human serum to bacterial infection. J Clin Invest 39:72-81
36. Rowley D (1968) Sensitivity of rough gram-negative bacteria to the bactericidal action of serum. J Bacteriol 95:1647-1650

37. Schoolnik GK, Buchanan TM, Holmes KK (1976) Gonococci causing disseminated infection are resistant to the bactericidal action of normal human serum. J Clin Invest 58:1163-1173
38. Shafer WM, Joiner K, Guymon LF, Cohen MS, Sparling PF (1984) serum sensitivity of *Neisseria gonorrhoeae:* the role of lipopolysaccharide. J Infect Dis 149:175-183
39. Simberkoff MS, Ricupero I, Rahal JJ (1976) Host resistance to *Serratia marcescens* infection: serum bactericidal activity and phagocytosis by normal blood leukocytes. J Lab Clin Med 87:206-217
40. Steele NP, Munson RS Jr, Granoff DM, Cummins JE, Levine RP (1984) Antibody-dependent alternative pathway killing of *Haemophilus influenzae* type b. Infect Immun 44:452-458
41. Tarr PI, Hosea SW, Brown EJ, Schneerson R, Sutton A, Frank MM (1983) The requirement of specific anticapsular IgG for killing of *Haemophilus influenzae* by the alternative pathway of complement activation. J Immunol 128:1772
42. Taylor PW, Parton R (1977) A protein factor associated with serum resistance in *Escherichia coli*. J Med Microbiol 10:225-232
43. Taylor PW, Robinson MK (1980) Determinants that increase the serum resistance to *Escherichia coli*. Infect Immun 29:278-280
44. Vosti KL, Randall E (1970) Sensitivity of serologically classified strains of *Escherichia coli* of human origin to the serum bactericidal system. Am J Med Sci 259:114-119
45. Young LS, Armstrong D (1972) Human immunity to *Pseudomonas aeruginosa:* I. *In vitro* interaction of bacteria, polymorphonuclear leukocytes, and serum factors. J Infect Dis 126:257-276

Discussion

(pp. 122-136)

The main question concerned how one could form an idea of non-acting C5b-9 complexes in serum-resistant bacteria. Different models have been offered. One assumes that certain nonfluctuating zones on the bacterial surface must be hit in order to kill bacteria. On this hypothesis, bactericidal antibodies could direct the C5b-9 complex to the right place on the surface. One possible objection to this hypothesis is the fact that these antigenic areas are of high density and low molecular weight (20 000-40 000). A more likely explanation could be the clustering of the C5b-9 complex around the antibody. The antibodies used in the experiments were of the same isotype. It seems to be clear, however, that bactericidal antibodies cluster C5b-9 complexes which have a different association with outer membrane constituents, a different profile on sucrose density ultracentrifugation, and different bactericidal efficiency.

Bayer-Symposium VIII
The Pathogenesis of Bacterial Infections, 138-145 (1985)

Gram-Negative Septicemia: Antibody Deficiency and Specific Protection*

L. S. Young

Summary

Gram-negative rod bacteremias are a major component of nosocomial infections. Studies in humans and experimental animals support a protective role for opsonic antibodies directed against bacillary surface antigens. These include somatic (O, lipopolysaccharide) capsular (K), and protein antigens. A role for antitoxic immunity cannot be excluded as well, and antibodies to substances such as *Pseudomonas* exotoxin A may give additive protection. Augmented levels of opsonic antibodies in humans at onset of sepsis correlate with protection and conversely, antibody deficiency with poor prognosis. Such results must be cautiously interpreted because these antibodies are often a reflection of underlying disease and/or presence of chronic infection. Definitive evidence for protection must come from antibody supplementation or augmentation and there have been few well-designed human studies of immunoprophylaxix/or therapy. Animal studies indicate that monoclonal antibodies against type-specific lipopolysaccharides of *P. aeruginosa* are both opsonic and protective. The functional capacity of antibodies directed against common core regions of lipopolysaccharide deserve further evaluation.

Introduction

Most of the gram-negative bacilli that cause invasive disease in humans or animals are either part of the normal fecal flora or are readily isolated from environmental sources [1]. It is not surprising that natural antibodies to these disease-causing organisms can readily be found in sera of adults [2]. In newborns, the transplacental transfer of IgG antibodies confers protection against many potentially invasive pathogens. A major exception to this observation is gram-negative bacillary neonatal septicemia, which in most studies is caused by *Escherichia coli* possessing the K1 polymeric sialic acid capsule [3]. The sera of many adults is relatively deficient in antibody activity against K1 organisms. Further, more of the antibody that can be measured against K1 in human sera is of the IgM class. Trans-

*This study was supported in part by Grant No. A11271 from the National Institute of Allergy and Infectious Diseases

placental passage of antibody of the IgM class seems negligible and this may be a factor predisposing neonates to overwhelming *E. col* K1 septicemia.

Even with advancing age, individuals who are immunologically intact may fail to form antibodies against antigens like K1. The poor immunogenicity of this polysaccharide antigen persists into the adult years. Purified K1 material, in the form of the immunochemically identical group B meningococcal polysaccharide have been notoriously unsuccessful as a means of immunizing military volunteers [4]. The decreased incidence of meningococcal (group B) and K1 bacteremia in individuals above the young adult age range and the corresponding increase in the prevalence of bactericidal antibody against group B *Meningococcus* [5] has led to the inference that with increasing age bactericidal and/or opsonic antibodies develop against surface determinants other then the sialic acid capsule.

Role of Anti-Somatic (O Antigen) Immunity in Gram-Negative Bacillary Infections

There is ample evidence from a host of animal studies that immunization with a killed or boiled gram-negative rod will protect against a subsequent lethal challenge with viable bacilli. The protection can be passively transferred with heat-inactivated serum and is thought to be primarily, though not exclusively, due to opsonic antibodies against the heat-stable O or somatic lipopolysaccharide antigens. Actually, the evidence from systemic gram-negative rod infections in humans that antibodies to specific cell surface components of invading organisms are protective is still largely inferential.

Beginning in 1972, McCabe and colleagues offered some evidence that type-specific and cross-reactive antibodies against the lipopolysaccharide (endotoxin) antigens of gram-negative bacilli measured the onset of bacteremia in humans correlated with survival [6,7]. The first study was limited to bloodstream infections due to a variety of enteric bacteria. Antibody levels were measured by passive hemagglutination against antigens derived from homologous infecting organisms. One of the major findings was that antibody directed against the Re chemotype determinant of the core glycolipid moiety of endotoxin (KDO-lipid A) correlated with protection against shock and death. This gave impetus to the development of such an antigen as a possible immunogen for the prevention of gram-negative infections and for the production of antiserum which could be administered therapeutically or prophylactically.

Several years later, a follow-up study was published by Zinner and McCabe using many of the same serologic specimens initially employed for the earlier studies [7]. Again, there was evidence for an inverse correlation between the magnitude of the antibody titer at the onset of septicemia and the likelihood of survival. Correcting for such important factors as the nature of the underlying disease, Zinner and McCabe used a different antibody test, namely indirect immunofluorescence, to demonstrate that high levels of IgG antibodies measured at the onset of septicemia were statistically associated with recovery from shock and death. The protective role of antibodies against the core glycolipid of enterobacterial endotoxin (Re determinant) was also reaffirmed in this latter study.

Our own investigations have evaluated the potential protective role of antibody by a different technique and have involved not only infections due to enteric bacteria, but to *Pseudomonas aeruginosa*. In an initial study with serum samples from immunocompromised patients, we recognized that patients who developed fatal *Pseudomonas* infections often had negligible titers of opsonic antibodies against infecting isolates [2]. At that time, a prospective, controlled evaluation of *Pseudomonas* immunization with type-specific lipopolysaccharide demonstrated that failures following immunization (breakthrough infections) were associated with low or negligible levels of opsonic antibody against infecting strains [8].

We subsequently studied another group of patients (146 examples) in whom we were fortunate to have serum or plasma samples collected within 48 h of the onset of gram-negative rod bacteremia. In the majority of individuals, specimens were obtained simultaneously with culture-positive blood. Infections were due to both *P. aeruginosa* and enteric bacilli. After heat inactivation and titering of serum samples, we combined this patient material with an exogenous complement source free of opsonic antibodies, the homologous infecting strain, and measured opsonic activity. The relationship of this activity to eventual outcome is shown in Table 1 [9]. Mortality was 60% in patients with negligible opsonic antibody titers, but almost 90% of patients who had initial opsonic antibody titers in excess of 1:80 recovered ($P<0.0001$). Thus, initial opsonic activity correlated strongly with the likelihood of clinical recovery.

Table 1. Initial opsonic titer and mortality in 146 cases of gram-negative rod bacteremia (adapted from [9])

Group	Reciprocal opsonic titer	Patients	Case fatality ratio
I	< 10	40	60%*
II	20-40	39	35%
III	⩾ 80	67	11%*

*$P < 0.0001$.

The studies reported by Zinner and McCabe [7] and by ourselves [9] offer several challenges in interpretation. There are at least three issues which must be confronted. First, any measurement which relates antibody titer at onset of bacteremia to survival or complications can assess protection only after bacteremia has developed. It cannot determine the ability of antibody to prevent infections or bacteremia. Second, a critical question is how or under what circumstances a patient develops high levels of antibody prior to bacteremia. A strong possibility is that these antibodies are a marker for host immunologic competence. Zinner and McCabe [7] studied no patients with "rapidly fatal" underlying disease, while our study had many individuals who could be categorized as such. Third, related to the issue of host competence is whether patients having high antibody titers were "autoimmunized" by chronic localized infections prior to sepsis. The bacteremia, then, could be a transient or self-limited process superimposed on chronic infection (as in the urinary tract) in an immunocompetent patient. Of the 146 patients studied in the material summarized in Table 1, 46 had *P. aeruginosa* bacteremia. Correlation of clinical results with heat-stable opsonic titer for these patients is summarized in Table 2. The trends parallel the data shown in Table 1 which includes patients with other types of gram-negative bacteremia.

Table 2. Heat-stable opsonins and prognosis in P. aeruginosa bacteremia

Group	Reciprocal opsonic titer	patients	Case fatality ratio
I	10	20	75%
II	20-40	8	50%
III	⩾ 80	18	17%

Of direct relevance to the issue of the relationship between antibody titer and host immune competence is the information summarized in Table 3. Patients with negligible opsonic titers against homologous infecting *Pseudomonas* strains were usually receiving immunosuppressive or cytotoxic therapy and had a hematologic malignancy or bone marrow failure. Only a quarter had chronic infection and/or urinary tract origin of sepsis. In contrast, the group III patients with initial opsonic titers ⩾ 1:80 were significantly less immunosuppressed and two-thirds had a chronic infection and/or urinary tract origin of septicemia. The evidence seems clear from this study that opsonic antibodies versus homologous infecting strains are dependent variables and a reflection of host immune competence. In yet another study of *P. aeruginosa* bacteremia, we were fortunate to have serum or plasma samples obtained simultaneously with culture-positive blood [10]. We examined the potential protective role of antibodies against both somatic (O lipopolysaccharide antigens) of *P. aeruginosa*, as well as against exotoxin A. Patients with high levels of antibodies against either antigen had a better prognosis, but the effect was additive and independent of such factors as neutropenia. The best prognosis was clearly in those individuals who had high levels of antibodies against both lipopolysaccharide and exotoxin A antigen. Conversely, mortality was greatest in patients who had negligible levels of antibody against both heat-stable (O antigens) and the protein heat-labile exotoxin A antigen elaborated by most invasive strains of *P. aeruginosa*.

Table 3. Host factors in *Pseudomonas* Septicemia[a]

Group[b]	Patients	Cytotoxic or immunosuppressive therapy	Leukemia, lymphoma, marrow failure	Chronic infection and/or urinary tract origin
I	20	17 (85%)	16 (80%)	5 (25%)
III	18	6 (33%)	5 (28%)	12 (67%)

[a]All differences significant, $P < 0.01$.

[b]Grouping of patients by opsonic titer as indicated in Table 2.

The Clinical Challenge of Antibody Augmentation

It seems obvious that controversy about the protective role of antibodies will be best resolved by experimental and clinical studies that attempt antibody supplementation to levels that appear protective (as inferred from the serologic studies). Unfortunately, active immunization has led to somewhat disappointing results [11]. Immunocompromised patients, particularly those at risk for developing *P. aeruginosa* bacteremia are often so intensely immunosuppressed that antibody responses are poor. The results of active immunization look best in patients who have sustained thermal injuries and do not have a hematologic malignancy. Other studies in burns have combined active immunization with antibody prophylaxis or therapy, but these are hard to interpret. Prior to the development of modified immunoglobulin for intravenous therapy, the administration of IgG fractions was restricted to intramuscular injection. The new preparations modified for intravenous infusion are particularly interesting because they can be enriched with specific antibodies such as against *P. aeruginosa*. However, we must await the results of properly controlled trials before conclusions that such forms of antibody supplementation are truly useful.

A recent human study has given hope to a therapeutic approach in which antiserum to core glycolipid antigens of gram-negative enteric bacteria is administered therapeutically. Statistically significant differences were observed in survival between patients who received human antiserum against the J5 mutant of *E. coli* O111 [12] and a control antiserum. No attempt was made, however, to assess both specific and nonspecific protection. In this report, no information was provided on type-specific antibody titers in recipients against their infecting strains, as well as antibody titers against the J5 antigen, either before or after the infusion of antiserum.

There are clearly other antigens present on the bacterial cell wall that serve as important virulence factors, and against which specific antibodies may confer protection. Capsular antigens render many strains of *E. coli* and *Klebsiella* inagglutinable to typing serum. It has been shown in experimental studies that antibodies directed against K or capsular antigens are actually more protective than antibodies against O antigens [13]. Anti-K antigens are opsonic and may well be the major surface structure of some gram-negative rods that are initially recognized by the host immune system. Certain capsular antibodies are, however, poorly immunogenic, and attempts to render them more immunogenic could result in serious sequelae like autoimmune disease.

Monoclonal Antibodies for the Assessment of Protective Antibodies Against Gram-Negative Bacilli

Studies carried out employing pooled human serum or animal serum after immunization may lead to confusing results in protection studies because of the diversity of antibodies present (including natural antibodies). Monoclonal antibodies against specific antigens represent a powerful tool for dissecting out the potential protective role of specific antibodies. One of the crucial issues that could be resolved is the relative protective role of type-specific versus cross-reactive antibodies against the endotoxin core region. In a series of experiments that we have recently reported, antibodies against the widely shared core region of enteric bacteria have been used both prophylactically and therapeutically [14,15]. Protection was directly related to the nature of the challenging organisms. Monoclonal antibodies against the Re antigen of *S. minnesota* R595 and the J5 antigen of *E. coli* O111 are, we believe, directed against the lipid A component. They failed to protect against a challenge due to highly encapsulated enteric organisms like those bacteria with a K13 capsule. On the other hand, if the challenge organism was poorly encapsulated, serum-sensitive, and therefore "rough", statistically significant protection could be demonstrated by pretreatment with antibody before challenge. This protection could be increased by the use of larger quantities of antibody and the protective effect could be overcome by augmenting the challenge dose of viable organisms. Type-specific protection, in the form of animal antiserum against the somatic or O antigen seem to be more protective for the more encapsulated or more virulent microorganisms. The same type of protective activity was also true for *Pseudomonas aeruginosa* serotypes. We have produced many monoclonal antibodies against somatic antigens of *P. aeruginosa* and they have opsonic and protective activity. Furthermore, the presence of two epitopes on a single organism and the use of two monoclonal antibodies against these different epitopes increased clinical effectiveness. We were unable to demonstrate that anti-J5 monoclonal antibodies (which would be considered non-specific protection) could enhance the results of intra-abdominal challenge by live *P. aeruginosa*. However, when a dose of antibiotic was used which was subtherapeutic, the additional use of anti-core J5 monoclonal antibody produced a significant increase in survival. Presumably, these antibodies against the core region of gram-negative endotoxin are neutralizing toxic effects, but have little effect on the multiplication of organisms.

Conclusions

The diversity of organisms causing gram-negative bacteremia has certainly been a limiting factor in the serologic approach toward prevention and treatment. Delivery of exogenously produced antibodies in a therapeutic or prophylactic setting overcomes the problem of poor immunogenicity, but there may be a quantitative problems to antibody administration. One concern is that insufficient quantities of functioning antibodies could be delivered either by an intramuscular or intraperitoneal route. Other concerns relate to use of animal antisera (such as monoclonal antibodies produced in rodent cell lines), the low yields, and low avidity of antibodies produced in vitro. Notwithstanding the many problems that would limit the immediate application of these procedures, we must also recognize that resistance to an invasion by opportunistic microorganisms probably has a multifactorial basis. The mere supplementation of antibodies, even in the presence of a functional reticuloendothelial system, may not be sufficient to engender protection. While granulocyte transfusions have fallen into considerable disrepute because of their complications, augmentation of numbers of phagocytic cells seems desirable if we are also attempting to supply exogenous antibodies.

References

1. Young LS (1981) Nosocomial infections in the immunocompromised adult. Am J Med 70:398-402
2. Young LS, Armstrong D (1972) Human immunity to *Pseudomonas aeruginosa:* 1. In vitro interaction of bacteria, polymorphonuclear leukocytes, and serum factors. J Infect Dis 126:257-276
3. Weinstein RJ, Young LS (1978) Phagocytic resistance of *Escherichia coli* K-1 isolates and relationship to virulence. J Clin Microbiol 8:748-755
4. Liu TY, Gotschlich EC, Egan W, Robbins JB (1977) Sialic acid containing polysaccharides of *Neisseria meningitidis* and *Escherichia coli* strain BOS-12. Structure and immunology. J Infect Dis 136(Suppl):S71-S77
5. Goldschneider I, Gotschlich EC, Artenstein MS (1969) Human immunity to the meningococcus: I. The role of humoral antibodies. J Exp Med 129:1307-1326
6. McCabe WR, Kreger BE, Johns M (1972) Type-specific and cross reactive antibodies in gram-negative bacteremia. N Engl J Med 287:262-267
7. Zinner SH, McCabe WR (1976) Effects of IgM and IgG antibody in patients with bacteremia due to gram-negative bacilli. J Infect Dis 133:37-45
8. Young LS, Meyer RD, Armstrong D (1973) *Pseudomonas aeruginosa* vaccine in cancer patients. Ann Intern Med 79:518-527
9. Young LS (1980) Immunoprophylaxis and immunotherapy of opportunistic infections in the compromised host. In: Verhoef J, Peterson PK, Quie PG (eds) Infections in the immunocompromised host: Pathogenesis, prevention and therapy. Elsevier, North Holland, pp 283-299
10. Pollack M, Young LS (1979) Protective activity of antibodies to exotoxin A and lipopolysaccharides of *Pseudomonas aeruginosa* at onset of septicemia in man. J Clin Invest 63:276-286
11. Young LS (1984) Immunoprophylaxis and serotherapy of bacterial infections. Am J Med 76:664-671

12. Ziegler EJ, McCutchan JA, Fierer JA, Glauser MP, Sadoff JC, Douglas H, Braude AI (1982) Treatment of gram-negative bacteremia and shock with human antiserum to a mutant *Escherichia coli*. N Engl J Med 307:1225-1230
13. Young LS (1979) Gram-negative sepsis. In Mandell G, Douglas JG, Bennett JE (eds) Principles and practice of infectious diseases. Wiley, New York, pp 571-608
14. Young LS (in press) Monoclonal antibodies: Technology and application to gram-negative infections. Infection
15. Young LS (1984) Functional activity of monoclonal antibodies against lipopolysaccharide antigens of gram-negative bacilli. Clin Res 32:518A

Discussion

(pp. 138-145)

Concerning the mouse protection experiments with monoclonal antibodies of two different isotypes, it seems to be likely that protection is enhanced because they are directed against two different determinants. It did not matter if the antibodies were administered before or after the animals were challenged with bacteria. Therefore, one could speculate that nature must have a reason for the polyclonal response. The more sites that are recognized on bacterial surfaces, the more the likelihood of protection of the host increases.

Chemiluminescence was used as a rapid method. In a system without luminol, doubling or tripling of chemiluminescence correlates with a 70%-90% kill of the inoculum using normal phagocytes. Therefore, one can determine some crude relationship between chemiluminescence and opsonic activity in a test system with antibody and normal phagocytes. Animal studies indicate that monoclonal antibodies against type specific lipopolysaccharides of *P. aeruginosa* are both opsonic and protective. Furthermore, if the animals are treated with subtherapeutic doses of antibiotics together with the antibody, an increased survival rate of the animals can be demonstrated.

Bayer-Symposium VIII
The Pathogenesis of Bacterial Infections, 147-156 (1985)

Mechanisms for Evasion and Survival of Bacteria by Perturbation of Phagocytes

P. G. Quie

Summary

Phagocytic cells are essential for host defense against invading bacteria and most pathogens have evolved mechanisms for evading phagocytosis. One of these mechanisms may be avoidance of attachment to a surface and persistence in the fluid phase. The recognition, uptake and killing of bacteria attached to plastic or bacterial colonies on the surface of agar were efficiently phagocytosed by human polymorphonuclear leukocytes and peritoneal macrophages. Other examples of nonopsonic phagocytosis included: opsonic effect of polyamines, and uptake of protein A positive *S. aureus* by human alveolar and peritoneal macrophages. Association of protein A with cytophilic IgG on peritoneal macrophages and alveolar macrophages appear to be the basis for attachment. The role of bacterial capsules in avoiding phagocytosis may be its ability to "hide" opsonically active molecules on the bacterial cell wall. The cell wall of *S. aureus* contains abundant C3b after incubation in normal human serum but specific anticapsular antibodies are necessary for phagocytosis.

Other methods of bacterial evasion of the phagocytic system include ability to survive intracellularly. Survival may be a consequence of bacterial inhibition of lysosome-phagosome fusion. A good example of this is *M. tuberculosis* which produces an acid sulfatide.

The expected oxidative responses of phagocytes during phagocytosis is also inhibited by certain microbial species including *Legionella pneumophila*.

Introduction

The normally peaceful coexistance between microbes which colonize mucous membranes and skin of their host results from a dynamic, complex balance between microbial aggression and host defense. Microbial factors which improve adherence, persistence, and possibly invasion are met by host factors which inhibit these factors such as mucous, ciliary action, fatty acids, lysozyme, lactoferrin, and specific antibodies of the IgA immunoglobulin class. A change in host physiology or break in surface integrity is usually necessary before bacteria and fungi are able to become established in tissue which is normally sterile.

Bacterial Evasion of Phagocytosis

Bacterial strategy for evading host surface defenses include secretion of IgA cleaving enzymes and successful competition for available nutrients and trace elements such as iron. *Neisseria meningitidis* and *N. gonorrhoeae* are good examples of bacterial species which have both of these properties [25]. When bacteria successfully breech surface barriers, nonimmunologically specific defenses usually localize and clear the invaders. Host factors include the bacteriocidins, i.e., natural or IgM antibodies which, together with activated terminal components of the serum complement system, cause lysis of certain bacteria. However, because of protective surfaces, most bacterial species are resistant to bacteriocidins. Gram-positive bacteria, for example, have thick cell walls of peptidoglycan and gram-negative bacteria are protected by surface lipopolysaccharide which hinder bacteriocidin association with bacterial membranes. A rich mosaic of bacterial surface proteins, capsules, and loosely associated "slime" contribute to survival and aggression of disease-producing bacteria. These bacterial antiphagocytic surface factors require opsonization for efficient phagocytosis. An intact phagocytic system is essential for defense against bacteria that have invaded and colonized tissues which are normally sterile.

Staphylococcus aureus

Peptidoglycan from *Staphylococcus aureus*, when separated from the rest of bacterial structures, has the same opsonic requirement as intact organisms before efficient phagocytosis occurs. Therefore, peptidoglycan is a primary bacterial surface antiphagocytic factor which requires opsonization for efficient uptake and killing by host phagocytes [18]. *Staphylococcus aureus* also has a unique surface protein, protein A, which reacts with the Fc portion of immunoglobulin without immunologic specificity and interferes with opsonic activity of specific anti-*Staphylococcus* antibodies.

Most strains of *Staphylococcus aureus* are opsonized efficiently by normal human serum since these sera contain anti-peptidoglycan antibodies and complement which compete successfully with the antiphagocytic influence of peptidoglycan protein A. Certain strains of *S. aureus* however, possess a stable capsule and encapsulated *S. aureus* strains are not phagocytized efficiently in the presence of normal human serum [19]. We found that encapsulated *S. aureus* were poorly opsonized in a variety of serum sources (fresh, chelated, and immunoglobulin-depleted) which effectively opsonized nonencapsulated strains [29]. The capsule, thetherefore, appears to interfere with phagocytic cell recognition of bacteria opsonized with either IgG or C3b.

When rabbits are immunized with encapsulated staphylococci and sera from these animals are used as sources of opsonin, encapsulated strains of staphylococci are efficiently phagocytized. Therefore, specific anticapsular antibodies which associate with the bacterial capsule (the true surface of the bacterium) provide ligands for phagotic cells.

The biologically activated component of complement, C3b, was found to be associated with the cell wall of encapsulated strains of *S. aureus*, however, presence of a capsule prevented these molecules from functioning as ligands, and phagocytosis did not occur [30]. Although the capsular structure did not inhibit deposition of C3b on the bacterial cell wall, the opsonic function of these molecules was prevented. The peptidoglycan cell wall of *S. aureus* is an "activating" surface, which allows C3 to be converted to C3b by the alternative pathway and function as opsonic ligands without participation of antibodies. Encapsulated *S. aureus*, however, have a "nonactivating" surface and specific antibacterial antibodies are necessary for conversion of C3 to C3b by the classical pathway. Human alveolar and peritoneal macrophages phagocytize protein-A-positive staphylococci without opsonins as a consequence of cytophilic IgG on the macrophage surface [26]. Therefore, human tissue macrophages in environments with little available opsonins may have adapted so that certain bacteria such as staphylococci with protein A surface factors are efficiently phagocytized.

Staphylococcus epidermidis

Staphylococcus epidermidis bacteremia is a serious complication of indwelling plastic lines and other devices in the vascular system. Catheters isolated from patients with *S. epidermidis* bacteremia have bacteria associated with the catheter embedded in a matrix of slime. This bacterial slime or glycocalyx with its adhesive and protective properties may be important in the adherence of organisms to plastic [14]. Plastic catheters removed from patients with *S. epidermidis* bacteremia contain staphylococcal organisms tightly adhering to the plastic surface embedded in a matrix of slime, suggesting that this slime substance may be important in bacterial adherence and persistence.

The slime produced by *S. epidermidis* may be fractionated after phenol extraction by DEAE column chromatography. A single fraction affects lymphoproliferation [12]. When human peripheral blood lymphocytes are incubated with *S. epidermidis* slime, the lymphocyte proliferative response to polyclonal stimulators phytohemagglutinin and streptococcal blastogen A is inhibited [12]. Slime appears to suppress normal host responses which may in turn contribute to the prolonged course of *S. epidermidis* infections associated with intravascular foreign bodies and increase the risk of patients with these infections to opportunistic pathogens.

Streptococcus pneumoniae

Pathogenic strains of *Streptococcus pneumoniae* have polysaccharide capsules which require specific anticapsular antibodies for efficient uptake by granulocytes. The capsule is a major virulence factor for these organisms since they are not toxigenic and they are rapidly killed after phagocytosis. Opsonic requirements of different serotypes of pneumococci have great heterogeneity in opsonic requirements which may account for the propensity of certain serotypes to predominate in human disease. The kinetics of uptake of four different serotypes of *S. pneumoniae* by human granulocytes was measured using radiolabeled bacteria and a variety of serum sources including normal serum, heat-inactivated serum, IgG-deficient serum, C2-deficient serum, and MgEGTA-chelated serum. All four serotypes were opsonized by the alternative pathway of complement activation, but there were striking differences in the quantity of serum necessary for effective opsonization [11]. Efficient rapid phagocytosis occurs when anti-pneumococcal antibodies are present. This requirement of specific anti-polysaccharide capsule antibodies may also explain the predisposition of patients with antibody or complement deficiencies to suffer severe pneumococcal disease. Furthermore, patients with overwhelming pneumococcal septicemia may have depleted serum opsonins because of alternative pathway activation of serum complement by circulating pneumococcal polysaccharide.

Evidence has been presented which suggests that antibody response to bacterial polysaccharide antigens may be of a single immunoglobulin subclass, IgG2 [24]. A direct correlation was found between IgG2 concentrations in serum and antibody response to 11 pneumococcal polysaccharides and *Hemophilus influenzae* type B antigen. There was no correlation between IgG2 and antibody response to protein antigens. Patients with Hodgkin's disease did not respond to pneumococcal polysaccharide antigens and had profoundly depressed levels of IgG2 subclass immunoglobulin in their serum. The antibodies that develop after polysaccharide immunization are restricted to a subclass of IgG immunoglobulin, suggesting a subclass-specific regulating mechanism for response to polysaccharide antigens. This abnormality of a highly specialized antibody response control system may be the reason why normal immunoglobulin levels and antibody responses to protein antigen, but poor antibody responses to polysaccharide antigens are found in patients with Wiskott-Aldrich syndrome, Hodgkin's Disease, recurrent sinopulmonary infections, and in infants less than 18 months of age.

Escherichia coli

Stools from normal human neonates contain a large variety of *E. coli* strains, although a single type, *E. coli* with K1 capsular antigen, is found in the blood or spinal fluid of approximately 80% of neonates with *E. coli* meningitis. *E. coli* with K1 capsular antigens are more virulent in experimental animals and are more resistant to phagocytosis by human granulocytes than strains without K1 antigen [5]. This virulence is related to inhibition of complement deposition on the bacterial surface by K1 antigen [7]. The K1 strains are rapidly phagocytized in the presence of specific antibody to K1 antigen.

Streptococcus pyogenes

The M protein of group A streptococci is another example of a highly specialized bacterial antiphagocytic structure. These organisms are also poorly opsonized in sera without specific antibodies [17]. The antiphagocytic effect of M protein was evaluated using radiolabeled bacteria which allowed simultaneous, independent evaluation of the process of opsonization, attachment to phagocytic cells, ingestion, and intracellular killing of bacteria [27]. Uptake of the labeled bacteria by phagocytes was determined at several time points to determine kinetics of phagocytosis. Using this method with chelated serum or C2-deficient serum allows measurement of the alternative pathway of complement activation. Bacteria were more slowly opsonized via the alternative pathway, i.e., opsonization via the classical pathway was complete within 5 min while 60 min are necessary for opsonization via the alternative pathway [17]. Once C3b is attached to the bacterial surface, either by the alternative or the classical pathway, organisms are efficiently phagocytized. Bacteria opsonized without complement were not only less efficiently attached to the phagocyte, but more slowly engulfed. Opsonization of an M-positive strain of *Streptococcus pyogenes* and an M-negative variant of this strain was studied using sera from several sources. The M-negative strain of streptococci was rapidly opsonized in the absence of immunoglobulin and in chelated serum, showing that these streptococci were efficiently opsonized via the alternative complement pathway. The M-positive streptococcal strain was poorly opsonized in fresh serum [17]. When specific M protein antibodies were present there was efficient opsonization of M-positive streptococci. The alternative complement pathway plays a major role in promoting phagocytosis of streptococci without M protein and this evidence suggests that cell surface M protein is a virulence factor for streptococci by inhibiting opsonization via the alternative complement pathway.

Pseudomonas aeruginosa

Six strains of *Pseudomonas aeruginosa* recovered from the blood of septicemia patients were efficiently opsonized, phagocytized, and killed by human granulocytes in the presence of normal human serum [16]. When complement-deficient sera and immunoglobulin-deficient sera were used as opsonin sources, a great heterogeneity of opsonic requirements for these six *Pseudomonas* strains was found. Assays with immunoglobulin-deficient serum suggested that immunoglobulins were necessary for alternative pathway opsonization of most strains of *Pseudomonas aeruginosa*.

More recently, it has been reported that certain *Pseudomonas* strains are phagocytized by human granulocytes in the absence of opsonin [3]. Only nonmucoid strains have this property. Mucoid strains require opsonin for uptake by phagocytic cells.

Robinson et al. [22] investigated the C1 response of normal human PMN to several bacterial species and to *Candida albicans* and zymosan. They found two distinct kinds of response with different microbial species. A prompt exponential response was found with *Staphylococcus*, *Candida*, the cell wall of *Saccharomyces cerevisiae* (zymosan), *Salmonella*, and *Shigella*. A slower response without a clearly defined peak was found with *Pseudomonas*, *Klebsiella*, *Proteus*, and *Streptococcus*.

When different *Pseudomonas* strains were studied, i.e., with an exopolysaccharide glycocalyx (slime) layer, with a capsule, without slime or capsule, different chemiluminescence results were obtained. Presence of a capsule inhibited the chemiluminescence response, but slime actually enhanced chemiluminescence. The peak chemiluminescence was higher in the slime-positive strains of *Pseudomonas*. These findings may relate to observations in our laboratory. Johnson, W.E. Regelmann and E.D. Gray (1984, unpublished work) found that slime from *S. epidermidis* stimulated chemiluminescence and degranulation of normal human PMN.

There were no consistent differences in chemiluminescence response to gram-positive organisms which contain a thick cell wall of peptidoglycan and teichoic acids and gram-negative bacteria containing lipopolysaccharides. Therefore, other mechanisms may be related to the chemiluminescence response of PMN and great differences exist between serotypes of the same bacterial species.

Association between bacteria and phagocytic cells may also be enhanced by products of inflammation which alter the electrostatic forces of cell surfaces. Peterson et al. [15] investigated the potential of three cationic polyamino acids: protamine, poly-l-arginine, and poly-l-lysine on *Staphylococcus aureus*, *S. epidermidis*, and *E. coli*. The predominant site of action was on the bacterial cell and these cationic polyamino acids functioned as opsonic ligands. Chemiluminescence responses were less prompt and blunted compared with response to bacteria opsonized in normal human serum, suggesting that the PMN respiratory burst is stimulated more efficiently via opsonic receptors than via surface electrostatic force alteration. After 30 min incubation, killing of intracellular bacteria was as efficient when bacteria were opsonized with polyamino acids as when normal human serum was used as opsonin. Changes in physiochemical surface properties may be the common denominator when bacteria are not opsonized and engulfed by surface phagocytosis, opsonized by cationic amino acids, activated components of the complement systems, and specific antibacterial antibodies.

Evasion of Intracellular Killing

Most bacterial species are rapidly killed after phagocytosis, however, some have evolved a remarkable capacity to survive in phagocytic cells by actively disturbing phagocyte function. Effects of toxins on cells are well known. For example, the lecithinases and phosphorylases of staphylococci, cytotoxins of *Pseudomonas*, and lysins of streptococci kill phagocytes. However, other bacterial species have more subtle effects such as inhibition of lysosome-phagosome fusion or alteration of the phagocytes metabolic response during engulfment.

Mycobacterium tuberculosis

Many years ago, Armstrong and Hart showed that azurophile granules remain intact in phagocytic cells containing *Mycobacterium tuberculosis* [4]. The viable mycobacteria produce an acidic sulfatide which prevents lysosome-phagosome fusion. This mycobacterial sulfatide accumulates in azurophile granules of infected macrophages. *Histoplasma capsulatum* and *Toxoplasma gondii* also inhibit phagosome-lysosome fusion. *Chlamydia* also inhibit lysosome-phagosome fusion and have the additional capacity to survive within the cytoplasm of epithelial cells [30].

Legionella pneumophila

A dramatic oxidative respiratory metabolic response occurs in granulocytes during phagocytosis. The oxygen radicals resulting from these reactions are usually lethal for bacteria, however, certain bacteria have evolved mechanisms for inhibiting the oxidative burst during phagocytosis. For example, *Legionella pneumophila* produce a factor which inhibits the respiratory oxidative burst of phagocytic cells. These organisms replicate within macrophages [10]. *Listeria monocytogenes* produces an iron-dependent dismutase which detoxifies oxygen radicals formed during the respiratory burst, which may be related to the ability of *Listeria* to survive intracellularly [28].

Bordetella pertussis

Patients infected with *Bordetella pertussis*, the etiologic agent of whooping cough, have little fever, normal neutrophil numbers, marked lymphocytosis, and a susceptibility to secondary bacterial pneumonia [9]. *Bordetella pertussis* produce a variety of toxins, including an adenylate cyclase toxin which binds to host phagocytic cells and bacterial adenylate cyclase is introduced into these cells. Human neutrophils exposed to *Bordetella* adenylate cyclase generate high levels of adenosine-3'5'-monophosphate (cyclic AMP) and become impotent [6]. Functional defects include: inhibited superoxide generation, inhibited chemotaxis, and decreased bactericidal capacity. Phagocyte impotence induced by microbial adenylate cyclase may be related to pathogenesis of whooping cough.

Influenza A Virus

Abramson et al. demonstrated that influenza A virus (an H_3N_2 strain) inhibits human neutrophils oxidative response and furthermore, other strains of influenza A virus inhibit lysosome-phagosome fusion as well as oxidative metabolism [1,2]. It is tempting to speculate that the greatly increased susceptibility of patients with influenza A virus infection secondary to bacterial infection may be related to the capacity of influenza viruses to inhibit phagocytic cell oxidative metabolism, lysosome-phagosome fusion, and ability to kill bacteria.

Patients with Increased Susceptibility to Infection

Balance between bacteria and host may be profoundly disturbed in patients with genetically transmitted or acquired abnormalities of their immunologic system. Hyperimmunoglobulin E-recurrent infection (Job's) syndrome and chronic granulomatous disease are examples of abnormalities of the phagocytic systems. Mononuclear cells from patients with the hyperimmunoglobulin E-recurrent infection syndrome produce, without stimulation, excessive amounts of an inhibitor of neutrophil chemotaxis [8]. Subtle defects in granulocyte locomotion compromise host defense in patients with Job's syndrome because prompt response to inflammatory stimuli is necessary for effective localization of invading bacteria. Delay of just a few hours in accumulation of phagocytes at a site of inoculation of bacteria may enhance the capacity of bacteria to produce clinically significant lesions by several thousand fold [13].

Patients with chronic granulomatous disease are born with a phagocyte membrane defect which prevents their cells from responding to stimuli with an oxidative response [21]. An ineffective membrane oxidase is believed responsible for this defect, but a majority of male patients with chronic granulomatous disease also lack a membrane-associated cytochrome *b* which contributes to this electron transfer [23]. As a consequence of this defective oxidase response during phagocytosis, superoxide and other reactive oxygen radicals are not produced by phagocytic cells from these patients and the cidal components of the oxidative burst do not accumulate within phagocytic vacuoles. Bacteria ordinarily killed rapidly by normal granulocytes remain viable. Certain bacteria such as streptococcal species provide their own toxic oxygen radicals in excess and are killed normally by CGD granulocytes, however, *Staphylococcus*, *Serratia*, or *Aspergillus* produce serious disease and granulomatous lesions [20].

Conclusions

More virulent microbes have evolved mechanisms for evading host defenses in general and the phagocytic system in particular by developing cell walls with specialized antiphagocytic or capsular structures. Fortunately, the host's specific adaptive immune antibody response to microbial surface antigens provides the host with opsonic antibodies for efficient phagocytosis by granulocytes and macrophages. When microbes are efficiently opsonized and engulfed the phagocytes' granule disruption, phagosome formation and oxidative burst usually result in host superiority. Prolonged coexistence does occur when microbial species successfully evade the intracellular antimicrobial armamentarium of host phagocytes.

References

1. Abramson JS, Lewis JC, Lyles DS, Heller KA, Mills EL, Bass DA (1982) Inhibition of neutrophil lysosome phagosome fusion associated with influenzae virus infection in vitro: role in depressed bactericidal activity. J Clin Invest 69:1393-1397
2. Abramson JS, Mills EL, Giebink GS, Quie PG (1982) Depression of monobyte and polymorphonuclear leukocyte oxidative metabolism and bactericidal capacity by influenzae A virus. Infect Immun 35:350-355
3. Apwwer SP (1984) Nonopsonic phagocytosis of strains of *Pseudomonas aeruginosa* from cystic fibrosis patients. Infect Immun 43:1006-1011
4. Armstrong JA, Hart PD (1971) Response of cultured macrophages to *Macrobacterium tuberculosis* with observations on fusion of lysosomes with phagosomes. J Exp Med 134:713-740
5. Bortolussi R, Ferrieri P, Bjorksten B, Quie PG, Wannamaker LW (1979) Capsular K1 polysaccharide of *E. coli:* Relationship to virulence in newborn rats and resistance to phagocytosis. Infect Immun 25:293-298

6. Confer DL, Eaton JW (1982) Phagocyte impotence caused by an invasive bacterial adenylate cyclase. Science 217:948-950
7. Cross AS, Gemski P, Sadoff JC, Orskov F, Orskov I (1984) The importance of the K1 capsule in invasive infections caused by *Escherichia coli*. J Infect Dis 149:184-193
8. Donabedian H, Gallin JI (1983) Two inhibitors of neutrophil chemotaxis are produced by hyperimmunoglobulin E recurrent infections sydrome mononuclear cells exposed to heat killed staphylococci. Infect Immun 40: 1030-1037
9. Eller J (1982) Pertussis (Whooping Cough). In Hoekelman RA, Blatman S, Brunell PA, Friedman SB, Seidel HM (eds) Principles of Pediatrics. McGraw-Hill, New York, pp 1211-1212
10. Friedman RL, Lochner JE, Bigley RH, Iglewski BH (1982) The effects of *Legionella pneumophilia* toxin on oxidative processes and bacterial killing of human polymorphonuclear leukocytes. J Infect Dis 146:328-334
11. Giebink GS, Verhoef J, Peterson PK, Quie PG (1977) Opsonic requirements for phagocytosis of *S. pneumoniae* types VI, SVIII, XXIII, and XXV. Infect Immun 18:291-297
12. Gray ED, Peters G, Verstegen M, Regelmann WE (1984) Effect of extracellular slime substance from *Staphylococcus epidermidis* on the human cellular immune response. Lancet 1:365-367
13. Miles AA, Miles EM, Burke J (1957) The value and duration of defense reactions of the skin to the primary lodgement of bacteria. Br J Exp Pathol 38:79-96
14. Peters G, Locci R, Pulverer G (1982) Adherence and growth of coagulase-negative staphylococci on surfaces of intravenous catheters. J Infect Dis 146:479-482
15. Peterson PK, Gekker G, Shapiro R, Freiberg M, Keane W (1984) Polyamino acid enhancement of bacterial phagocytosis by human polymorphonuclear leukocytes and peritoneal macrophages. Infect Immun 43:561-566
16. Peterson PK, Kim Y, Schmeling D, Lindemann M, Verhoef J, Quie PG (1978) Complement-mediated phagocytosis of *Pseudomonas aeruginosa*. J Lab Clin Med 92(6):883-894
17. Peterson PK, Schmeling D, Cleary PP, Wilkinson BJ, Kim Y, Quie PG (1979) Inhibition of alternative complement pathway opsonization by group A streptococcal M protein. J Infect Dis 139:575-585
18. Peterson PK, Verhoef J, Sabath LD, Quie PG (1976) Extracellular and bacterial factors influencing staphylococcal phagocytosis and killing by human polymorphonuclear leukocytes. Infect Immun 14:496-501
19. Peterson PK, Wilkinson BJ, Kim Y, Schmeling D, Quie PG (1978) Influence of encapsulation on staphylococcal opsonization and phagocytosis by human polymorphonuclear leukocytes. Infect Immun 19:943-949
20. Quie PG (1983) The phagocytic system and associated diseases. In: Behrman RE, Vaughan VC (eds) Nelson's Textbook of pediatrics, 12th edn. Saunders, Philadelphia, pp 518-523
21. Regelmann W, Hayes N, Que PG (1983) Chronic granulomatous disease: Historical perspective and clinical experience at the University of Minnesota Hospital. In: Gallin JI, Fauci AS (eds) Advances in host defense mechanisms, vol 3. Raven, New York, pp 3-23
22. Robinson P, Wakefield D, Breit SN, Easter JF, Penny R (1984) Chemiluminescent response to pathogenic organisms: Normal human polymorphonuclear leukocytes. Infect Immun 43:744-752
23. Segal AW, Cross, AR, Garcia RC, Borregaard N, Valerius NH, Soothill JF, Jones OTG (1983) Absence of cytochrome b in chronic granulomatous disease. A multicentre European evaluation of its incidence and relevance. N Engl J Med 308:245-250

24. Siber GR, Schur PH, Aisenberg AC, Weitzman SA, Schiffman G (1980) Correlation between serum IgG-2 concentrations and the antibody response to bacterial polysaccharide antigens. N Engl J Med 178:178-182
25. Sparling PG (1983) Bacterial virulence and pathogenesis: An overview. Rev Infect Dis *5*(suppl. 4):S637-S646
26. Verbrugh HA, Hoidal JR, Nguyen BT, Verhoef J, Quie PG, Peterson PK (1983) Human alveolar macrophage cytophilic immunoglobulin G mediated phagocytosis of protein A positive staphylococci. J Clin Invest 69:63-71
27. Verhoef J, Peterson PK, Quie PG (1977) Kinetics of staphylococcal opsonization attachment, infection, and killing by human polymorphonuclear leukocytes: A quantitative assay using (^3H) thymidine labelled bacteria. J Immunol Methods 14:303-311
28. Welch DF, Sword CP, Brehm S, Dusanic D (1979) Relationship between superoxide dismutase and pathogenic mechanisms of *Listeria monocytogenes*. Infect Immun 23:863-872
29. Wilkinson BJ, Peterson PK, Quie PG (1979) Cryptic peptidoglycan and the anti-phagocytic effect of *Staphylococcus aureus* capsule: A model for the anti-phagocytic effect of bacterial cell surface polymers. Infect Immun 23:502-512
30. Wyrick PB, Brownridge EA (1978) Growth of *Chylamydia psittaci* in macrophages. Infect Immun 19:1054-1060

Discussion

(pp. 147-156)

Cytophilic IgG using fluorescein-labeled anti-IgG was found only on peritoneal and alveolar macrophages, but not on peripheral blood polymorphs or monocytes. In addition, alveolar macrophages from experimental animals did not have cytophilic IgG. As nonspecific opsonins, polyamines seem to increase the hydrophobicity of bacteria. The relationship of protein A to virulence of *S. aureus* is not clear, since protein A-positive *S. aureus* associate with and are killed by macrophages; therefore, protein A on staphylococci favors the host rather than bacteria.

Bayer-Symposium VIII
The Pathogenesis of Bacterial Infections, 158-165 (1985)

Interacting T Cell Functions Elicited by Facultative Intracellular Bacteria

H. Hahn and H. Näher

Summary

Immunity to facultative intracellular bacteria (FIB) rests upon collaboration between antigen-specific T cells and macrophages. Work mostly done in the *Listeria* infection model in mice has yielded that granulomas are formed and macrophages activated under the influence of specific T lymphocytes which, upon antigen stimulation, secrete lymphokines. Macrophages are activated by MAF (γ interferon) which is secreted both by naturally produced and by cloned Ly 1^+T cells, whereas granuloma formation is due to the activity of Ly 12^+T cells. Both macrophage activation and granuloma formation contribute to the effective buildup of immunity to FIB, granuloma formation being the more important part. Ly 1^+2^-T cells are H2-I-A restricted whereas granuloma-inducing Ly 12^+T cells are H2-K restricted. The former recognize dead bacterial antigen whereas the latter need antigen produced by viable bacteria. Ly 1^+2^-T cells with *Listeria* specificity have been cloned and shown to produce γ interferon, transfer delayed-type hypersensitivity, and transfer systemic macrophage activation.

Introduction

Infections by facultative intracellular bacteria (FIB) (Table 1) are characterized by the formation of granulomatous lesions in infected tissue, macrophage activation, and delayed-type hypersensitivity (DTH). FIB are trapped within granulomatous lesions and in these lesions macrophages become activated; in this way they acquire a heightened antibacterial activity which enables them to deal more effectively with the bacterial parasite (for review see [1]). For many years, little was known about the underlying mechanisms of granuloma formation and macrophage activation. Likewise, the role of DTH in immunity to these infections remained a matter of dispute [2]. In particular, it could not be decided whether DTH plays a causative role in anti-infective immunity or whether it is a totally unrelated phenomenon.

Mackaness [3] in 1969, using the listeriosis model of mice, showed that macrophage activation and granuloma formation are the consequences of specific immune reactions involving viable lymphocytes and antigen. This observation was based on the results of adoptive transfer experiments in which viable lymphocytes

Table 1. Facultative intracellular bacteria

Mycobacterium tuberculosis	*Yersinia* species
Mycobacterium leprae	*Francisella* species
Brucella species	*Salmonella typhi*
Listeria monocytogenes	*Salmonella paratyphi*
Erysipelothrix rhusiopathiae	*Treponema pallidum*
	Legionella pneumophila

from infected and immune animals were able to transfer to non-immune recipients a specific form of antibacterial immunity. Antibodies, on the other hand, were completely ineffective. Later on, it was established [4-6] that the cells transferring protection were T cells. Zinkernagel and Doherty [7] showed that, in mice, recognition of antigen by T cells is restricted by the major histocompatibility locus (MHC). Zinkernagel et al. [8] claimed that T cell-antigen interactions in immunity to FIB were restricted by products coded by the H2-I locus whereas Cheers and Sandrin [9] provided evidence that these interactions were restricted by the H2-K locus. In this paper, results mostly from our laboratory will be summarized which deal with the role of T cell subpopulations in the generation of immunity to FIB, especially in granuloma formation and macrophage activation. The relative importance of macrophage activation and of granuloma formation will be evaluated, and it will be shown that these two phenomena are differently regulated and are induced by different T cell subpopulations.

T Cell Subpopulations in Adoptive Transfer of Specific Immunity and Delayed-Type Hypersensitivity in Murine Listeriosis

Both DTH and specific immunity to the FIB, *Listeria monocytogenes*, can be transferred by specific T cells from peritoneal exudates induced in mice with a 7-day-old *Listeria* infection. The cells which transferred protection and DTH were sensitive to in vitro treatment with an antiserum to Ly 1 plus complement and also to treatment with antiserum to Ly 2 plus complement. Thus, the protection and DTH transferring T cells carry both the Ly 1 and the Ly 2 markers [10] (Table 2).

From these experiments, the following alternative conclusions were considered:

Ly 12^+T cells activate macrophages directly
Ly 12^+T cells attract macrophages to form granulomatous lesions
Ly 12 T cells recruit other subpopulations of T cells (either Ly 1 and/or Ly 2) which in turn are responsible for macrophage activation and/or granuloma formation
Ly 12^+T cells are precursors and, after transfer into recipients develop into Ly 1^+2^- and/or Ly 2^+T cells which in turn are responsible for the buildup of an effective immunity.

Table 2. Ly-Phenotype of T cell subsets involved in antibacterial protection and DTH[a]

Group	Treatment of PETL	T cell subset	$\log_{10}$ protection	DTH (0.1 mm footpad swelling)
1	Nil	Unselected	3.68	8.8
2	C	Unselected	2.59	9.2
3	Anti Thy 1.2 + C	No	0.65	2.4
4	Anti Ly 1.2+C	Ly 1^-2^-	0.62	2.2
5	Anti Ly 2.2, 3.2 + C	Ly 1^+2^-	0.78	4.4
6	Mixture (1:1) of groups 4 and 5	Ly 1^+2^-		
7	No PETL			2.2

[a]PETL were treated with anti-Ly antisera plus C and equivalents of 3×10^6 PETL were injected intravenously into recipients which received live *L. monocytogenes* intravenously for evaluation of protection or soluble listerial antigen subcutaneously for evaluation of DTH (from [10]).

In Vitro Studies

In order to decide between these possibilities, in vitro studies were performed using an assay first described by Farr et al. [11]. This assay allows one to measure T cell proliferation, interleukin-1 (LAF) production by stimulated macrophages, and interleukin-2 (TCGF) production by stimulated T cells. Interaction of *Listeria* antigen (heat-killed *Listeria monocytogenes*) in the presence of antigen-presenting normal macrophages and listeria-specific peritoneal exudate T lymphocytes (PETL) revealed that antigen-specific proliferation, interleukin-2 production, and induction of interleukin-1 production by macrophages all are functions of Ly 1^+2^-T cells (Table 3) [12-14].

Experiments with Cloned T Cells

Listeria-specific T lymphocytes were cloned [15] using the method of Sredni et al. [16]. These cloned cells carried the Ly 1 marker and were able to adoptively mediate both DTH and a certain degree of protection (Table 4). In addition, *Listeria*-specific cloned T cells were able to produce γ interferon [14] and macrophage activating factor (Sperling et al. in press). Likewise, when supernatants from antigen-stimulated, cloned T cells were injected into normal mice, the latter exhibited some degree of protection after subsequent challenge with *Listeria monocytogenes*, most likely owing to systemic activation of macrophages [18].

Table 3. Ly phenotype of T cell subsets involved in T cell proliferation and interleukin production

Group	Treatment of PETL[a]	T cell subset	Proliferation (^{3}HTdR uptake (cpm))[b]	Interleukin-1 activity (^{3}HTdR uptake of thymocytes (cpm))[c]	Interleukin-2 activity (% specific lysis of ^{51}Cr-labeled P815)[d]
1	None	Unselected	38 400	8500	70
2	C	Unselected	39 900	8200	63
3	Anti-Thy 1.2 + C	No	320	130	0
4	Anti-Ly 1.2 + C	Ly 1^+2^-	280	180	0
5	Anti-Ly 2.2,3.2+C	Ly 1^-2^+	40 100	100	67
6	Mixtures of groups 4 and 5	Ly 1^-2^+ + Ly 1^+2^-	44 600	4100	68
7	no PETL		1400	11o	66

[a]PETL were treated with anti-Ly antisera plus C and equivalents of 1×10^6/ml PETL were cocultured with normal macrophages and heat-killed *L. monocytogenes*.

[b]Proliferative response after 3 days, last 18 h with 0.1 µCi ^{3}HTdR (from [12]).

[c]Proliferative response of thymocytes in presence of 25% cell-free supernatant after 3 days, last 18 h with 0.1 µCi ^{3}HTdR (from [13]).

[d]Cytotoxic activity of alloreactive cytotoxic T cells after coculture with 50% supernatant. Killer: target cell ratio 10:1 (from [14]).

Table 4. Adoptive antibacterial protection and DTH after systemic transfer of cloned *L. monocytogenes*-specific T cells[a]

T cell line	Cell number	$\log_{10}$ protection in spleen	DTH (0.1 mm footpad swelling)
9-6	2×10^4	0.13	1.0
9-6	2×10^6	1.06	6.4
	No cells		0.8
9-16	5×10^4	0.24	2.0
9-16	5×10^6	1.87	Not detectable
	No cells		1.0

[a]Cloned T cells were injected intravenously into recipients which received live *L. monocytogenes* intravenously for evaluation of protection or soluble listerial antigen subcutaneously for evaluation of DTH (from [10]).

Role of T Cells in Granuloma Formation

From these observations, at first sight a discrepancy seemed to exist between the in vitro findings and the transfer of protection and DTH in vivo, both of which required Ly 12^{+}T cells. Therefore, the possibility was entertained that macrophage activation and granuloma formation might be phenomena which rest upon different underlying mechanisms and are possibly due to different T cell subpopulations. In order to elucidate this question, a model of adoptive granuloma formation was devised (Näher et al., manuscript submitted). *Listeria*-specific T cells from peritoneal exudates of *Listeria*-immune mice were adoptively transferred to normal recipients. The latter were subsequently challenged with *Listeria monocytogenes* and the numbers of granulomas in the infected liver determined by light microscopy. Adoptive granuloma formation was abolished when the transferring T cells were subjected in vitro to treatment with anti-Ly 1 antiserum and also by treatment with anti-Ly 2 antiserum and complement (Fig. 1). Thus, granuloma formation, as is the case with protection as a whole, depends on a critical T cell which bears both the markers Ly 1 and Ly 2. When only Ly $1^{+}2^{-}$T cells were transferred, no granulomas were formed.

Furthermore, employing point-mutated mice, it could be shown (H. Näher et al., unpublished) that compatibility at the K, but not I, locus of the maior histocompatibility gene complex was necessary and sufficient for the adoptive transfer of granuloma formation (Table 5). Thus, granuloma formation is restricted by H2-K, and not by H2-I-A. In addition, the transfer of granuloma formation was critically dependent on the presence of living bacteria in recipients whereas the in vitro observations

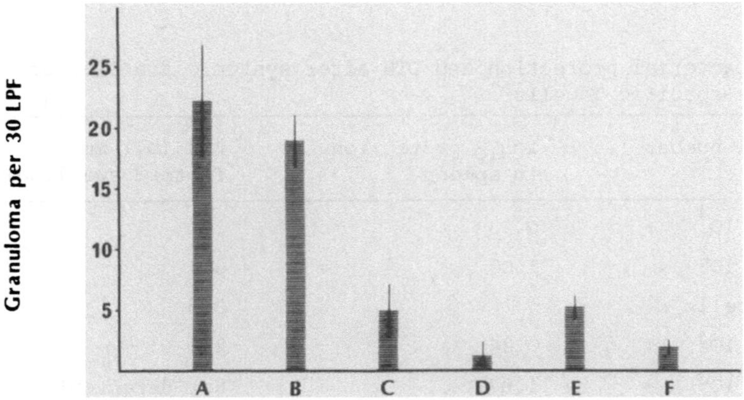

Fig. 1. Effect of anti-Ly antisera plus C treatment on the capacity of *L. monocytogenes*-immune PETL to transfer systemic granuloma formation; 5×10^6 unselected PETL (*A*), treated with C alone (*B*), equivalent numbers of anti-Ly 1.2 antiserum plus C (*C*), anti-Ly 2.2 antiserum plus C (*D*) treated PETL, or a mixture of *C* and *D* in a ratio 1:1 (*E*), were injected intravenously together with 5×10^4 *L. monocytogenes*. Injection of 5×10^4 *L. monocytogenes* alone (*F*). Mean ± standard deviation of five mice per group

Table 5. Genetic restriction of adoptive transfer of granuloma formation

Recipient[a]	H2 complex K I D / A B J E C	Homology	Granulomas per 30 LPF ± standard deviation
C 57Bl/6			2.0 ± 1.4
C 57Bl/6	bbbbbbb	All	33.2 ± 8.4
B 10.A (4R)	kkbbbbb	I-B, I-J, I-E, I-C, D	2.4 ± 1.7
B 10.A (5R)	bbbkkdd	K, I-A, I-B	30.8 ± 7.3
B 10.MBR	bkkkkkq	K	36.4 ± 5.7
C 57Bl/6			1.8 ± 1.3
C 57Bl/6	bbbbbbb	All	32.7 ± 9.7
B 10.A (4R)	kkbbbbb	I-B, I-J, I-E, I-C, D	2.3 ± 1.2
B 6.C-H-2^{bm12}	b.bbbbb	All except I-A	29.5 ± 6.3
B 6.C-H-2^{bm1}	.bbbbbb	All except K	2.5 ± 1.3

[a] 5×10^6 *L. monocytogenes*-immune PETL were injected intravenously into congeneic or point-mutated recipients which received live *L. monocytogenes* for evaluation of granuloma formation (from H. Näher et al., unpublished work).

could easily be made by using heat-killed *Listeria* organisms. Thus, only "living" antigen is seen by *Listeria*-specific T cells (Table 6) (H. Näher et al., unpublished work).

Conclusions

From the experiments described, it is concluded that both macrophage activation and granuloma formation contribute to the effective buildup of an antibacterial defense. Macrophage activation is a function of H2-I-A-restricted Ly 1^+2^-T cells which secrete γ interferon which is activating macrophages and in this way achieves some degree of protection. Granuloma formation, on the other hand, is a function of Ly 12^+T cells. Ly 12^+T cells are restricted by the H2-K locus of the MHC, whereas the macrophage-activating T cells are restricted by the H2-I-A locus of the MHC. Granuloma-forming Ly 12^+T cells, in order to function properly, must recognize living antigen, whereas for the Ly 1^+2^- cell-dependent functions, dead antigen suffices.

Table 6. Effect of live and heat-killed *L. monocytogenes* organisms on the expression of granuloma formation in adoptively immunized mice

Number of immune PETL transferred[a]	*Listeria* antigen	Granulomas per 30 LPF
	5×10^4 live	2.8 ± 1.6
5×10^6	5×10^4 live	26.4 ± 5.1
	1×10^5 heat-killed	3.4 ± 2.7
5×10^6	1×10^5 heat-killed	2.8 ± 1.9
	1×10^6 heat-killed	1.7 ± 2.1
5×10^6	1×10^6 heat-killed	2.4 ± 2.2
	1×10^7 heat-killed	2.9 ± 1.4
5×10^6	1×10^7 heat-killed	3.7 ± 2.5
	1×10^8 heat-killed	2.2 ± 1.7
5×10^6	1×10^8 heat-killed	1.9 ± 1.3

[a] *L. monocytogenes*-immune PETL were injected intravenously into recipients which received either live or graded doses of heat-killed *L. monocytogenes* for evaluation of granuloma formation (from H. Näher et al., unpublished work).

References

1. Hahn H, Kaufmann SHE (1981) The role of cell-mediated immunity in bacterial infections. Rev Infect Dis 3:1232-1250
2. Youmans GP (1975) Relation between delayed hypersensitivity and immunity in tuberculosis (editorial). Am Rev Respir Dis 111:109-118
3. Mackaness GB (1969) The influence of immunologically committed lymphoid cells on macrophage activity in vivo. J Exp Med 129:973-992
4. Blanden RV, Langman RE (1972) Cell-mediated immunity to bacterial infection in the mouse. Thymus-derived cells as effectors of acquired resistance to Listeria monocytogenes. Scand J Immunol 1:379-391
5. Lane FC, Unanue ER (1972) Requirement of thymus (T) lymphocytes for resistance to listeriosis. J Exp Med 135:1104-1112
6. North RJ (1973) Importance of thymus-derived lymphocytes in cell-mediated immunity to infection. Cell Immunol 7:166-176
7. Zinkernagel RM, Doherty PC (1974) Restriction of in vitro T cell-mediated cytotoxicity in lymphocyte choriomeningitis within a syngeneic or semiallogeneic system. Nature 248:701-702
8. Zinkernagel RM, Althage A, Adler B, Blanden RV, Davidson WF, Kees U, Dunlop MBC, Shreffler DC (1977) H-2 restriction of cell-mediated immunity to an intracellular bacterium. Effector T cells are specific for Listeria antigen in association with H-2I region coded self-markers. J Exp Med 145:1353-1367
9. Cheers C, Sandrin MS (1983) Restriction in adoptive transfer of resistance to Listeria monocytogenes: II. Use of congenic and mutant mice shows transfer to be H-2K restricted. Cell Immunol 78:199-205
10. Kaufmann SHE, Simon MM, Hahn H (1979) Specific Lyt 123 T cells are involved in protection against Listeria monocytogenes and in delayed-type hypersensitivity to listerial antigens. J Exp Med 150:1033-1038

11. Farr AG, Kiely J-M, Unanue ER (1979) Macrophage-T cell interactions involving Listeria monocytogenes - Role of the H-2 gene complex. J Immunol 122:2395-2404
12. Kaufmann SHE, Simon MM, Hahn H (1982) Regulatory interactions between macrophages and T-cell subsets in Listeria monocytogenes-specific T-cell activation. Infect Immun 38:907-913
13. Kaufmann SHE, Hahn H, Simon MM (1982) T-cell subsets induced in Listeria monocytogenes-immune mice. Scand J Immunol 16:539-542
14. Kaufmann SHE, Hahn H, Simon MM, Röllinghoff M, Wagner H (1982) Interleukin 2 induction in Lyt $1^{+}23^{-}$T cells from Listeria monocytogenes-immune mice. Infect Immun 37:1292-1294
15. Kaufmann SHE, Hahn H (1982) Biological functions of T cell lines with specificity for the intracellular bacterium Listeria monocytogenes in vitro and in vivo. J Exp Med 155:1754-1765
16. Sredni B, Tse HY, Chen C, Schwartz RH (1981) Antigen-specific clones of proliferating T lymphocytes: I. Methodology, specificity, and MHC restriction. J Immunol 126:341-347
17. Kaufmann SHE, Hahn H, Berger R, Kirchner H (1983) Interferon γ production by Listeria monocytogenes-specific T cells active in cellular antibacterial immunity. Eur J Immunol 13:265-268
18. Kaufmann SHE (1983) Effective antibacterial protection induced by a Listeria monocytogenes-specific T cell clone and its lymphokines. Infect Immun 39:1265-1270

Discussion

(pp. 158-165)

Listeria- specific T cell clones are Ly 1^+ and recognize only class 2 antigens. Class 1 antigens are recognized by Ly 1^+2^+ T cells that form granuloma, but these have not yet been cloned. Two types of transfer experiments were done. In the first type, T cells from mice immunized 7 days before inducing peritoneal exudates were collected. After 3 days, the cells were harvested and run over a nylon wool column, an enriched T cell population was thus obtained. These cells were immediately transferred. In the second type of experiment, cloned T cells were expanded by keeping them in vitro for several days. There are two elements of protection: 1 granuloma formation macrophage activation. First, there is recruitment of monocytes to form granuloma in which the reaction between T cells and antigen leads to macrophage activation. If irradiated recipients have enough monocytes to make a granuloma, transfer experiments with those sets of T-cells can be made. Both DTH and protection need the cooperation of recipient mononuclear phagocytes.

Session 3

Features of Bacterial Virulence

Chairman: V. Braun

Bayer-Symposium VIII
The Pathogenesis of Bacterial Infections, 168-176 (1985)

Iron Supply as a Virulence Factor

V. Braun

Summary

Iron, an essential nutrient for bacteria, is withheld by the host by binding to transferrin of the serum and to lactoferrin in secretory fluids. Bacteria have developed elaborate iron supply systems to overcome iron deprivation. Usually, they synthesize and secrete compounds of low molecular weight, termed siderophores, that complex Fe^{3+} with extremely high affinity and specificity. The iron-siderophore complexes are taken up by specific transport systems. In *Escherichia coli*, at least five different transport systems exist, controlled by about 30 genes. They effectively compete with the iron limitation devices of the host.

Synthesis of a number of exotoxins is induced by iron limitation, including a cell-bound hemolysin of various *Serratia* strains. Lysis occurs within 30 min after contact of living *Serratia* cells with human erythrocytes (cell ratio 1:1). Surprisingly, erythrocyte membrane proteins are hydrolyzed at a few sites. The hemolysin resides in the membrane fraction of *Serratia* and can be inactivated by incubating cells with proteases under conditions such that they remain viable, suggesting that the hemolysin is exposed at the cell surface.

Introduction

The role iron plays in host-parasite interactions is multifold. Iron is probably the only nutrient that is generally available in very limited amounts to pathogens. Iron(III) ion is insoluble at pH 7, in serum it is strongly bound to transferrin, and in secretory fluids to lactoferrin. The concentration of free iron in equilibrium with the polymeric iron(III) hydroxide, or with the iron binding proteins, is only a few ions per milliliter which is certainly not sufficient to support growth of 10^8 bacterial cells per milliliter, each of which contains about 10^6 iron ions. Under these conditions, only those microbes can multiply which contain very efficient iron supply systems. They require iron as an essential component of the electron transport chains and of various indispensable cytoplasmic enzymes.

If iron is a growth-limiting factor, the host may actively reduce its availability as a defense against microbial infections. In fact, numerous studies cite as responses to infections iron withdrawal by deposition in storage compartments, decreased intestinal absorption, enhanced synthesis of transferrin, stationing of lactoferrin at sites of inflammation by discharge from neutrophils, inhibition of iron mobilization from hemoglobin by binding of haptoglobin, and hormonal induction of hypoferremia by the leukocytic endogenous mediator (LEM), to mention only the most obvious mechanisms. In contrast, hyperferremia increases the incidence and the intensity of infections. For detailed accounts of these findings, the reader is referred to recent discussions [7, 21, 23] and to the book *Microbiology – 1983* (see, e.g., reference [15]) which contains 22 contributions concerning various aspects of iron metabolism in microorganisms and their hosts. This paper will briefly review two subjects: (a) the way bacteria overcome iron deprivation; and (b) regulation of toxin production by iron.

Acquisiton of Iron by Bacteria

Under iron-limiting growth conditions, many bacterial strains synthesize and release compounds of low molecular weight, called siderophores, that complex iron(III) with high affinity and specificity. In addition, they express very effective transport systems so that an iron concentration of 0.1 μM is sufficient for growth. Iron assimilation of *Escherichia coli* has been studied in most detail. About 30 genes are involved which specify at least five iron transport systems. The transport systems are defined by different siderophores and by specific transport components confined to one particular iron(III)-siderophore compound [2]. Figure 1 illustrates the present-day knowledge of iron supply systems of *E. coli*. They are different from all the other transport systems of nutrients studied so far. Iron is not transported as a metal ion, but only as a siderophore complex. This must first be bound by a receptor protein in the outer membrane. It looks as if the scarce iron(III)-siderophores are extracted from the medium, and concentrated at the cell surface, from which they are translocated further into the cell. Outer membrane proteins that are synthesized in response to iron limitation were also found in *Salmonella typhimurium* [1, 3], *Shigella flexneri* [16], various strains of *Vibrio* [15], *Pseudomonas aeruginosa* [14, 19] and *Neisseria gonorrhoeae* [13]. Their regulation by iron suggests their participation in iron uptake in these strains as in *E. coli*. For all gram-negative strains for which outer membrane proteins were related to the iron supply, siderophores of the hydroxamate and/or the phenolate type were identified [15].

However, the picture may look more uniform than it is in reality. For example, meningococci require direct contact with human transferrin in order to acquire transferrin-bound iron [20]. A surface protein with an apparent molecular weight of 69 000 has been implicated in the use of transferrin iron. No siderophores produced by *Yersinia* were found, but pathogenic species could use hemin [17]. In cases where several iron transport sys-

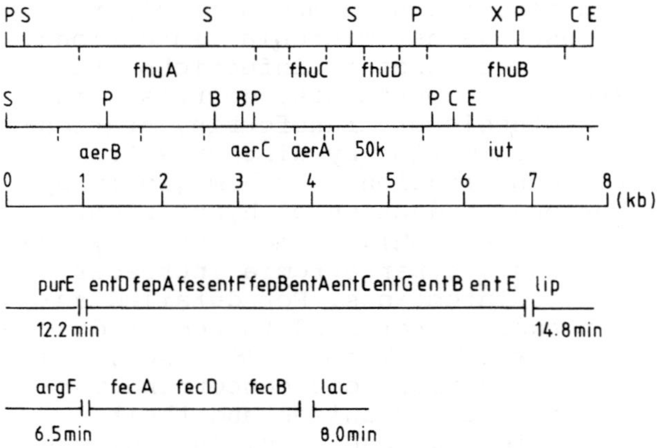

Fig. 1. Gene arrangement of *E. coli* iron supply systems. The *first line* shows the chromosomal genes for the uptake of iron hydroxamate compounds [6]. *fhuA* encodes an outer membrane receptor protein that is required for the transport of ferrichrome and its derivatives. Additional receptor proteins were defined for the uptake of hydroxamate-bound iron via aerobactin and coprogen. Iron uptake via all of these compounds depends on functional *fhuC, D, B* genes. The *second line* indicates the order of genes for aerobactin synthesis *aerA, aerB, aerC* [10], and for iron(III) aerobactin transport (50*k*, *iut*) encoded by certain ColV plasmids. The *iut* gene specifies the outer membrane receptor protein. In *lines 1* and *2*, the direction of transcription is from left to right. The *broken lines* indicate the outermost sites of mutations, obtained either by the insertion of transposons or by cleavage with restriction enzymes that inactivate the genes. Restriction sites are denoted as follows: *Pst*I (P), *Sal*I (S), *Cla*I (C), *Eco*RI (E), *Xho*I (X), *Bam*HI (B). The *third line* gives a schematic view of the linkage map of the genes that participate in the uptake of iron via enterochelin (enterobactin) [9]. *fepA* specifies the outer membrane receptor protein, *fepB* an additional transport function [18]. The *ent* genes encode proteins for enterochelin synthesis, the *fes* gene product(s) hydrolyze enterochelin. The *fourth line* gives the linkage map of genes that are involved in ferric dicitrate transport [25]. An outer membrane protein is encoded by the *fecA* gene, *fecB* specifies an additional transport component, and *fecD* mutants prevent induction of the *fecA* and the *fecB* gene by ferric dicitrate

tems exist in one organism, one may speculate that they operate under different ecological conditions. Strains of *E. coli* that express the iron(III)-aerobactin transport system rapidly multiply in undiluted calf serum. Within 22 h, they grow from 10^3 to 5×10^8 cells per milliliter [2]. Neither the iron(III)-enterochelin nor the iron(III)-dicitrate transport system support growth. It was not studied whether the serum contained antibodies against enterochelin, as has been found in human serum [12], or whether antibodies directed against cell surface structures impaired iron supply via enterochelin [8]. Citrate is probably not a strong enough ligand to release enough iron from transferrin to support growth. However, the concentration of citrate in serum is sufficient (0.1 m*M*) to induce the iron(III)-dicitrate transport system of *E. coli*. On the other hand, it has clearly been shown in mice that the production of enterochelin by *S. typhimurium* SR-11 reduced the 50% lethal dose 2-3 logarithmic units compared with an enterochelin-negative derivative [24]. Although knowledge on iron assimilation is still fragmentary even for the best studied microorganism, *E. coli*, it may safely be predicted that bacteria have developed various mechanisms for adaptation to different environmental conditions. As frequently observed in host-parasite relations, both organisms successfully compete for the elusive iron.

Regulation of Toxin Production by Iron

Diphtheria is the best studied case of a toxin produced only at iron-limiting growth conditions. Additional toxins have since been found to be under iron regulation (Table 1). Those most recently added to the list are the α-hemolysins of *Listeria monocytogenes* and of *E. coli*. *Listeria* released hemolysin when grown in dialyzed brain-heart infusion broth containing 1 μ*M* iron. Supplementation with increasing amounts of ferric citrate (1:6) reduced the hemolysin titer at 8 μ*M* iron to values between 5% and 10%, depending on the strain investigated [5]. Nephropathogenicity of an *E. coli* strain for mice disappeared in a nonhemolytic derivative and could be restored by simultaneous injection of hemolysin, intraperitoneal administration of hemoglobin, or iron sulfate before intravenous challenge with the nonhemolytic strain [22]. The amount of released hemolysin in the culture

Table 1. Protein virulence factors that are subject to regulation by iron

Virulence factor	Species	References
Diphtheria toxin	*Corynebacterium diphtheriae*	[11]
Toxin A	*Pseudomonas aeruginosa*	[11]
Elastase	*Pseudomonas aeruginosa*	[11]
Alkaline protease	*Pseudomonas aeruginosa*	[11]
Hemagglutinin	*Pseudomonas aeruginosa*	[11]
Shiga toxin	*Shigella dysenteriae* 1	[11]
Tetanus toxin	*Clostridium tetani*	[11]
α-Toxin	*Clostridium perfringens*	[11]
α-Toxin	*Listeria monocytogenes*	[5]
α-Toxin	*Escherichia coli*	[22]
Toxin	*Legionella*	B. Iglewski
β-Toxin	*Serratia marcescens*	This study
β-Toxin	*Serratia kiliensis*	This study

medium decreased from a titer of 2^9 (highest dilution that lysed more than 25% of sheep erythrocytes) at 0.1 μM iron to 2^1 at 3 μM iron.

In a study on the effect of a protease on erythrocytes, which is secreted in large amounts (175 mg/l) by four *Serratia* strains from different sources, we observed that all four strains rapidly lysed human erythrocytes independent of their blood group. Since the purified protease [4] and the culture supernatant were inactive, we investigated the requirement for erythrocyte lysis in more detail. Growth of *Serratia* in a glycerol minimal medium resulted in no exoprotease formation, but in a full hemolysis activity. A mutant that formed no exoprotease was hemolytically as active as the parent strain. These results show that the exoprotease was not active in hemolysis.

Lysis required contact between *Serratia* cells and erythrocytes. Lysis of the entire erythrocyte population was obtained with a 1:1 ratio of bacterial to red blood cells (Fig. 2). A higher ratio accelerated the onset and rate of lysis. Treatment with pronase E or proteinase K of the *Serratia* cells abolished hemolysis, but had no effect when the erythrocytes were incubated with the proteases prior to addition of the bacteria. A cell homogenate of *Serratia* was active. The activity resided in the membrane fraction. Although the soluble fraction was inactive, its addition to the membrane fraction increased the hemolytic activity.

A surprising result was obtained when the proteins of erythrocyte ghosts obtained by lysis with an exoprotease-deficient strain of *Serratia* were compared with those of osmotically lysed erythrocytes (Fig. 3). The amounts of the major membrane proteins were very much reduced, and instead several bands with a high electrophoretic mobility appeared. This result indicates that hemolysis was accompanied by a substantial cleavage of the major erythrocyte membrane proteins. This result is especially noteworthy when one compares the surface area of an erythrocyte (100 μm^2) with that of a *Serratia* cell (6 μm^2). However, complete lysis of erythrocytes by an equal number of *Serratia* cells has to take into account that the *Serratia* strains employed do not hemagglutinate so that binding to the erythrocytes is probably not permanent. Since no hemolysin was detectable in a cell-free form, it is assumed that the hemolysin acted either from the surface of the *Serratia* cells or went over into the erythrocyte membrane during contact between the two cell types. At present, it is unknown whether degradation of the erythrocyte proteins is achieved by the hemolytic activity itself or whether it is a consequence of hemolysis that activates proteases of the red blood cell.

The hemolytic activity of *Serratia* is mainly expressed at iron-limiting growth conditions (Fig. 4). Therefore, not only α-hemolysins released into the culture medium are subject to regulation by iron, but also cell-bound β-hemolysins. Control by iron may indicate that hemolysins render intracellular iron resources available for microorganisms such as hemoglobin and ferritin.

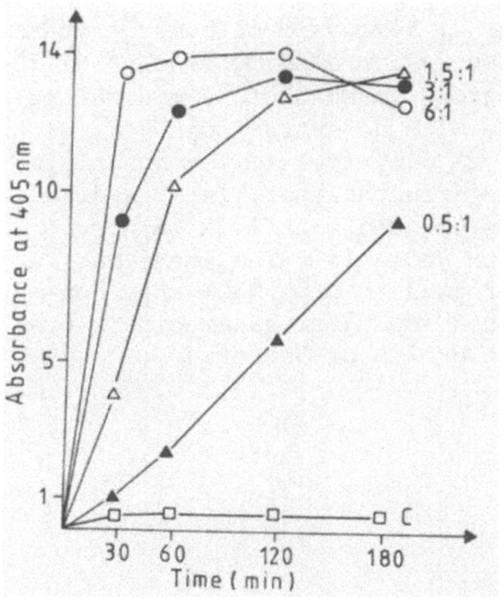

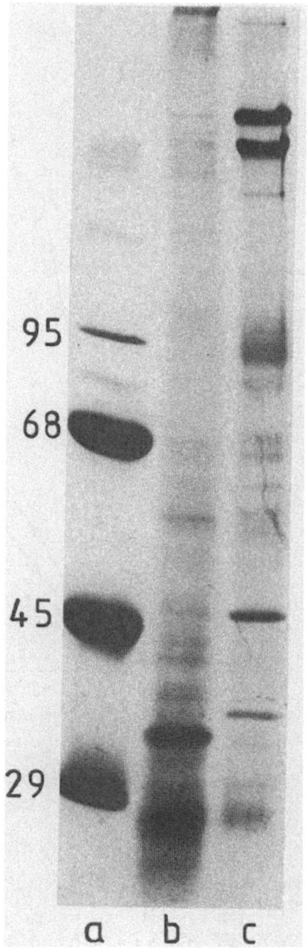

Fig. 2. Lysis of human erythrocytes (5×10^8/ml) of blood group A by various concentrations of *Serratia marcescens* W1436 cells which is an exoprotease and exolipase-negative mutant of W1128 (from U. Winkler, University of Bochum). The ratio of *Serratia* to erythrocyte cells is indicated on the curves. *C* denotes the control consisting of an eryhthrocyte suspension without added *Serratia* or with added *E. coli* cells

Fig. 3. Electropherogram of erythrocyte ghost proteins obtained after hemolysis with *Serratia* (*lane b*), and after osmotic shock (*lane c*). The membrane proteins were separated on polyacrylamide slab gels in the presence of 0.1% sodium dodecylsulfate. 95, 68, 45, and 29 indicate the molecular weights of the standard proteins (*lane a*) α-gelatin (95 000), bovine serum albumin (68 000), ovalbumin (45 000), and carboanhydrase (29 000)

However, iron could also function as an indicator of a general deprivation. Consequently, lysins for host cells would be synthesized which in turn make available nutrients that are released from the cells. When sufficient nutrients, including iron, are present, synthesis of the lysins by the bacteria is shut off until the next deprivation period is encountered. Such a mechanism would contribute to a balanced relationship between

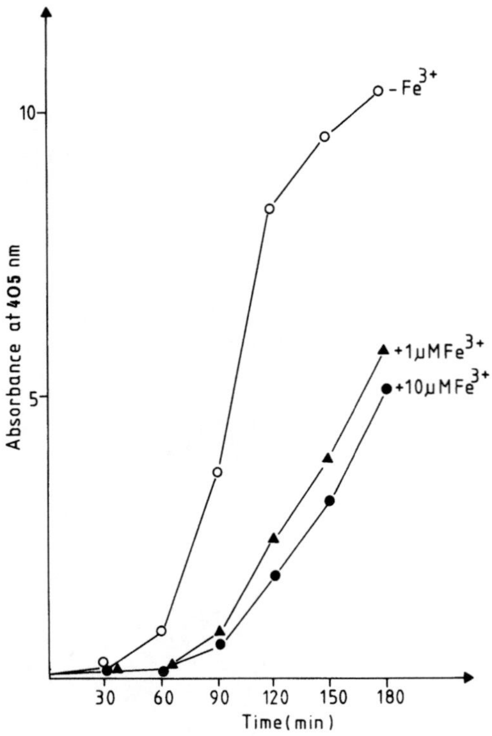

Fig. 4. Hemolysis of human erythrocytes by *Serratia marcescens* W1128 pregrown in M9 glucose minimal medium with no extra added (O), with 0.2 m*M* dipyridyl (O), a nonutilizable iron chelator, in M9 medium supplemented with 1 μM (▲) or 10 μM $FeCl_3$ (●). The assay was performed in 0.9% NaCl that contained 100 μg/ml kanamycin to prevent growth of *Serratia*

the host and the pathogen and lengthen the life of the host in favor of the pathogen.

Perspectives

Nutritional factors certainly play a role in the outcome of a bacterial infection. They are difficult to study experimentally since the microorganisms frequently colonize rather narrow and specific sites where the nutritional conditions are unknown. Iron is perhaps the only nutrient that is generally lacking in sufficient amounts. The mechanisms employed by mammals to reduce the available iron further upon infection are worthy of study. Furthermore, interference with the iron supply systems of microorganisms by inhibiting synthesis of siderophores with drugs would support the defense system of the host based on iron withdrawal. Synthetic analogs of siderophores that cannot supply iron to microorganisms, but are very effective in iron binding may not only be suitable to treat iron overload diseases, but also reduce the available iron to a level unsuitable to support microbial growth.

The iron supply is a suitable model to study the competition between the host and the invader for a component essential for both. The defense line of the host that consists mainly of the iron binding proteins transferrin and lactoferrin, and the storage protein ferritin (which are only partially loaded and therefore can immediately withdraw iron without an increase in protein synthesis) is overcome by the invading microorganism that synthesize siderophores and iron siderophore transport systems in response to iron deprivation. Further studies on the influence of iron concentration and of siderophores on the immune system, complement, and especially on the phagocytic cells (respiratory burst) are indicated.

Acknowledgments. The author thanks G. Braun, H. Günther, W. Köster, B. Neuss, C. Tautz, and L. Zimmermann for providing data prior to publication. This work was supported by the Deutsche Forschungsgemeinschaft (SFB 76, Br 330/8-1).

References

1. Bennet RL, Rothfield LI (1976) Genetic and physiological regulation of intrinsic proteins of the outer membrane of *Salmonella typhimurium*. J Bacteriol 127:498-504
2. Braun V (1984) The iron transport systems of *Escherichia coli*. In: Martonosi A (ed) The enzymes of biological membranes, vol. 3. Plenum, New York, pp 617-652
3. Braun V, Hantke K, Stauder W (1977) Identification of the *sid* outer membrane receptor protein in *Salmonella typhimurium* SL1027. Mol Gen Genet 155:227-229
4. Braun V, Schmitz G (1980) Excretion of a protease by *Serratia marcescens*. Arch Microbiol 124:55-61
5. Cowart RE, Foster BG (1981) The role of iron in the production of hemolysin by *Listeria monocytogenes*. Curr Microbiol 6:287-290
6. Fecker L, Braun V (1983) Cloning and expression of the *fhu* genes involved in iron(III)-hydroxamate uptake by *Escherichia coli*. J Bacteriol 156: 1301-1314
7. Finkelstein RA, Sciortino CV, McIntosh MA (1983) Role of iron in microbe-host interactions. Rev Infect Diseases 5 (Suppl. 4):759-777
8. Fitzgerald SP, Rogers H (1980) Bacteriostatic effect of serum: role of antibody to lipopolysaccharide. Infect Immun 27:302-308
9. Fleming TP, Nahlik MS, McIntosh MA (1983) Regulation of enterobactin iron transport in *Escherichia coli*: characterization of *ent*: Mu d(Ap^r *lac*) operon fusions. J Bacteriol 156:1171-1177
10. Gross R, Engelbrecht F, Braun V (1984) Genetic and biochemical characterization of the aerobactin synthesis operon on pColV. Mol Gen Genet 196:74-80
11. Holmes RK, Russel LM (1983) Role of iron in regulatory synthesis of bacterial toxins. In: Schlessinger D (ed) Microbiology – 1983. American Society of Microbiology, Washington, pp 359-362
12. Moore DG, Earhart CF (1981) Specific inhibition of *Escherichia coli* ferrienterochelin uptake by a normal serum immunoglobulin. Infect Immun 31: 631-635
13. Norquist A, Davies J, Norlander L, Normark S (1978) The effect of iron starvation on the outer membrane protein composition of *Neisseria gonorrhoeae*. FEMS Microbiol Lett 4:71-75
14. Okkawa I, Shiga S, Kageyama M (1980) Effect of iron concentration in the growth medium on the sensitivity of *Pseudomonas aeruginosa* to pyocin S 2. J Biochem (Tokyo) 87:323-331
15. Payne S (1983) Siderophores and acquisition of iron by gram-negative pathogens. In: Schlessinger D (ed) Microbiology – 1983. American Society of Microbiology, Washington, pp 346-349

16. Payne SM, Niesel DW, Peixotto SS, Lawlor KM (1983) Expression of hydroxamate and phenolate siderophores by *Shigella flexneri*. J Bacteriol 155: 949-955
17. Perry RD, Brubaker RR (1979) Accumulation of iron by *Yersinia*. J Bacteriol 137:1290-1298
18. Pierce JR, Pickett CL, Earhard CF (1983) Two *fep* genes are required for ferrienterochelin uptake in *Escherichia coli* K-12. J Bacteriol 155: 330-336
19. Simonson C, DeVoe JW (1983) Removal of iron from transferrin at the meningococcal surface. In: Schlessinger D (ed) Microbiology — 1983. American Society of Microbiology, Washington, pp 350-353
20. Sokol PA, Woods DE (1983) Demonstration of an iron-siderophore-binding protein in the outer membrane of *Pseudomonas aeruginosa*. Infect Immun 40:665-669
21. van Asbeck RS, Verhoef J (1983) Iron and host defence. Eur J Clin Microbiol 2:6-10
22. Waalwijk C, MacLaren DM, de Graaff J (1983) In vivo function of hemolysin in the nephrophathogenicity of *Escherichia coli*. Infect Immun 42:245-249
23. Weinberg ED (1984) Iron withholding, a defense against infection and neoplasia. Physiol Rev 64:65-107
24. Yancey RJ, Breeding SA, Lankford CE (1979) Enterochelin (enterobactin): virulence factor for *Salmonella typhimurium*. Infect Immun 24:174-180
25. Zimmermann L, Hantke K, Braun V (1984) Exogenous induction of the iron-dicitrate transport system of *Escherichia coli* K-12. J Bacteriol 159: 271-277

Bayer-Symposium VIII
The Pathogenesis of Bacterial Infections, 177-191 (1985)

The Relationship Between Iron Utilization and Virulence of the Pathogenic *Neisseria*

D. W. Dyer, S. E. H. West, and P. F. Sparling

Summary

All pathogenic *Neisseria* (meningococci, gonococci) can utilize transferrin as a sole source of essential iron, probably by a non-siderophore-mediated mechanism. Most gonococci and all meningococci also can utilize partially iron-saturated lactoferrin for growth on iron-depleted media. Mechanisms for utilization of these iron proteins are unknown, but may involve binding to surface receptors. Iron depletion results in increased amounts of several membrane proteins. Streptonigrin selection is useful for selecting mutants unable to utilize various sources of iron, which should allow better insights into the role of iron utilization in pathogenicity, and the biochemical mechanisms of iron uptake.

Introduction

The pathogenesis of bacterial infections is nearly always multifactorial, and the gonococci and meningococci are no exception. Several contributions to these proceedings address the functions of various gonococcal cell surface components (pili, outer membrane proteins PI and PII, lipopolysaccharide) which are involved in infection. There is intense interest in developing vaccines based on some of these antigens, and although a clinically useful gonococcal vaccine, or group B meningococcal vaccine has not been achieved yet, exciting progress is being made.

A different strategy for prevention of infection by the pathogenic *Neisseria* might be based on specific interference with bacterial uptake of essential iron from the host. This is a highly speculative approach, since there is no precedent for successful immune blockade of microbial nutrient uptake. Our reasons for thinking this might be feasible and pertinent preliminary results are the basis of this paper.

Iron and Virulence

Background

The relationship between iron and microbial virulence, with particular reference to enteric bacteria, is discussed elsewhere in this volume by Braun. To recapitulate briefly: ferric iron is quite insoluble, and most bacteria make iron-solubilizing compounds (siderophores) to help scavenge essential iron from the environment. The problem that confronts a pathogen upon entry into the human host is not scarcity of ferric ion, but the relative inaccessibility of the nutrient owing to its tight binding to various host iron-binding proteins. Presence of siderophores enhances virulence of many bacteria for mammalian hosts [11, 12, 35, 36, 47], probably by increasing availability of protein-bound iron [35]. Iron-siderophore complexes are recognized by specific bacterial outer membrane protein receptors which vary in size in *Escherichia coli* from 74K to 81K [37]. Iron is removed from the siderophore by mechanisms which vary, depending on the type of siderophore [35]. Production of siderophores and their outer membrane protein receptors is repressed by iron, and derepressed by iron starvation. Thus, many bacteria have specific, rather complicated high affinity systems either for solubilizing iron in an inanimate environment, or for removing iron bound very tightly to soluble carrier proteins in animal hosts.

In humans, iron in serum is found principally on transferrin, which ordinarily is only partially saturated. An uncertain amount of iron in serum is complexed to heme or hemoglobin, although specific binding of heme to hemopexin and of hemoglobin to haptoglobin usually results in rapid clearing of these iron sources from serum [17, 33]. Most bacteria require at least 0.4 μM iron for growth, but the serum concentration of free (non-protein-bound) iron is only 10^{-18} M. Since iron bound to transferrin is present in concentrations of about 15 μM, bacteria which can utilize transferrin as a sole source of iron might be expected to be more systemically invasive. On mucosal surfaces, most iron probably is bound to the related glycoprotein, lactoferrin. Polymorphonuclear leukocytes also contain abundant lactoferrin in their specific granules, and an early response of neutrophils to contact with piliated gonococci is release of specific granule lactoferrin [16]. Bacteria which can utilize lactoferrin as a sole iron source might be expected to be better pathogens of mucosal surfaces than those which are growth inhibited or killed [5-7] by lactoferrin.

Relatively little work has been done on mechanisms of iron utilization by obligate human pathogens such as gonococci or meningococci, but virulence in the *Neisseria* may be related in part to their ability to scavenge iron. The evidence is of two sorts: epidemiologic correlations, and studies of the effects of iron on virulence in animal models.

Epidemiologic Correlations

Transferrin

Using an agar plate bioassay, Mickelsen and Sparling found that all (21/21) meningococci and all (29/29) gonococci could utilize 25% iron-saturated transferrin as a sole source of iron for growth, whereas only a minority of nonpathogenic *Neisseria* could do so [30]. Among the nonpathogens, ability to utilize transferrin-bound iron was common in certain species (5/6 *N. lactamica*, 3/3 *N. flavescens*), but was rare (2/46) among other tested nonpathogenic *Neisseria* [30]. None of 13 locally isolated pharyngeal isolates of nonpathogenic *Neisseria* was able to utilize transferrin as an iron source [30]. Those isolates which grew in response to transferrin were able to take up ^{55}Fe from transferrin, in contrast to those which could not use transferrin for growth stimulation. These observations suggest that transferrin iron utilization may be one of several pathogenic mechanisms required for neisserial virulence.

Lactoferrin

In a similar study, Mickelsen et al. [31] found that 100% (15/15) tested meningococci could use 20% saturated partially purified human lactoferrin for growth on an iron-depleted agar medium, whereas only 24% (8/33) commensal *Neisseria* could do so. Gonococci occupied an intermediate position in this survey: only 14% (4/28) of isolates with the arginine$^-$, hypoxanthine$^-$, uracil$^-$ auxotype (AHU$^-$) were able to use lactoferrin for growth on Desferal agar, as compared with 86% (19/22) of all other gonococci. Ability to utilize lactoferrin for growth was correlated with ability to take up ^{55}Fe from lactoferrin [31]. Piliation had no effect on utilization of either transferrin or lactoferrin. Since AHU$^-$ gonococci previously were shown to be particularly associated with asymptomatic male urethral infection [13], the hypothesis was raised that strains of gonococci which cannot compete with lactoferrin for iron may be unable to grow to sufficient density in the urethra to cause symptoms [31]. These epidemiologic correlations in ability of gonococci and meningococci to use partially purified, 20% iron-saturated lactoferrin for growth are consistent with a role of lactoferrin iron utilization in pathogenicity, but considerable uncertainty remains. Other work [19] suggests gonococci and meningococci may not be able to grow in the presence of apo- (iron-free) lactoferrin; the degree of saturation of lactoferrin by iron at mucosal sites is unknown. The effect of lactoferrin on microbial growth may be influenced by secretory IgA concentrations (R. Arnold 1984, personal communication), which were not controlled in these experiments. More work with highly purified lactoferrin and IgA is needed, as is a careful prospective study of the effect of coexistent *Chlamydia trachomatis* infection and other variables on asymptomatic local gonococcal infection.

Animal Models

In a chick embryo model of bacteremic gonococcal infection, Payne and Finkelstein observed a correlation between iron levels and LD_{50} [40, 41]. Gonococci which were thought to be particularly virulent (piliated, isolated from patients with bacteremic disease) had very low LD_{50} (were chick virulent) even if available iron in the chick was reduced by infusion of conalbumin. In contrast, other isolates were relatively less virulent unless supplemental iron was added to the chick [41]. The most convincing evidence for a relationship of iron to *Neisseria* virulence in an animal model was provided by Holbein [22, 23], who studied meningococcal bacteremia in mice. As levels of iron saturation of transferrin began to decline in response to infection, bacteremia was abruptly terminated [22], whereas provision of increments of additional iron-transferrin resulted in more prolonged and intense bacteremia and a roughly linear increase in infection-related mortality [23]. Interestingly, bacteremia was terminated well before all iron was removed from transferrin to intracellular iron pools [22], suggesting that simple inaccessibility of serum iron may not have been the sole reason for cessation of bacteremia.

If ability to scavenge iron in vivo is related to local and systemic virulence of the *Neisseria*, how do they accomplish this? Do they produce siderophores? Do they have specific surface-exposed receptors for transferrin or other potential iron sources? How can definitive answers to these questions be obtained?

Neisserial Mechanisms for Iron Uptake

Siderophore Production?

Conflicting reports exist regarding siderophore production by either gonococci or meningococci. Payne and Finkelstein [41] initially reported the production of siderophores by both species. Later, Yancey and Finkelstein [49] reported that, when grown in GC-conalbumin biphasic medium, both organisms produce a hydroxamate siderophore, though in exceedingly small quantities (100- to 1000-fold less than other hydroxamate-producing microorganisms). In contrast to this, Archibald and DeVoe searched extensively for meningococcal siderophores in concentrated (20×) and unconcentrated culture supernatants (*Neisseria* defined medium) and ethyl acetate extracts of these supernatants using several bioassays, two chemical assays [8, 14], and a physical assay, with entirely negative results [2, 3]. In similar experiments, Norrod and Williams [39] also were unable to detect siderophore activity in spent culture supernatants of a *N. gonorrhoeae* strain grown in a chemically defined medium containing EDDA.

Simonson et al. [45] found that spent meningococcal culture supernatants could not remove iron from transferrin immobilized on Sepharose beads. When grown in an iron-limiting medium, neither the meningococcus nor the gonococcus was able to remove iron from transferrin within a dialysis sac ([2]; unpublished work). Mickelsen and Sparling showed that the gonococcus could not grow in a chemically defined medium containing Desferal and excess $FeCl_3$, unless minimal amounts of an exogenous iron-solubilizing compound such as citrate, pyrophosphate, oxalacetate, or nitrilotriacetate were present [30]. Culture filtrates of iron-limited gonococci did not stimulate the growth of gonococci in the absence of these iron-solubilizing compounds. In the same low-chelate medium, hemin and transferrin stimulated growth. These results showed that the gonococcus did not produce sufficient quantities of a siderophore under these conditions to facilitate the use of insoluble iron compounds.

Siderophores in Culture Media

One significant difference that may help to explain these conflicting experimental results is that investigators in Finkelstein's laboratory utilized a complex proteose-peptone-based medium to assay for siderophore production, whereas DeVoe's group, Norrod and Williams, and our laboratory used chemically defined media. Accordingly, we repeated the experiments of Yancey and Finkelstein [49]. Thirtyfold concentrated uninoculated proteose-peptone broth (GC base) medium and culture supernatants from strains F62 and FA19 in the same medium were tested for siderophore activity using the *Salmonella typhimurium* LT-2 *enb7* [28] and *Arthrobacter flavescens* JG-9 [49] bioassays. *S. typhimurium* LT-2 *enb7* is a mutant which requires either a hydroxamate or phenolate siderophore for growth in the presence of citrate; *A. flavescens* JG-9 has an absolute requirement for either hemin or an exogenously supplied hydroxamate siderophore. Uninoculated culture medium contained small amounts of siderophore-like activity, which stimulated growth of both test organisms. Proteose-peptone 3 (Difco) was the medium component which contributed the majority of this activity. We did not detect an increase in siderophore activity in spent culture medium used for growth of strains F62 and FA19. These results indicate that the gonococcus does not produce detectable amounts of a hydroxamate or phenolate siderophore, but crude culture media contain variable, small amounts of a hydroxamate-type siderophore. This observation has been confirmed by Finkelstein and Sciortino (1984, personal communication).

Possible Non-Siderophore-Mediated Transferrin Iron Uptake

Although it seems unlikely, we cannot totally rule out the possibility that gonococci (or meningococci) produce a novel siderophore not detected by these various assays. For instance, recent work has shown that *Corynebacterium diphtheriae* produces a novel siderophore of unknown chemical composition, but clearly different from classical phenolate or hydroxamate types [44]. We also note, however, that *Bordetella pertussis* [4], *Legionella pneumophila* [43], and *Yersinia pestis* [42] do not produce siderophores detectable by a battery of chemical or biologic assays, yet are able to acquire essential iron by still unknown means. It is interesting that several of the pathogens which do not produce classical siderophores (including gonococci and meningococci) are obligate parasites of the human host, which raises the question of whether obligate human pathogens have evolved non-siderophore-mediated mechanisms of iron utilization. Humans, for instance, have solved the problem of acquisition of iron from transferrin in the absence of siderophores very well, by an elegant system which depends on recognition of transferrin by specific cellular receptors [15, 24, 25].

Intimate contact between the neisserial cell surface and host iron carriers (such as transferrin) probably is required for utilization of these iron sources. Gonococci and meningococci cannot utilize transferrin-bound iron contained within a dialysis sac (as discussed previously). Simonson et al. [45] demonstrated that transferrin binds to the meningococcal cell surface. Since apotransferrin is bound as effectively as diferritransferrin, the meningococcal surface seems to recognize the transferrin molecule itself, rather than the transferrin-bound iron [45]. In double-label experiments, both meningococci and gonococci ([45]; unpublished work) accumulate iron from diferritransferrin, but transferrin is not internalized. Removal of iron from transferrin by meningococci is energy dependent, and digestion of the meningococcal surface with trypsin inhibits transferrin-iron utilization [45]. The suggestion that emerges from these studies is that meningococci and gonococci may have surface receptors for transferrin (and perhaps other host iron carriers), and the *Neisseria* obtain iron from these sources without the use of soluble siderophores.

Iron-Repressible Outer Membrane Proteins

In Gonococci

In a variety of microorganisms, iron-limited growth derepresses the synthesis of a variety of outer membrane proteins (OMP) that have critical roles in iron utilization [37]. By analogy, the appearance of iron-stress-related gonococcal and meningococcal OMP may uncover critical components of the iron-uptake systems of these two species. Early work by Norqvist et al. [38] showed that iron-limited gonococci produced OMP of 97, 86, and 76 k-daltons. We have just completed an extensive survey of gonococcal OMP associated with iron limitation. In a typical experiment, log-phase gonococci were diluted into fresh medium containing 50 μM Desferal (a siderophore that neither gonococci nor meningococci can use as an iron source). In Fig. 1 are shown the results of one such experiment, in which *N. gonorrhoeae* F62 was iron stressed, and an aliquot of cells was surface labeled (by iodination) at 1-h intervals following introduction into the iron-limited medium. Three iron-repressible proteins of approximately 90, 70, and 19.5 kdaltons appeared with increasing iron stress. The susceptibility of iron-repressible proteins to iodination is a good indication of the degree of surface exposure of these proteins, and is consistent with the possibility that these proteins are involved in iron acquisition. An iron-repressible protein of 36 kdaltons was also seen in purified membrane preparations of F62, although not apparent on this autoradiogram. By several criteria, the 36 kdaltons iron-repressible protein is different from the serotype-specific OMP,PI. In addition, several proteins (71, 33, 33.5, and 20 kdaltons) that are expressed in iron-sufficient conditions were expressed poorly or not at all in iron-deficient media.

The appearance of iron-repressible OMP in gonococci is both qualitatively and quantitatively different between gonococcal strains Strain FA19, for instance, produces additional iron-repressible OMP of 104 and 76 kdaltons, and much less of the 70 kdaltons

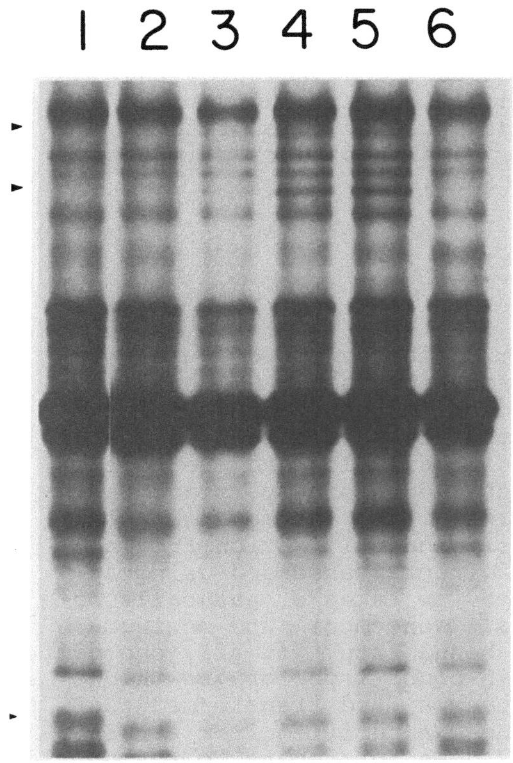

Fig. 1. Autoradiogram of *N. gonorrhoeae* F62, iodinated after growth under iron-limiting conditions. Log-phase gonococci were diluted into fresh GC base medium (Difco) containing 50 μM Desferal. At each time interval, approximately 10^9 CFU was removed from the culture and iodinated according to the procedure of Markwell [29]. Whole cells were then solubilized and electrophoresed according to the procedure of Laemmli [27] in a 15% polyacrylamide gel. *Lane 1*, cells iodinated at the start of the experiment. *Lanes 2-5* show the iodination patterns of cells grown for 1, 2, 3, and 4 h in the iron-limited medium. *Lane 6* shows the iodination pattern of cells grown for 4 h in iron-sufficient medium. Iron-repressible proteins are identified by *arrows*; some iron-repressible proteins were not resolved in this experiment

protein than strain F62. In a survey of 12 recent clinical isolates from symptomatic and asymptomatic urogenital disease, and from disseminated infection, no particular iron-repressible OMP profile could be correlated with auxotype, serotype, or type of infection. Each of these 12 strains produces the 36 kdaltons OMP under iron-limited conditions, which has also been observed by T. Meitzner and S. Morse using other strains (1984, personal communication). Interestingly, certain of the iron-repressible OMP are expressed differentially, depending on the iron source in which the gonococcus is grown, indicating that these proteins are not subject to the simple coordinate control implied by their simultaneous expression in a Desferal-containing medium.

In Meningococci

Meningococcal iron-repressible OMP were first demonstrated by Brener et al. [10], and their appearance was associated with an increased virulence of strain SD1C for the mouse. When iron limited by addition of EDDA to the growth medium, strain SD1C produced new OMP of 69 and 31 kdaltons, and a third of 28 kdaltons when the cells were grown at pH 6.6 in addition to iron limitation. Susceptibility to lactoperoxidase-catalyzed iodination demonstrated that the 69 and 31 kdaltons proteins were surface exposed. Meningococci also produce a 37 kdaltons protein when iron stressed (T. Meitzner and S. Morse 1984, personal communication). The observation of Brener et al. [10] that the appearance of these OMP is associated with an increase in virulence strengthens the proposition that these proteins may be important in the pathobiology of the meningococcus, and indicates that these OMP warrant further study. This is particularly true in light of the recent observation that at least some of these proteins appear to be expressed in the human host during infection (J. Black 1984, personal communication).

Genetic Approaches to Iron Acquisition

Naturally Occurring Mutants

Our initial approach to the problem of mechanisms of neisserial iron acquisition and function of iron-repressible OMP has been to isolate meningococcal and gonococcal mutants unable to utilize specific iron sources. These mutants should then be useful for examining the mechanism of iron acquisition and the role of iron-repressible OMP in this process. Additionally, since the mouse has proven to be a useful animal model for meningococcal disease, the role in pathogenesis of iron utilization from a carrier such as transferrin can be directly assessed using appropriate mutants. Some advantage may be taken of naturally occurring gonococcal mutants. While all gonococci (and meningococci) are able to use transferrin-bound iron, not all gonococci are capable of utilizing lactoferrin-bound iron for growth. We have taken strain F62 (an LF^- gonococcus) and transformed the ability to utilize lactoferrin using DNA purified from strain FA19 (an LF^+ isolate). Although F62 does not revert to the LF^+ phenotype at detectable frequency (less than 10^{-7}), F62 is transformed to LF^+ at a frequency of approximately 10^{-3}, which is suggestive of a lesion in a single locus that impairs lactoferrin utilization. We compared membranes from both the LF^+ (FA19) and LF^- (F62) parents with membranes isolated from an LF^+ transformant of F62 (Fig. 2), but there were no ostensible changes in the OMP profiles of the LF^+ transformant in iron-replete or iron-depleted media. (The 36 kdaltons iron-repressible OMP is well resolved on this gel.) A more careful examination of the F62 LF^+ transformants is certainly required to understand the lesion in F62 which abrogates lactoferrin utilization.

A problem with an experiment of this type is that it makes the assumption that iron assimilation mechanisms in different gonococcal strains are similar enough for information to be gained by genetic crosses between different isolates. Although this seems reasonable, it may introduce unwanted problems in understanding the results. In addition, there are no naturally occurring transferrin or hemin mutants. As a consequence, it is necessary to generate laboratory-derived mutants of a single gonococcal or meningococcal strain, in order to dissect the process of iron acquisition.

Streptonigrin Selection of Iron Uptake Mutants

We have developed a strategy for isolating iron-uptake mutants of both meningococci and gonococci, using the antitumor agent streptonigrin. Streptonigrin is bactericidal for *E. coli*, and the killing effect of streptonigrin is dependent upon the concentration of intracellular iron [50]. Streptonigrin was recently

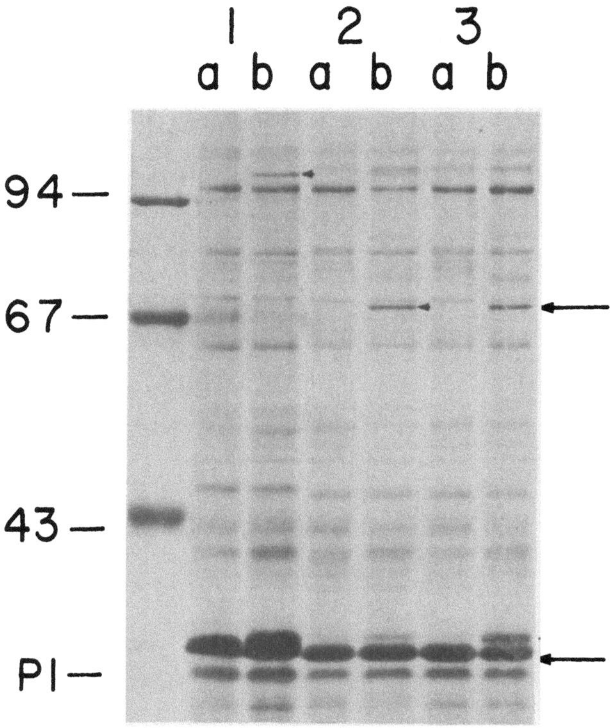

Fig. 2. Gonococcal membranes analyzed by electrophoresis in a 10% polyacrylamide gel; Coomassie blue stain. In each pair of samples, *lane a* designates membranes from cells grown in iron-sufficient conditions, and *lane b* designates membranes isolated from cells after iron-limited growth. Sample 1, strain FA19 (lactoferrin-utilizing, LF^+); sample 2, strain FA6028 (an LF^+ transformant of F62); sample 3, strain F62 (LF^-). Iron-repressible proteins are identified by *arrows*

used by Braun et al. [9] to isolate *E. coli* mutants unable to utilize ferriaerobactin. Iron-replete bacteria (*E. coli* or *Neisseria*) are highly sensitive to streptonigrin, whereas iron-depleted cells are quite refractory to killing ([50]; unpublished work). This suggests that, in a culture growing rapidly with a particular iron source such as transferrin, mutants which are unable to utilize transferrin will become iron depleted by continued growth. If this culture is then exposed to levels of streptonigrin sufficient to kill the iron-replete wild-type cells, one should be able to produce a dramatic enrichment of iron uptake mutants that are minimally susceptible to the bactericidal effects of streptonigrin.

Meningococcal Iron Mutants

We have isolated mutant meningococci compromised in the ability to utilize a specific iron source (transferrin) as well as other mutants which may be blocked in a pathway common to all iron sources available to meningococci. Preliminary results with one such mutant, FAM11, are representative. FAM11 was isolated from a streptonigrin enrichment of ethylmethanesulfonate-mutagenized meningococci that were presented with transferrin as an iron source in a complex medium containing 50 μM Desferal. Iron uptake assays (Fig. 3) indicate that FAM11 is severely limited in the amount of iron that can be internalized from either $FeCl_3$ or

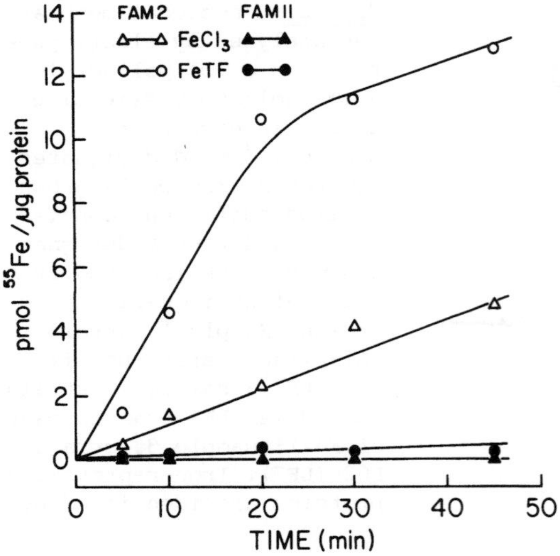

Fig. 3. Iron uptake by *N. meningitidis* FAM2 (wild-type) and FAM11 (mutant of FAM2). Uptake assays were performed as described by Mickelsen and Sparling [30]

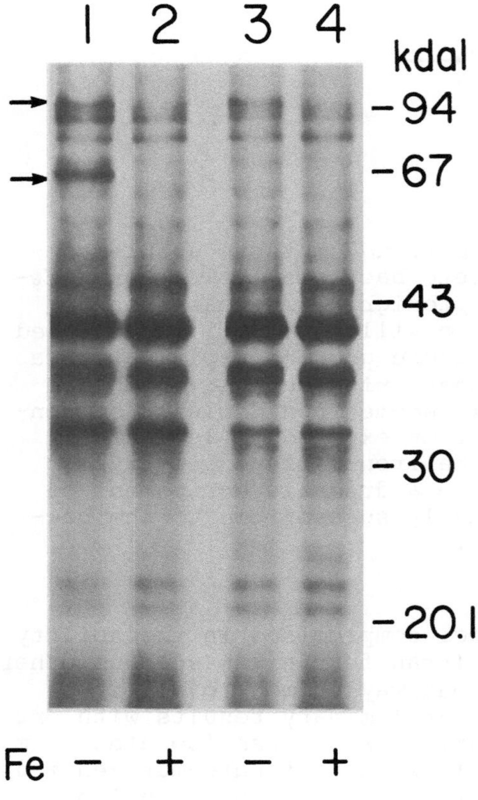

Fig. 4. Iodination profiles of FAM2 (*lanes 1, 2*) and FAM11 (*lanes 3, 4*). Molecular weight standards are indicated on the right. Cells were grown in defined deferrated liquid medium [30], without (*lanes 1, 3*) and with (*lanes 2, 4*) added iron (2 μ*M* Fe $(NO_3)_3$), and iodinated. Cells were then solubilized and analyzed by electrophoresis in a 15% SDS-polyacrylamide gel. Iron-repressible proteins are identified by *arrows*. FAM11 did nct produce the approximately 70 kdaltons iron-repressible protein under iron-limiting conditions

transferrin, when compared with the wild-type parent, FAM2. Surface iodination of outer membranes of FAM11 shows that FAM11 has lost the ability to express the major 70 kdaltons iron-repressible OMP (Fig. 4). Curiously, FAM11 appears to grow normally in defined media (without an iron chelator) when presented with either transferrin or inorganic iron ($Fe(NO_3)_3$) as the sole iron source. It is difficult to reconcile the kinetics of iron uptake and growth at this point, but these results suggest the 70 kdaltons OMP may be involved in a common step of iron uptake.

FAM11 was originally identified by a plate assay in which a complex medium was supplemented with transferrin as the sole iron source, and Desferal was added to chelate the available inorganic iron. Since Desferal may introduce artifacts that complicate our ability to identify mutants unable to use a specific iron source, we have switched to a low-iron-containing defined medium [30] for assessing iron utilization in plate assays. Using this defined medium, we have recently been able to isolate mutants of a group C meningococcus specifically compromised in the ability to use human transferrin. Preliminary results show that these mutants are reduced about 90% in their ability to take up iron from transferrin, but are normal in their ability to use iron as lactoferrin or as soluble inorganic iron salts. Additionally, these mutants grow much more slowly in heat-inactivated murine and human serum than the parental strain; supplementation of serum with soluble inorganic iron restores normal growth. Much more work needs to be done before any firm conclusions can be drawn. However, the relative inability of mutants with reduced rates of uptake of transferrin-bound iron to grow in serum is consistent with the thesis that the ability to use transferrin as an iron source is crucial to pathogenicity. The biochemical basis for reduced ability of this mutant to utilize transferrin-bound iron is presently unknown.

Summary and Concluding Remarks

The ability to obtain iron from human sources is probably an important factor determining the course of gonococcal and meningococcal infection. All gonococci and meningococci use human transferrin as an iron source, and Holbein [22, 23] has shown that the course of experimental meningococcal infection in the mouse is closely correlated with the levels of iron saturation of serum transferrin. Since no effective gonococcal or group B meningococcal vaccines have been developed, it is reasonable to investigate the potential of neisserial iron acquisition systems as a target for immunoprophylactic measures. However, much needs to be learned before the possibility of reaching such a goal can be assessed.

A second reason for studying gonococcal and meningococcal iron acquisition is that the mechanisms may be unusual. The general conclusion, from both published studies and our own experiments, is that the *Neisseria* do not produce siderophores. Less clear is whether these organisms utilize siderophores produced by other microorganisms. *E. coli* can utilize heterologous siderophores [20, 21], and it is possible that the *Neisseria* do this as well.

In fact, one report suggests that gonococci are capable of utilizing ferriaerobactin for growth [48], which deserves further attention.

An interesting but poorly understood area is the question of how bacteria acquire iron on mucosal surfaces, and the role of lactoferrin in host defense. Lactoferrin probably is not highly iron saturated in vivo, and some data suggest iron-poor lactoferrin may be growth inhibitory for most gonococci and meningococci [19]. In addition, evidence collected in R. Arnold's laboratory shows that lactoferrin may be bactericidal for a variety of microorganisms [5-7]. The bactericidal effect is most pronounced at low iron saturation levels, and at low pH, conditions which exist at many mucosal surfaces. If unsaturated lactoferrin does not donate iron to the *Neisseria* in vivo, what iron sources support growth of these organisms on the mucosal surface? Most commensal *Neisseria* do not use either transferrin or lactoferrin as iron sources [30, 31], yet they persist and presumably grow on mucosal surfaces.

Other possible mucosal iron sources include hemin and hemoglobin. We have examined the ability of gonococci to use hemin and hemoglobin as iron sources: growth with each of these iron sources is extremely slow. However, in serum, each is quickly bound by a specific glycoprotein (hemin by hemopexin and hemoglobin by haptoglobin [17, 33]) which rapidly direct these iron compounds to sites in the RES [17, 33]. The hemin-hemopexin and hemoglobin-haptoglobin complexes may donate iron more efficiently than the uncomplexed compounds, although no data on this point are available.

The mechanisms of removal of iron from host iron proteins by pathogenic *Neisseria* is totally unknown. Transferrin and lactoferrin are related in both structure and function [1, 32], and might be expected to donate iron by a common pathway. However, isolation of natural and laboratory-derived mutants which discriminate between these sources indicates transferrin and lactoferrin are processed differently. There probably is an outer membrane receptor for transferrin, but its identity is obscure. Why is uptake of iron from transferrin apparently inducible, while binding is not [45]? Does the cell modify transferrin in some way (by proteolysis, for example) which releases the bound iron? Is the iron removed by reduction (to ferrous iron) or by a localized drop in pH (analogous to the removal of iron from transferrin by the eukaryotic endocytic vesicle [15, 24])? Since pyrophosphate is known to remove iron from transferrin [26], does the capsular polyphosphate found on most *Neisseria* [34] play a role in removing transferrin-bound iron? We have even less information on how other iron sources are utilized.

Our preliminary results with one iron-uptake mutant of meningococci indicate that iron-repressible OMP may be involved in iron uptake. In addition to characterizing more mutants, another strategy for understanding the roles of the iron-repressible OMP would be to generate antisera against each of these proteins. These could then be used to determine the effect of antibody binding on iron uptake; a monoclonal antibody against the eukaryotic transferrin receptor blocks iron uptake from transferrin [46]. Mouse protection experiments could also be performed with appropriate antisera, and they might be useful both for generating mutants lacking specific iron-repressible OMP, and for cloning the loci responsible for these proteins. However, we believe that the first efforts should focus on mutants compromised in function, hoping to determine, among many questions, whether these mutations result in observable changes in iron-repressible OMP. The future looks bright. We are confronted with what may be a novel method of microbial iron assimilation, whose outlines are only crudely defined. Better understanding of these biologic phenomena will have both basic and applied significance.

Acknowledgments. We thank E. Blackman for excellent technical assistance, and L. Brooks for typing the manuscript. The author's unpublished work was supported by Public Health Service grant AI15036 and National Research Service award AI07001, both from the National Institute of Allergy and Infectious Diseases.

References

1. Aisen P (1980) The transferrins. In: Jacobs A, Wormwood M (eds) Iron in biochemistry and medicine, vol 2. Academic, London, pp 87-129
2. Archibald FS, DeVoe IW (1979) Removal of iron from human transferrin by *Neisseria meningitidis*. FEMS Microbiol Lett 6:159-162
3. Archibald FS, DeVoe IW (1980) Iron acquisition by *Neisseria meningitidis* in vitro. Infect Immun 27:322-324
4. Armstrong SK, Parker CD (1984) Effects of iron starvation on *Bordetella pertussis*. Abstr Ann Meet Am Soc Microbiol, p 14
5. Arnold RR, Brewer M, Gauthier JJ (1980) Bactericidal activity of human lactoferrin: sensitivity of a variety of microorganisms. Infect Immun 28:893-898
6. Arnold RR, Cole MF, McGhee JR (1977) A bactericidal effect for human lactoferrin. Science 197:263-265
7. Arnold RR, Russell JE, Champion WJ, Brewer M, Gauthier JJ (1982) Bactericidal activity of human lactoferrin: differentiation from the stasis of iron deprivation. Infect Immun 35:792-799
8. Arnow LE (1937) Colorimetric determination of the components of 3,4-dihydroxyphenylalanine-tyrosine mixtures. J Biol Chem 118:2810-2815
9. Braun V, Gross R, Koster W, Zimmermann L (1983) Plasmid and chromosomal mutants in the iron(III)-aerobactin transport system of *Escherichia coli*. Use of streptonigrin for selection. Mol Gen Genet 192:131-139
10. Brener D, DeVoe IW, Holbein BE (1981) Increased virulence of *Neisseria meningitidis* after in vitro iron-limited growth at low pH. Infect Immun 33:59-66
11. Bullen JJ (1981) The significance of iron in infection. Rev Infect Dis 3:1127-1138
12. Bullen JJ, Rogers JH, Griffiths E (1978) Role of iron in bacterial infection. Curr Top Microbiol Immunol 80:1-35
13. Crawford G, Knapp JS, Hale S, Holmes KK (1977) Asymptomatic gonorrhoeae in men: caused by gonococci with unique nutritional requirements. Science 196:1352-1353
14. Csaky TZ (1948) On the estimation of bound hydroxylamine in biological materials. Acta Chem Scand 2:450-454

15. Dautry-Varsat A, Ciechanover A, Lodish HF (1983) pH and the recycling of transferrin during receptor-mediated endocytosis. Proc Natl Acad Sci USA 80:2258-2262
16. Densen P, Mandell GL (1978) Gonococcal interactions with polymorphonuclear neutrophils. Importance of the phagosome for bactericidal activity. J Clin Invest 62:1161-1171
17. Eaton JW, Brandt P, Mahoney JR, Lee JT Jr (1982) Haptoglobin: a natural bacteriostat. Science 215:691-693
18. Emery T (1982) Iron metabolism in humans and plants. Am Sci 70:626-632
19. Finkelstein RA, Sciortino CV, McIntosh MA (1983) Role of iron in microbe-host interactions. Rev Infect Dis 5:S759-S777
20. Hantke K (1983) Identification of an iron uptake system specific for coprogen and rhodotorulic acid in *Escherichia coli* K12. Mol Gen Genet 191: 301-306
21. Hartman A, Braun V (1980) Iron transport in *Escherichia coli*: uptake and modification of ferrichrome. J Bacteriol 143:246-255
22. Holbein BE (1980) Iron-controlled infection with *Neisseria meningitidis* in mice. Infect Immun 29:886-891
23. Holbein BE (1981) Enhancement of *Neisseria meningitidis* infection in mice by addition of iron bound to transferrin. Infect Immun 34:120-125
24. Klausner RD, Ashwell G, van Renswoude J, Harford JB, Bridges KR (1983) Binding of apotransferrin to K562 cells: explanation of the transferrin cycle. Proc Natl Acad Sci USA 80:2263-2266
25. Klausner RD, van Renswoude J, Ashwell G, Kempf C, Schechter AN, Dean A, Bridges KR (1983) Receptor-mediated endocytosis of transferrin in K562 cells. J Biol Chem 258:4715-4724
26. Konopka K, Mareschal J-C, Crichton RR (1980) Iron transfer from transferrin to ferritin mediated by pyrophosphate. Biochem Biophys Res Commun 96:1408-1413
27. Laemmli UK (1970) Cleavage of structural proteins during the assembly of the head of bacteriophage T4. Nature 227:680-685
28. Luckey M, Pollack JR, Wayne R, Ames BN, Neilands JB (1972) Iron uptake in *Salmonella typhimurium*: utilization of exogenous siderochromes as iron carriers. J Bacteriol 111:731-738
29. Markwell MAK (1983) A new solid-state reagent to iodinate proteins: I. Conditions for the efficient labeling of antiserum. Anal Biochem 125: 427-432
30. Mickelsen PA, Sparling PF (1981) Ability of *Neisseria gonorrhoeae Neisseria meningitidis*, and commensal *Neisseria* to obtain iron from transferrin and iron compounds. Infect Immun 33:555-564
31. Mickelsen PA, Blackman E, Sparling PF (1982) Ability of *Neisseria gonorhoeae*, *Neisseria meningitidis*, and commensal *Neisseria* species to obtain iron from lactoferrin. Infect Immun 35:915-920
32. Morgan EH (1974) Transferrin and transferin iron. In: Jacobs A, Wormwood M (eds) Iron in biochemistry and medicine. Academic, London, pp 29-71
33. Muller-Eberhard U (1970) Hemopexin. N Engl J Med 283:1090-1094
34. Noegel A, Gotschlich EC (1983) Isolation of a high molecular weight polyphosphate from *Neisseria gonorrhoeae*. J Exp Med 157:2049-2060
35. Neilands JB (1981) Microbial iron compounds. Ann Rev Biochem 50:715-731
36. Neilands JB (1981) Iron absorption and transport in microorganisms. Ann Rev Nutr 1:27-46
37. Neilands JB (1982) Microbial envelope proteins related to iron. Ann Rev Microbiol 36:285-309
38. Norqvist A, Davies J, Norlander L, Normark S (1978) The effect of iron starvation on the outer membrane protein composition of *Neisseria gonorrhoeae*. FEMS Microbiol Lett 4:71-75

39. Norrod P, Williams RP (1978) Growth of *Neisseria gonorrhoeae* in media deficient in iron without detection of siderophores. Curr Microbiol 1:281-284
40. Payne SM, Finkelstein RA (1975) Pathogenesis and immunology of experimental gonococcal infection: role of iron in virulence. Infect Immun 12:1313-1318
41. Payne SM, Finkelstein RA (1978) The critical role of iron in host-bacterial interactions. J Clin Invest 61:1428-1440
42. Perry RD, Brubaker RR (1979) Accumulation of iron by Yersiniae. J Bacteriol 137:1290-1298
43. Reeves MW, Pine L, Neilands JB, Balows A (1983) Absence of siderophore activity in *Legionella* species grown in iron-deficient media. J Bacteriol 154:324-329
44. Russell LM, Holmes RK (1984) Novel siderophore produced by *Corynebacterium diphtheriae*. Abstr Ann Meet Am Soc Microbiol, p 14
45. Simonson C, Brener D, DeVoe IW (1982) Expression of a high-affinity mechanism for acquisition of transferrin iron by *Neisseria meningitidis*. Infect Immun 36:107-113
46. Trowbridge IS, Lopez F (1982) Monoclonal antibody to transferrin receptor blocks transferrin binding and inhibits human tumor cell growth in vitro. Proc Natl Acad Sci USA 79:1175-1179
47. Weinberg ED (1971) Role of iron in host-parasite interactions. J Infect Dis 124:401-410
48. Yancey RJ, Finkelstein RA (1981) Assimilation of iron by pathogenic *Neisseria* spp. Infect Immun 32:592-599
49. Yancey RJ, Finkelstein RA (1981) Siderophore production by pathogenic *Neisseria* spp. Infect Immun 32:600-608
50. Yeowell HN, White JR (1982) Iron requirement in the bactericidal mechanism of streptonigrin. Antimicrob Agents Chemother 22:961-968

Discussion

(pp. 168-191)

With regard to the cell-bound hemolysin of *Serratia*, the question arose whether its presence could be related to the high incidence of *Serratia* infections in patients with chronic granulomatous disease lacking an oxidative response and the metabolites involved in killing. Since iron is essential for killing, the improvement of the iron supply of *Serratia* by hemolysin could have an as yet unknown effect. However, one has to bear in mind that hemolysins are cytolysins so that their function may go beyond their mobilization of iron resources. A question concerning the determination of the extreme formation constants between iron(III) and siderophores was referred to the work of Ken Raymond at the Organic Chemistry Department, Berkely, California, most of which has been published in the *Journal of the American Chemical Society*.

Additional findings were presented that showed that bacteria isolated from various hosts contained strongly expressed outer membrane proteins related to iron and that experiments in iron-limited chemostats support the in vivo results. In this regard, it is of interest that sera of convalescent patients with meningococcal disease, but not of acute or pure normal human serum react with the 70 kdaltons protein that is derepressed under iron limitation. This suggests an immunologic importance, even for vaccine development.

In gonococci and meningococci, there is no direct proof of the participation of the iron-related protein in iron supply via transferrin nor is any other function (porin) known. Antibodies against receptor proteins binding with sufficient affinity to compete for iron(III)-siderophore adsorption have not been described for any system. However, antibodies against enterochelin (enterobactin) have been found in human serum. Concern was expressed regarding the use of mutants for virulence studies unless they are precisely defined genetically.

Bayer-Symposium VIII
The Pathogenesis of Bacterial Infections, 193-207 (1985)

Binding of Microbial Pathogens to Connective Tissue Fibronectin: An Early Step in Localized and Invasive Infections

T. Wadström, L. Switalski, P. Speziale, K. Rubin, C. Rydén, G. Fröman, A. Faris, M. Lindberg, and M. Höök

Summary

Fibronectin (fn) is a major protein of plasma and connective tissue which binds to *Staphylococcus aureus* and strains of other staphylococcal species often isolated from pyogenic infections. Strains of pyogenic streptococci (group A, C, and G strains) also bind fn in a similar time-dependent, saturable, and functionally irreversible way. Fibronectin-binding components released from staphylococcal and streptococcal cells after treatment with bacteriolytic or proteolytic enzymes are sensitive to protease degradation. Cross-absorption experiments with fn peptides show that the major binding for both organisms occurs to the NH_2 terminal (29 kdalton) fragment while enterotoxigenic *E. coli* strains of the O6 serogroup show binding to one or two fn fragments outside the NH_2 terminal domain. *S. aureus* cells bind to fn immobilized on plastic surfaces, suggesting that binding to biomaterials is an important portal of entry for pyogenic cocci to invade subepithelial tissues. Recent observations that other pathogens such as *Treponema pallidum*, tissue invasive parasites, and *Candida albicans* also bind fn indicate that many microbial pathogens may invade tissues by first binding to fn, or other connective tissue matrix proteins such as collagens or laminin. We recently defined uropathogenic *E. coli* and *S. pyogenes* strains binding to laminin or collagen. Finally, one protein A mutant of *S. aureus* (SA113-spA26) which is low in fn binding has a low virulence in experimental infections, indicating that fn binding is an important step in colonization of tissues and development of localized tissue infections.

Introduction

Some 70 years ago, Much discovered that staphylococci isolated from infections are able to clump in the presence of plasma. Some decades later, it was shown that fibrinogen is the plasma protein responsible for rapid clumping of *Staphylococcus aureus* cells in plasma (for review see [31]). However, some strains clumping was also observed in fibrinogen-depleted plasma, indicating that fibrinogen is the major, but not the only plasma protein interacting with staphylococci.

Four decades later, Morrison and co-workers described the proteins designated as cold insoluble globulins which precipitate in plasma at 4°C. The role and nature of these proteins remained unclear for two decades. In the early 1970s, several groups of researchers using various techniques observed that fibroblasts grown in tissue culture possess a high molecular weight surface protein shown to be immunologically identical or closely related to cold insoluble globulin. Fibronectin (fn) is now a widely accepted designation for both the plasma (soluble) and cell associated (insoluble) forms of this protein as illustrated by several reviews [23, 24, 40].

Immunoglobulins were the first plasma proteins other than fibrinogen shown to bind to *S. aureus* (Table 1). Kuusela [13] first reported on fn binding to heat- and formalin-killed staphylococci. Interactions of fn with bacterial cells of *S. aureus* first reported by Kuusela [13] remained unnoticed for a few years. However, new observations assigning plasma fn the role as a third opsonin (besides IgG and complement factors) initiated new studies. Fibronectin was considered as both an opsonin, i.e., a component of plasma involved in host defense in infections and an adhesion factor (an adhesin) which enable staphylococci and streptococci to colonize mucosal surfaces and wound tissues.

On the other hand, other pyogenic gram-positive cocci such as group A and C streptococci were already known to bind various plasma proteins such as fibrinogen, albumin, aggregated β2-mic-

Table 1. Binding of various serum and connective tissue proteins to *Staphylococcus aureus* and *Streptococcus pyogenes* (group A streptococci)

	Staphylococcus aureus	*Streptococcus pyogenes*
Immunoglobulins[a]	+	+
Albumin	-	+
Fibrinogen	+	+
Fibronectin	+	+
Haptoglobin	-	+
β2-Microglobulin	-	+
Collagen[b]	+	+
Laminin[c]	-	+

[a] Binding occurs to the Fc domain of immunoglobulin G.
[b] Type II collagen (P. Speziale, L. Switalski, M. Höök, and T. Wadström 1984, unpublished work).
[c] Laminin binds also to viridans streptococci (L. Switalski, T. Wadström, and M. Höök 1984, unpublished work).

roglobulin, and haptoglobin (Table 1). M protein was defined as the receptor for β2-microglobulin and fibrinogen and albumin proposed to bind to a specific cell surface amphiphile, i.e., lipoteichoic acid (LTA) [3]. The original observation by Kuusela [13] encouraged us to explore the possibility that pyogenic infections, mainly in wounds and skin lesions, start with an initial colonization of exposed connective tissue fn by organisms possessing surface components which interact with fn and possibly other connective tissue components.

Binding of Fibronectin to Staphylococci

Mosher and Proctor [16] showed that *S. aureus* cells bind specifically to the NH_2 terminal region of fn. This domain also has an affinity for heparin and fibrin and possibly other macromolecules [40]. However, it was shown that heparin and staphylococcal binding sites can be allocated to different peptides [16]. Binding of staphylococci could be inhibited by certain amino acids, monosaccharides, and polysaccharides such as heparin, which probably interfere with charge interactions [13, 34].

The binding of fn to cells of *S. aureus* (Fig. 1) is concentration dependent and occurs to both live and heat-killed cells [25]. Binding is irreversible and the dissociation constant $2 \times 10^{-10} M$ indicates a very strong affinity of binding (i.e., several orders of magnitude greater than binding to eukaryotic cells). The number of binding sites in the surface of *S. aureus* depends on the strain, growth conditions such as medium composition, and growth phase. The number of binding components ranges from 250 to 25 000 [19, 25].

Fibronectin binding components seem to reside with a glycoprotein faction that can be solubilized by lysostaphin digestion of the staphylococcal cells [25]. These components can be precipitated with ammonium sulfate (Fig. 2), and purified by affinity chromatography on Sepharose-immobilized fn [25]. This purification scheme was used to purify both low and high molecular

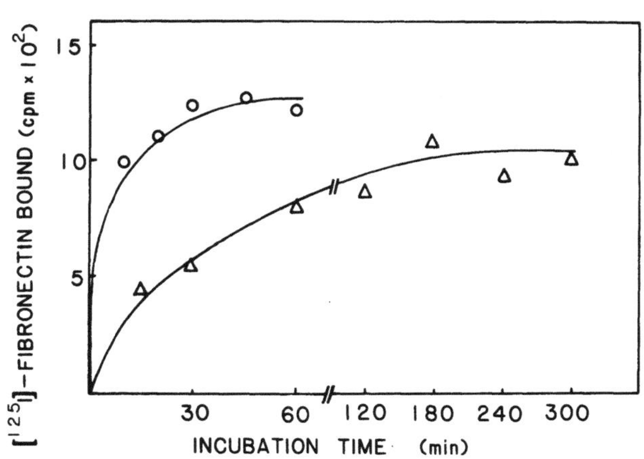

Fig. 1. Time course of binding of ^{125}I-labeled fn to strains *Streptococcus pyogenes* 1321 (*circles*) and *Staphylococcus aureus* Cowan 1 (*triangles*). Heat-killed cells of bacteria were incubated with ^{125}I-labeled fn for the periods of time indicated. Data refer to the sample containing 5×10^8 bacteria. Adapted from [25] and [30]

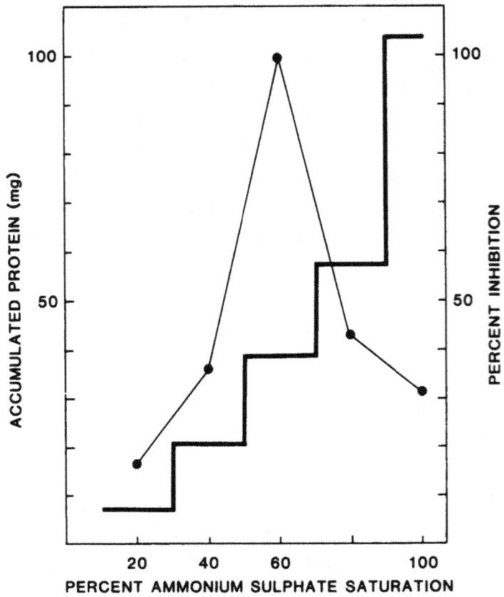

Fig. 2. Purification of solubilized fn-binding components of *S. aureus*, Cowan 1 strain by ammonium sulfate precipitation. 10 ml lysate obtained by lysostaphin digestion of *S. aureus* Cowan I with a protein concentration of 9.4 mg/ml was subjected to a stepwise ammonium sulfate precipitation. Precipitated protein was recovered by centrifugation at 20 000 *g* for 30 min and subsequently redissolved in phosphate-buffered saline and tested for inhibitory capacity of the binding of ^{125}-labeled fn to staphylococcal cells as described [25]

weight fragments that inhibit the binding of fn to intact staphylococcal cells or to immobilized crude lysostaphin lysates.

Others have reported on high molecular weight components (M_r <160 000) obtained after sonication of staphylococcal cells followed by affinity chromatography on fn immobilized on Sepharose [6]. The exact relationship between these components and substantially smaller peptides that is reported on herein is unclear, but it is likely that the lysostaphin digestion represents more thorough digestion of the staphylococcal cell envelope. The fn-binding components were proposed to be located on protein A, the main component of the cell wall of *S. aureus* [4]. This is unlikely since: (a) mutants of *S. aureus* that do not express protein A still bind fn; (b) strains of *S. aureus* producing protein A do not necessarily bind fn; (c) the solubilized components show affinity to immobilized fn on Sepharose gels, but not to IgG; (d) and purified protein A does not inhibit binding of ^{125}I-labeled fn to staphylococci and the purified fn-binding protein or proteins lack affinity for IgG [25, 32, 36, 38, 39]. Nitrosoguanidine mutagenesis of *S. aureus* strain 113 (83A) resulting in isolation of a whole set of protein A-negative mutants, but with capacity to bind fn (Table 2) gives further proof for the notion that the receptor for fn is different from protein A. Interestingly, none of the protein A-negative mutants showed a decrease in virulence in the mouse mastitis model, except SA113-spA-26 [38]. These studies are now expanded in order to isolate a set of well-characterized mutants lacking fn-binding protein or proteins. Additional studies in other animal models such as mouse septicemia-pyelonephiritis and a skin infection model in young pigs suggest that fn surface binding protein or proteins may be an important first step in the infectious process in different tissues ([38] T. Wadström, unpublished work).

Table 2. Virulence of mutants isolated from *Staphylococcus aureus* after mutagenesis with nitrosoguanidine[a] SA 113 (83A)

Strain	Fibronectin binding (%)	Virulence
SA113	100	+++
hPrA3	140	+++
PrA26	37	-
PrA303	108	+++
PrA304	120	+
PrA305	130	+
PrA347	120	+
PrA320	130	+
PrA346	120	+
Coa347	115	++
Coa143	120	++
Hla6	0	+
Hla5	68	++

[a]For details on isolation of mutants see references [11, 12]. Data on these experiments have been presented elsewhere [38]. In brief, mutants and parent strain were compared for virulence in a mouse mastitis model and the virulence scores estimated from both macroscopic and microscopic examination [11].

Our studies on fn binding to strains of ten different staphylococcal species also suggest that fn binding may be an important virulence determinant since species commonly isolated from different human infections such as *S. epidermidis*, *S. haemolyticus*, *S. warneri*, and *S. hyicus* will bind fn while a strain of a species rarely if ever isolated from infections (*S. xylosus*) and strains of different micrococcal species were unable to bind fn (Fig. 3). Preliminary experiments show that binding of fn to cells of strains of these species is commonly inhibited with solubilized fn receptors of *S. aureus*, Cowan 1 (C. Rydén, K. Rubin, and T. Wadström, unpublished work). These observations indicate that fn-binding receptor molecules on coagulase-negative staphylococci may be related to surface receptors of *S. aureus*. However, much work has to be performed to define if these surface components are genetically and immunologically identical or if different variants exist in analogy with different staphylococcal toxins such as α-, β-, γ-, and δ-hemolysins and enterotoxins [36].

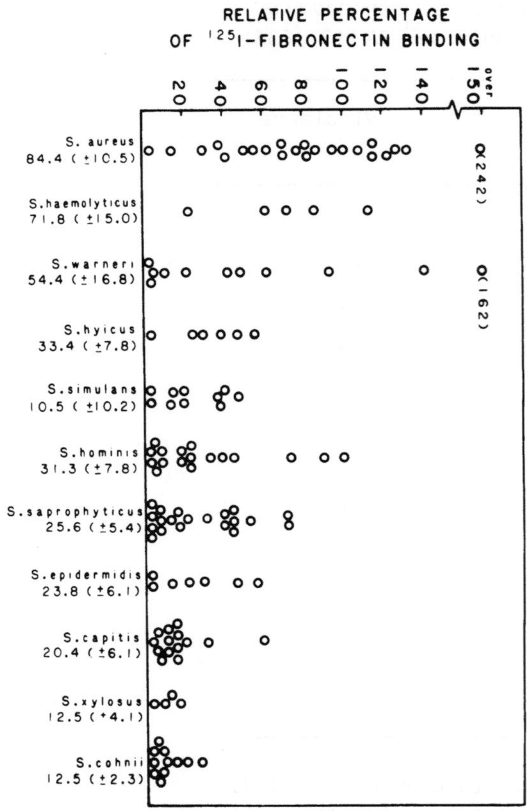

Fig. 3. Binding of fn (relative percentage) to staphylococcal strains of eleven different species. Binding of fn was calculated as described elsewhere [33]. Each *circle* indicates one staphylococcal strain

Binding of Fibronectin to Group A, C, and G Streptococci

Some three years after the discovery of fn binding to staphylococcal cells, it was first reported that group A, C, and G streptococci bind fn [27, 32]. The observation that fn promotes attachment of M protein negative but not M-positive cells of *S. pyogenes* to human polymorphonuclear leukocytes and studies showing that fn enhances uptake of latex beads into phagocytes have stimulated much research to explore the idea that fn may be an important natural opsonin in serum and tissue fluids [40]. The observation that M protein seems to inhibit binding suggests that this protein polymer probably specifically prevents binding to the cell receptor molecules [32].

The surface binding capacity of group A (*Streptococcus pyogenes*, Fig. 1), C, and G streptococci varies markedly between different strains. Since the surface antigen mosaic is quite complex in these three serotypes (see Table 1) and many strains produce hyaluronic capsule substances, it is tempting to speculate that binding of fn to the cell receptors can be inhibited by capsule polymers as well as by protein components such as M protein in group A strains.

Beachey and Simpson [2] have proposed a model of the *S. pyogenes* cell surface with fatty acid ligands (palmitic acid residues) of the amphiphilic lipoteichoic acid (LTA) molecule located at the surface as the receptor not only for albumin, but also for fn-mediated binding to human pharyngeal epithelial cells. It was shown that LTA inhibits binding of fn to streptococcal cells and that fn binds to the lipid domain of LTA [3].

Our studies indicate rather that the main component of the *S. pyogenes* cell wall involved in binding of fn is a surface-located protein [30] (Tables 3, 4; Fig. 4). Binding was found to be specific, functionally irreversible with an apparent K_d of $5 \times 10^{-9} M$, similar to that of *Staphylococcus aureus*. Moreover, the streptococcal binding site of the fn molecule is also located in the NH_2 terminal region.

Comparative binding studies with fn fragments to staphylococcal and streptococcal cells suggest that group A strains also bind additional fragments. In conclusion, our findings suggest that this strain has more than one class of receptors recognizing different regions of the fn molecule. One receptor is rapidly released by trypsin treatment of the cells whereas a second receptor seems to be trypsin resistant. It is tempting to speculate that this second class may interact with LTA via a more

Table 3. Inhibition of binding (specificity) of ^{125}I-labeled fn to *S. pyogenes* strain 1321 by some proteins. For details on experimental conditions see reference [30][a]

	Inhibition (%)	
	Amount of protein added	
	100 µg	500 µg
Control (no protein added)	0	0
Fetuin	10	9
α_1-acid glucoprotein	20	22
Fibrinogen	19	34
IgG	13	32
Fibronectin	89	100
Egg albumin	9	27

[a] Fetuin, α_1-acid glycoprotein, fibrinogen, IgG, fn, and egg albumin were tested as potential inhibitors of the binding of ^{125}I-labeled fn to streptococcal cells. Bacteria (~10^9) and 10^5 cpm ^{125}I-labeled fn in 1 ml PBS were incubated in the presence of 100 or 500 µg of each protein for 3 h at 22°C.

Table 4. Inhibition of ^{125}I-labeled fn binding to *S. pyogenes* strain 1321 by trypsin-released surface components of the same strain. For details on experimental conditions see reference [30][a]

Fractionation of trypsinate	Inhibition (%)
Crude	94.5
Adsorbed on:	
Sepharose 4B	86.0
Sepharose 4B-egg albumin	90.0
Sepharose 4B-fn	7.0

[a]Streptococcal cells (1 g wet weight) were digested with trypsin (25 µg/ml) in PBS for 1 h at 37°C. Trypsin was inactivated by addition of an excess of soybean trypsin inhibitor and the bacteria were removed by centrifugation. Material released from bacteria during incubation with trypsin was heated for 10 min at 100°C.

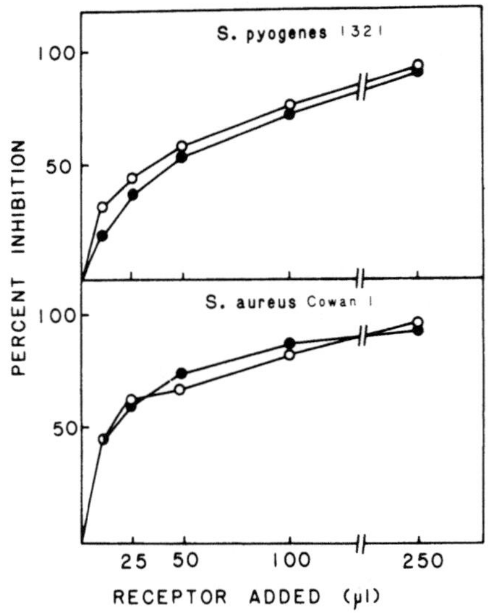

Fig. 4. Inhibition of ^{125}I-labeled fn binding to *S. pyogenes* strain 1321 and *S. aureus* Cowan I by fn fragments adsorbed with streptococcal (*full circles*) and staphylococcal cells (*open circles*). For details see [30]

centrally located part of the fn molecule, containing hydrophobic amino acid sequences.

Trypsin treatment releases initially a class of receptors which bind to immobilized fn, but not to a monoclonal LTA antibody, suggesting that the receptor molecule is not a protein-LTA complex. This class of receptors is rapidly degraded by papain or pronase, indicating that the receptor is indeed protein in nature [30]. The binding components of streptococci other than *S. pyogenes* have not been studied in detail. Preliminary observations suggest that the binding components of group A, C, and G strains are related since there is a cross-inhibition of binding by intact cells of one group by solubilized components from another [32]. Group B and D streptococci and pneumococci do not bind fn according to this study.

Binding of Fibronectin to Other Microbial Pathogens

Van de Water, Destree, and Hynes [34] suggest that other gram-positive organisms such as *Bacillus subtilis*, *Saccharomyces cerevisiae*, *Escherichia coli*, and *Salmonella typhimurium* may bind fn. Moreover, recent studies on *Treponema pallidum* [18] and *Trypanosoma cruzi* (Table 5) suggest that pathogens with tissue-invasive properties may have specific surface structures able to bind fn or other connective tissue proteins.

Table 5. Microorganisms shown to interact with fn[a]

	Reference
1. Gram-positive organisms	
Staphylococcus aureus	[13], [19], [25]
Other staphylococcal species	[33]
Group A, C, and G streptococci	[32], [27]
Treponema pallidum	[18]
2. Gram-negative organisms	
Escherichia coli	[8], [9]
3. Parasites	
Trichomonas vaginalis	[18]
Trypanosoma cruzi	[20]
Leishmania donovani	D. Wyler (unpublished work)
4. Fungi	
Candida albicans	[28]

[a]Binding of fn to other microorganisms such as *B. subtilis* and *Salmonella typhimurium* are not listed owing to lack of experimental evidence that the binding is of specific nature.

At the Interscience Conference on Antibiotics and Chemotherapy (ICAAC) 1982 it was reported by several groups that strains of *E. coli* isolated from urinary tract infections as well as from septicemia with invasive properties did not bind fn. Prototype strains of the F7, F8, etc. strains of *E. coli* isolated from urinary tract infections were shown to bind to laminin, which is a major constituent of basal membranes in the kidney and other tissues, but not to fn [29]. This observation encouraged us to screen *E. coli* strains from various infections for binding to fn, laminin, and other connective tissue components.

In this screening procedure, we found that four of 17 enterotoxigenic *E. coli* (ETEC) strains originally isolated from African children with diarrhea bound fn (^{125}I-labeled) [8]. The binding process was studied to exclude nonspecific binding as these fimbriated hemagglutinating strains show pronounced hydrophobic properties [7]. Unlabeled fn, in contrast to several other proteins, inhibited the binding, indicating that the process is specific [9]. It was shown that these ETEC strains bind to at least two distinct sites in the fn molecule; the NH_2 terminal, i.e., the binding site for staphylococci and streptococci, and one site outside this domain. When grown at 40 °C, a temperature known to suppress formation of hemagglutinating fimbriae at the surface of *E. coli*, ETEC strain 34289 c did not express fn receptor. This observation does not prove, however, that the receptor is located on the pili (fimbriae) since not all piliated strains bind fn.

Cells of *E. coli* strains expressing receptor adhere well to the extracellular matrix and the surface of fibroblasts in vitro. Bacteria grown at 40°C adhere to the fibroblasts to a much lesser extent.

Our previous studies suggest that some uropathogenic *E. coli* strains which bind to specific carbohydrate components on uroepithelial cells can also bind to a specific subepithelial tissue protein, i.e., laminin [29]. Since uropathogenic strains, in contrast to ETEC strains, commonly produce a cytolytic toxin (hemolysin), it is tempting to speculate that the binding to connective tissue components such as laminin could be an important step in local tissue invasion after destruction of epithelial cells by toxin (see Tables 1 and 4). However, since human ETEC strains, in contrast to strains from animal infections, do not produce cytolytic toxins in vitro and do not show local gut mucosal invasive properties, we cannot explain the possible role of these findings as to the virulence of ETEC in humans.

The recent concept that noninvasive pathogens are also actively taken up by M cells in the small bowel gut lining epithelium suggest that binding to fn may occur on such specific cells or upon deposition underneath the epithelial cells or around Peyer's patches. Since fn has been demonstrated between epithelial cells in the gut [21] and in the rectal mucosa [26] by ultrastructural immunochemistry, we propose that local invasive properties of ETEC as well as other intestinal microbial pathogens, i.e., *Giardia lamblia* and *Entamoeba histolytica* must be experimentally explored.

Binding of Microorganisms and Eukaryotic Cells to Artificial Surfaces Coated with Fibronectin

Plastic surfaces coated with fn facilitate adhesion and outgrowth of tissue culture cells such as hepatocytes [23]. Attachment of fibroblasts to native collagen proceeds in the presence of fn while other studies showed that attachment of other cells to type IV collagen and other matrix proteins such as laminin can proceed, even in the absence of fn [22].

We have studied the binding of *S. aureus* strain Cowan 1 which expresses to a high extent both cell bound protein A and fn-binding surface proteins [25] and strain Wood 46 which poorly expresses both these surface proteins to plain tissue culture plastic surfaces and to such surfaces coated with fn, albumin, or whole serum. Binding of these strains and a medium level fn-binding strain SA113 (83A) is shown in Fig. 5. Performing these experiments with high concentrations of albumin in the incubation mixture did not affect binding of these strains to uncoated or fn-precoated surfaces. This is interesting since strain Cowan 1, like most fresh *S. aureus* strains isolated from human and animal infections, showed pronounced hydrophobic (lipophilic) surface properties [11, 38] which certainly facilitates binding to most plastic surfaces. Certain coagulase-negative staphylococci isolated from infections can also bind to plastic surfaces [15]. In conclusion, we believe that further studies of binding to surfaces coated or uncoated with fn and other serum components simulates what happens in the patients who, for example, receive artificial vascular grafts and other artificial prostheses [14]. Furthermore, we have experimental evidence that similar events probably determine colonization of intravenous and other

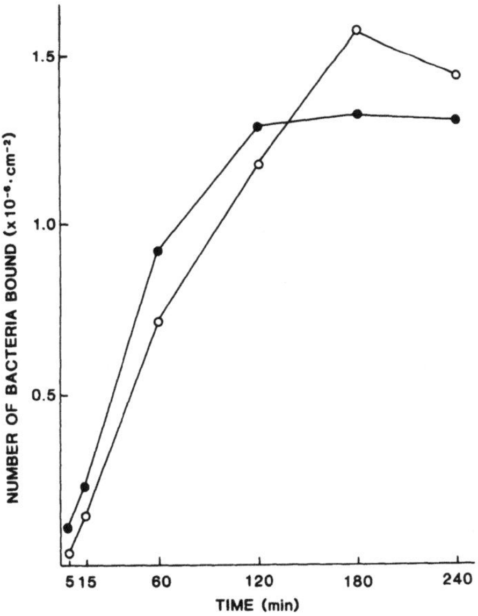

Fig. 5. Attachment of live cells of *S. aureus*, strain SA113 (83A) to fn immobilized on a plastic surface. Cells were allowed to attach at two different temperatures 37°C (*full circles*) and 22°C (*open circles*). The attachment was quantitated essentially as described by Ludwicka et al. [15]. The plastic surface was incubated overnight (Linbro tissue culture flask) with a solution of fn (20 mg/ml), and then incubated with bovine serum albumin (10 mg/ml) to block remaining hydrophobic sites on the plastic surface. A bacterial suspension (5×10^8 cells in PBS) were then incubated with plastic disks and organisms attaching determined by a bioluminescent assay [15]. Binding was a rapid process at both temperatures. No binding was observed to surfaces coated only with albumin while uncoated surfaces bind a high number of organisms owing to hydrophobic interactions [11, 15]

catheter material (such as Spitz Holter devices) and may also initiate such events as development of microabscesses around surgical sutures. We are now studying these processes at the molecular level in experimental systems to try to develop new preventive measures against graft- and catheter-induced infections.

It is also possible that other artificial materials (such as vaginal tampons which cause vaginal and cervical ulcers) also generate microtrauma on other mucosal surfaces and soft tissues which facilitate colonization of staphylococci and streptococci with fn-binding surface components [39]. Abraham, Beachey, and Simpson [1] recently showed that group A streptococci bind selectively to buccal cells, exposing fn on the surface, while Switalski et al. [33] recently demonstrated that such organisms also bind to laminin. The recent original discovery that certain streptococci as well as staphylococci also bind to specific collagen components such as type II collagen suggests that binding to several tissue components may also determine colonization of certain subchronic and chronic tissue infections, such as periodontal disease [39].

Future Perspectives

The biologic significance of specific as well as nonspecific binding of fn to microbial pathogens is not clear. Early studies suggested that such binding mediated an active uptake of bacterial cells into phagocytes. However, studies by Verbrugh et al [35] and others have failed to demonstrate that fn is an important natural opsonin, stimulating active uptake of bacteria into either human polymorphonuclear leukocytes, monocytes, or macrophages, i.e., C3b and IgG are the only major staphylococcal opsonins.

We would like to propose the following events in early colonization of wound tissues by staphylococci and streptococci. Since both organisms seem commonly to possess surface receptors for fn and fibrinogen, they are able to colonize traumatized tissues and blood clots. Recent studies in our laboratories also suggest that both pathogens can show specific binding to collagens and laminin, indicating alternative binding mechanisms in different strains as well as different tissues. We do not know at the moment if the binding process also involves biospecific protein-protein interactions of non-lectin-like type, such as fn binding to staphylococci and streptococci. Since laminin is a carbohydrate-rich glycoprotein, lectin-like interactions with group A streptococci cannot be excluded since these organisms possess a galactose-specific surface antigen [29, 37].

A recently improved understanding of the specific binding mechanisms of fimbriated ETEC in the gastrointestinal tract as well as uropathogenic *E. coli* strains to uroepithelium have initiated research along new lines to find alternative preventive and curative methods for these infections such as receptor therapy and new immunoprophylaxis. We believe that more research on mechanisms for binding of microorganisms to connective tissue components as an early step in tissue infections is a new fruitful area for exploitation. The recent discovery that binding to fn may also be an important early event in certain parasitic infections such as trypanosomiasis and leichmaniasis (see Table 4) suggests that a diverse group of tissue-invasive pathogens may use a similar mechanism for tissue invasion.

Acknowledgments. We want to thank D. Wyler for stimulating discussions on *Leishmania donovani* and other parasites binding fn. This work was supported by Public Health Service grants AM27807 from the National Institutes of Health and grants from the Swedish Medical Research Council (16x-04723 and K84 13P 70001 01), the Medical Board of the Swedish Armed Forces and a grant from the World Health Organization (WHO diarrheal disease control program) to Torkel Wadström.

References

1. Abraham SN, Beachey EH, Simpson WA (1983) Adherence of *Streptococcus pyogenes*, *Escherichia coli*, and *Pseudomonas aeruginosa* to fibronectin-coated and uncoated epithelial cells. Infect Immun 41:1261-1268
2. Beachey EH, Simpson WA (1982) The adherence of group A streptococci to oropharyngeal cells: the lipoteichoic acid adhesin and fibronectin receptor. Infection 10:107-110
3. Courtney HS, Simpson WA, Beachey EH (1983) Binding of streptococcal lipoteichoic acid to fatty acid-binding sites of human plasma fibronectin. J Bacteriol 153:763-770
4. Doran JE, Raynor RH (1981) Fibronectin binding to protein A-containing Staphylococci. Infect Immun 33:683-689
5. Espersen F, Clemmensen I (1981) Clumping of *Staphylococcus aureus* by human fibronectin. Acta Microbiol Scand 89:317-321
6. Espersen F, Clemmensen I (1982) Isolation of a fibronectin-binding protein from *Staphylococcus aureus*. Infect Immun 37:526-531
7. Faris A, Wadström T, Freer JH (1981) Hydrophobic adsorptive and hemagglutinating properties of *Escherichia coli* possessing colonization factor antigens (CFA/I or CFA/II), type 1 pili or other pili. Curr Microbiol 5:67-72
8. Faris A, Fröman G, Höök M, Wadström T (1983) Adhesion of enterotoxigenic *E. coli* with CFA/I and CFA/II antigens to human intestinal cells and binding to fibronectin. US Japan Cholera Conference, NIH, p 25
9. Fröman G, Switalski L, Faris A, Wadström T, Höök M (1984) *Escherichia coli* binding to fibronectin: Mechanisms for tissue adherence. J Biol Chem 259:14899-14905
10. Ichiman Y, Yoshida K (1981) The relationship of capsular-type of *Staphylococcus epidermidis* to virulence and induction of resistance in the mouse. J Appl Bacteriol 51:229-241
11. Jonsson P, Wadström T (1983) High surface hydrophobicity of *Staphylococcus aureus* as revealed by hydrophobic interaction chromatography. Curr Microbiol 8:347-353
12. Kinsman O, Jonsson P, Haraldsson I, Lindberg M, Arbuthnott JP, Wadström T (1981) Decreased virulence of α-haemolysin-negative and coagulase-negative mutants of *Staphylococcus aureus* in experimental infections in mice. In: Jeljaszewicz J (ed) Staphylococci and staphylococcal infections. Zentralbl Bakteriol (Suppl) 10:651-659
13. Kuusela P (1978) Fibronectin binds to *Staphylococcus aureus*. Nature 276: 718-720

14. Lowy FD, Chang DS, Neuhaus EG, Horne DS (1983) Effect of penicillin on the adherence of *Streptococcus sanguis* in vitro and in the rabbit model of endocarditis. J Clin Invest 71:668-675
15. Ludwicka A, Jansen B, Wadström T, Pulverer G (1984) Attachment of *Staphylococci* to various synthetic polymers. Zentralbl Bakteriol Microbiol Hyg 256:479-489
16. Mosher DF, Proctor RA (1980) Binding and factor XIII_a-mediated cross-linking of a 27-kilodalton fragment of fibronectin to *Staphylococcus aureus*. Science 209:927-929
17. Myhre EB, Kuusela P (1983) Binding of human fibronectin to group A, C, and G streptococci. Infect Immun 40:29-34
18. Peterson KM, Baseman JB, Alderete JF (1983) *Treponema pallidum* receptor binding proteins interact with fibronectin. J Exp Med 157:1958-1970
19. Proctor RA, Mosher DF, Olbrantz PJ (1982) Fibronectin binding to *Staphylococcus aureus*. J Biol Chem 257:14788-14794
20. Quaissi MA, Afchain D, Capron A, Grimaud JA (1984) Fibronectin receptors on *Trypanosoma cruzi trypomastigotes* and their biological function. Nature 308:380-382
21. Quaroni A, Isselbacher KJ, Ruoslahti E (1978) Fibronectin synthesis by epithelial crypt cells of rat small intestine. Proc Natl Acad Sci USA 75:5548-5552
22. Rubin K, Johansson S, Pettersson I, Ocklind K, Öbrink B, Höök M (1979) Attachment of rat hepatocytes to collagen and fibronectin; a study using antibodies directed against cell surface components. Biochem Biophys Res Commun 91:86-94
23. Ruoslahti E, Engvall E, Hayman EG (1981) Fibronectin: Current concepts of its structure and functions. Coll Relat Res 1:95-128
24. Ruoslahti E, Pierschbacher M, Engvall E, Oldberg Å, Hayman EG (1982) Molecular and biological interactions of fibronectin. J Invest Dermatol 79: 65-68
25. Rydên C, Rubin K, Speziale P, Höök M, Lindberg M, Wadström T (1983) Fibronectin receptors from *Staphylococcus aureus*. J Biol Chem 258:3396-3401
26. Scott DL, Morris CJ, Blake AE, Low-Beer TS, Walton KW (1981) Distribution of fibronectin in the rectal mucosa. J Clin Pathol 34:749-758
27. Simpson WA, Beachey EH (1983) Adherence of group A streptococci to fibronectin on oral epithelial cells. Infect Immun 39:275-279
28. Skerl KG, Calderone RA, Segal E, Sreevalsan T, Scheld WM (1984) In vitro binding of *Candida albicans* yeast cells to human fibronectin. Can J Microbiol 30:221-226
29. Speziale P, Höök M, Wadström T, Timpl R (1982) Binding of the basement membrane protein laminin to *Escherichia coli*. FEBS Lett 146:55-58
30. Speziale P, Höök M, Switalski LM, Wadström T (1984) Fibronectin binding to a *Streptococcus pyogenes* strain. J Bacteriol 157:420-427
31. Switalski LM (1976) Isolation and purification of staphylococcal clumping factor. Zentralbl Bakt Hyg Infekt Abt 1 Suppl 5:413-423
32. Switalski LM, Ljungh A, Rydên C, Rubin K, Höök M, Wadström T (1982) Binding of fibronectin to the surface of group A, C, and G streptococci isolated from human infections. Eur J Clin Microbiol 1:381-387
33. Switalski LM, Rydên C, Rubin K. Ljungh A, Höök M, Wadström T (1983) Binding of fibronectin to *Staphylococcus* strains. Infect Immun 42:628-633
34. van de Water L, Destree AT, Hynes RO (1983) Fibronectin binds to some bacteria but does not promote their uptake by phagocytic cells. Science 220:201-204
35. Verbrugh HA, Peterson PK, Smith DE, Nguyen BT, Hoidal JR, Wilkinson BJ, Verhoef J, Furcht LT (1981) Human fibronectin binding to staphylococcal surface protein and its relative inefficiency in promoting phagocytosis

by human polymorphonuclear leukocytes, monocytes, and alveolar macrophages. Infect Immun 33:811-819

36. Wadström T (1983) Biological effects of cell damaging toxins. In: Easmon CSF, Adlam C (eds) Staphylococci and staphylococcal infections. Academic, London, pp 671-704
37. Wadström T, Tylewska S (1982) Glycoconjugates as possible receptors for *Streptococcus pyogenes*. Curr Microbiol 7:343-348
38. Wadström T, Haraldson I, Jonsson P, Rydén C, Rubin K, Switalski LM, Höök M, Lindberg M (1981) Experimental infections with *Staphylococcus aureus*. In: Keusch GT, Wadström T (eds) Animal models for experimental bacterial and parasitic infections. Elsevier, Amsterdam, pp 91-96
39. Wadström T, Switalski S, Speziale P, Höök M (1984) In: Mergenhagen S, Rosen B (eds) Molecular interactions in oral microbial adherence and aggregation. American Society for Microbiology (to be published)

39a. Wadström T, Ljungh Å, Höök M, Switalski L (1984) Fibronectin and toxic shock syndrome. JAMA 252:343

40. Yamada KM (1983) Cell surface interactions with extracellular materials. Ann Rev Biochem 52:761-799

Bayer-Symposium VIII
The Pathogenesis of Bacterial Infections, 208-218 (1985)

Protective Immunogenicity of Chemically Synthesized Peptide Fragments of Group A Streptococcal M Proteins

E. H. Beachey

Summary

The M protein on the surface of group A streptococci contains epitopes that evoke type-specific protective immunity against subsequent encounters with the related serotypes of streptococci. Because some of the M proteins are closely associated with potentially harmful epitopes that give rise to antibodies cross-reactive with host tissues, especially the heart, we have undertaken studies of the covalent structures of M protein polypeptide fragments extracted with pepsin at pH 5.8 from rheumatogenic strains of group A streptococci. We have identified 35-residue peptide fragments of type 24 M protein that elicit protective, but not heart-cross-reactive antibodies. Chemically synthesized copies of a 35-residue peptide and subpeptides containing as few as 13 M protein amino acid residues were shown to be immunogenic when covalently conjugated to poly-L-lysine or tetanus toxoid. A 20-residue NH_2 terminal peptide of type 5 M protein was shown to be similarly immunogenic. The immune responses in each case were protective, but not tissue cross-reactive. These results show that the whole M protein molecule is not necessary for the production of protective immunity. Moreover, selected synthetic peptide copies of the natural M protein molecule provide effective immunogens without the potential fear of tissue damage.

Introduction

For many years, attempts have been made to develop safe and effective vaccines against strains of group A streptococci that give rise to acute rheumatic fever and rheumatic heart disease. Vaccination efforts have been hampered by toxic reactions to almost any streptococcal product injected into human subjects [1]. Moreover, a number of vaccine preparations have been associated with antigens that evoke antibodies that cross-react with host tissues, especially heart sarcolemmal membranes [2].

Protective immunity against group A streptococci is directed exclusively against the type-specific M protein on the surface of virulent organisms [3]. Since this protein is often tenaciously associated with antigens that evoke toxic reactions, or worse, immunologic cross-reactions with host tissues, efforts have been directed toward the isolation and purification of the protective M protein antigens free from potentially harmful antigens. Recent studies of the immunogenicity of polypeptide fragments of M protein liberated from whole type 24 group A streptococci by limited peptic digestion have been promising because the purified extracts lacked detectable heart-cross-reactive antigens, but retained protective determinants as demonstrated by vaccination of laboratory animals [4, 5] and in preliminary vaccine trials in human volunteers [6].

Animal trials with another serotype of M protein (pep M5) extracted with pepsin from "rheumatogenic" type 5 group A streptococci, however, resulted in the development of heart-cross-reactive antibodies in one of the first three rabbits immunized with the purified protein [7]. Detailed analyses revealed that the cross-reactive determinant resided in the M protein molecule itself rather than in a contaminant. Furthermore, antibody directed toward the heart-cross-reactive determinant was shown to be opsonic and protective against types 5 and 19 streptococci, both of which had been shown by Kaplan [2] to be associated with type-specific, heart-cross-reactive antigens. Cross-absorption studies showed that the cross-protective, heart-cross-reactive antigen represented only a minor determinant of the type 5 M protein molecule since other protective determinants (probably the majority) on the pep M5 molecule were clearly not heart-cross-reactive [7]. This raised the hope that one might be able to cleave M protein and eliminate potenially harmful regions of the molecule while retaining protective regions.

In this paper, we shall review studies of the chemistry and immunology of natural and chemically synthesized peptide fragments of streptococcal M proteins. Evidence is presented that selected regions of the M protein molecule consisting of as few as 12 amino acid residues contain epitopes that inhibit opsonic anti-streptococcal antibodies. Chemically synthesized peptide fragments as short as 13 amino acid residues, when covalently linked to tetanus toxoid, are capable of evoking protective antibodies against the related streptococci. Moreover, a synthetic copy of the NH_2 terminal 20-residue peptide of an M protein molecule (type 5) that contains heart-cross-reactive epitopes within its covalent structure was capable of eliciting protective anti-streptococcal antibodies without eliciting heart-cross-reactive immunity.

Immunogenicity of Native Peptide Fragments of M Protein

The notion that one might evoke protective immune responses by immunization with peptide fragments of M protein is based on several lines of evidence. First, the intact M protein molecule appears to be considerably larger than the polypeptide extracted by most methods from whole streptococci or cell walls [8]; thus far, most M protein vaccines extracted by a number of different methods [3, 5, 9-12] and studied for immunogenicity have consisted only of large polypeptide fragments of the M protein molecule. Second, several laboratories have presented evidence that individual M protein molecules contain many antigenic determinants, most of which are type specific [9, 11, 13-16], but some of which are cross-reactive with other M serotypes [17-21]. Third, purified subpeptides derived by cyanogen bromide cleavage of type 24 M protein each evoked protective antibodies against the homologous serotype of streptococci [22]. Finally, two chemically synthesized, 35-residue peptide fragments of pep M24 were shown to evoke similar type-specific protective antibodies without eliciting heart-reactive antibodies [23, 24].

Structure of M Protein

Recent studies of the primary structures of three different serotypes of M protein have revealed several remarkable features. First, although the amino acid sequences of each of three different M serotypes (types 5, 6, and 24) are unique, certain amino acids are conserved among all three [20, 25-27]. Second, the M protein molecules are composed in varying degrees of internally repeating covalent structures [15, 26, 28]. Third, the M proteins contain a seven-residue periodicity in their amino acid sequences which is reminiscent of α-tropomyosin of muscle tissue [26, 29]. The latter characteristic accounts for an α-helical coiled-coil structure of the M protein molecule (Fig. 1); it is the first such conformation to be demonstrated for any surface appendage of bacteria [8]. Electron microscopy of the rotary shadowed coiled coils of pepsin-, detergent-, and phage lysin-extracted M protein of type 6 streptococci suggested that the pepsin- and detergent-extracted M proteins represented the distal ends of these surface fibrillar structures, whereas the lysin-extracted M protein represented most, if not all, of these structures. Thus far, most of the primary structural studies have employed pepsin or detergent extracts of M protein. Our own studies

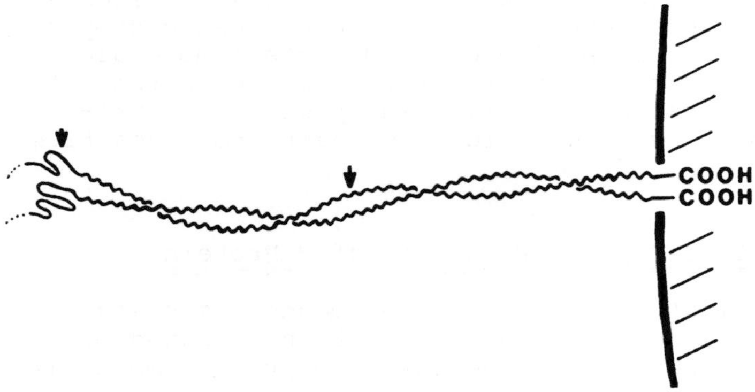

Fig. 1. Schematic drawing of the arrangement of the coiled-coil structure of M protein on the streptococcal surfaces. *Arrows* indicate probable sites of cleavage by limited pepsin digestion. Reproduced by permission of Phillips et al. [8]

of chemically synthesized fragments of M protein have been based on the covalent structures of pepsin-extracted M proteins (pep M).

Chemically Synthesized M Protein Fragments

The synthesis of M protein polypeptides was based on the covalent structures determined for the cyanogen bromide peptides of type 24 M protein (pep M24) and of the NH_2 terminal sequence analysis of type 5M protein. Since we had shown that at least one protective determinant resided in each of the seven purified repeating covalent structures of pep M24 [14, 21], and had established the immunogenicity of the 35-residue peptides whose sequences had been completed [22-24], we decided to chemically synthesize two of these, CB3 and CB7; the synthetic peptides being designated S-CB3 and S-CB7.

In addition, we synthesized subpeptides of the 35-residue S-CB7, including S-CB7(13-35), S-CB7(18-35), S-CB7(23-35)Cys, and S-CB7 (18-29). The latter peptide overlaps two subpeptides derived by digesting lysyl-blocked CB7 (see later discussion). A 20-residue peptide of pep M5, S-M5(1-20) also was synthesized. Each of the peptides was synthesized by the solid phase method of Merrifield [30] as previously described [23, 24, 31, 32]. The identity of the synthetic peptides was confirmed by amino acid analyses and automated Edman degradation [22].

When emulsified in complete Freund's adjuvant and injected as a single 25 nmol dose, S-CB7 evoked antibody titers at six weeks of 1:400, 1:1280, and 1:25 600, respectively, in each of three rabbits as determined by enzyme-linked immunosorbent assays (ELISA). Only the serum of the rabbit showing the highest ELISA titer was able to opsonize type 24 streptococci. In contrast, the same dose of S-CB7 covalently linked to polylysine and emulsified in complete Freund's adjuvant evoked strong ELISA as well as opsonic antibody titers in each of three rabbits (Fig. 2). The results obtained by using S-CB3 instead of S-CB7 were virtually identical (data not shown; see reference [24]). In opsonobactericidal assays using types 5, 6, and 24 streptococci, the immune sera were capable of promoting phagocytosis and killing of the type 24 streptococci only, indicating that the humoral immune responses to S-CB7 were type specific [22].

Immunodiffusion tests of the immune sera revealed precipitin arcs of identity between wells containing polylysine conjugates of native and synthetic CB7 as well as with the intact pep M24 (Fig. 3). There was no cross-reactivity of the anti-S-CB7 antiserum with pep M5 or pep M6. None of the S-CB7 immune sera reacted with the sarcolemmal membranes of frozen sections of human heart as determined by immunofluorescence [6]. The protective activity of the S-CB7 immune sera was tested by passive mouse protection tests. Mice were injected with 0.2 ml of a pool of the immune sera and 24 h later challenged with type 24 or type 6 streptococci. The immune sera clearly protected against the homologous type 24, but not against the heterologous type 6 streptococci (Table 1).

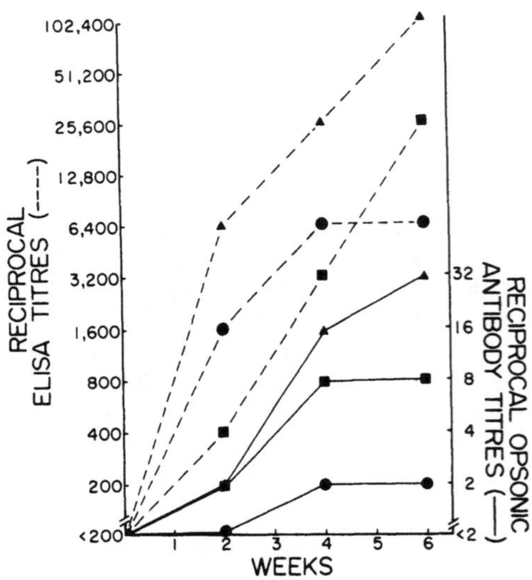

Fig. 2. Immune responses of three rabbits (*triangles*, *squares*, *circles*) immunized with 25 nmol S-CB7 conjugated to polylysine in complete Freund's adjuvant as measured by ELISA (*broken line*) or opsonophagocytic tests (*full line*). Reproduced by permission of Beachey et al. [23]

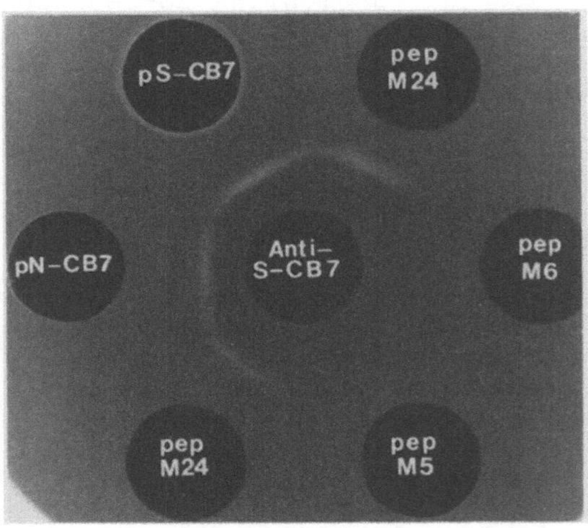

Fig. 3. Immunodiffusion in agar gel of S-CB7 immune rabbit serum (anti-S-CB7) against polylysine-conjugated native CB7 (pN-CB7), type 24 (pep M24), type 5 (pep M5), and type 6 (pep M6) M proteins. Virtually identical results were obtained with antisera against S-CB3 and the various subpeptides of S-CB7 [24, 32]

Having demonstrated that a protective determinant of M protein resides in a synthetic peptide as small as 35 residues, it was of interest to determine whether protective determinants were retained on even smaller peptide fragments. Therefore, we cleaved CB7 with trypsin after blocking lysine residues with maleic anhydride. Since CB7 contains only one arginine residue at position 23, the molecule was cleaved into a COOH terminal dodecapeptide and an NH_2 terminal 23-residue peptide (Fig. 4). After deblocking the lysine residues with pyridine/acetate, the subpeptides were separated and purified by HPLC reverse-phase chromatography [23]. The purified peptides were then tested for their abilities to inhibit opsonization by anti-S-CB7. In addition, we tested the synthetic overlapping peptide, S-CB7(18-29), for inhibitory activity. The results clearly showed that the

Table 1. Mouse protection against challenge infections with type 24 streptococci by sera of rabbits immunized with S-CB7

Serum used to passively immunize mice	LD_{50} in mice challenged with:	
	Type 6 streptococci	Type 24 streptococci
Preimmune serum	<500 (2/15)[a]	<500 (3/15)
Pooled (3 rabbits) immune anti-S-CB7 serum	<500 (2/15)	3500 000 (14/15)

[a]Figures in parentheses indicate the number of survivors/number of challenged mice. Three rabbits were immunized intracutaneously with 25 nmol S-CB7 conjugated to polylysine (molecular weight ~35 000) and emulsified in complete Freund's adjuvant as previously described. The initial immunizing dose was followed 1 week later by the same dose emulsified in incomplete Freund's adjuvant and injected subcutaneously. Preimmune and immune sera obtained before immunization and 6 weeks after the initial immunizing dose, respectively, were pooled and white Swiss mice injected intraperitoneally with 0.2 ml preimmune or immune serum; 24 h later the mice were challenged by the same route with various doses (ranging from 500 to 4×10^6 CFU) of type 6 or type 24 streptococci. The survivals were recorded over a 7-day period and are shown in parentheses. These data are from [22].

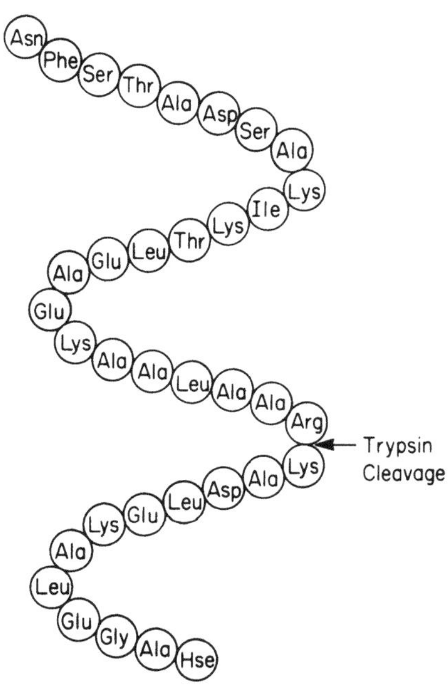

Fig. 4. Sequence of CB7 of type 24 M protein. After blocking the lysine residues with maleic anhydride, trypsin cleaves CB7 at the arginine residue as indicated into a COOH terminal dodecapeptide and an NH_2 terminal 23-residue peptide

NH_2 terminal 23-residue peptide and the COOH terminal 12-residue peptide were inhibitory although higher concentrations than that of the intact CB7 were required to achieve equal levels of inhibition. The overlapping 12-residue peptide, S-CB7(18-29), on the other hand, was without effect even at concentrations as high as 100 nmol [23].

These results indicated that a protective determinant of type 24 M protein resided in a peptide fragment containing only 12 residues. The inability of the overlapping synthetic peptide to block opsonization suggests that CB7 contains at least two distinct protective antigenic determinants neither of which resides in the overlapping peptide.

That protective epitopes resided in the subpeptides of CB7 was confirmed by studies of the immunogenicity of the synthetic peptides S-CB7(13-35), -(18-35), and -(23-35)Cys covalently linked to tetanus toxoid [32]. Each of these peptides evoked opsonic antibodies in rabbits (Fig. 5A-C). The substitution, however, of a single amino acid in the 13-residue M protein peptide, S-CB7(23-35)Cys, as position 33 (lysine substituted for glycine) rendered this protective peptide nonprotective (Fig. 5D).

In contrast to the high degree of type specificity of the humoral immune responses to each of the synthetic peptides, the cellular immune responses were highly cross-reactive. The lymphocytes of rabbits immunized with S-CB7 were equally responsive in mitogenic assays to heterologous pep M5 as they were to the homologous pep M24 (Table 2). Furthermore, immunization with S-CB7(18-29) covalently conjugated with polylysine, although failing to evoke effective humoral immunity, nevertheless induced non-type-specific cellular immunity similar to that of S-CB7. Neither of the synthetic peptides was of sufficient size to induce mitogenesis of lymphocytes from immunized rabbits [22].

These studies provided evidence in support of the hypothesis that limited peptide regions of the M protein molecule would suffice as protective immunogens, especially when covalently linked to carrier molecules, such as polylysine or tetanus toxoid. Furthermore, these findings suggested the possibility that one might select for synthesis small peptide regions of M protein that contain protective, but not tissue-cross-reactive, antigenic determinants. With this in mind, we examined the protective and heart-cross-reactivity of a 20-residue synthetic peptide of type 5 M protein, a molecule demonstrated to contain within its covalent structure an epitope (or epitopes) that raised antibodies cross-reactive with a protein in the sarcolemma of human heart tissue. When covalently linked to tetanus toxoid with glutaraldehyde, the synthetic peptide S-M5(1-20) evoked antibodies that were protective against the related type 5 streptococci [33]. Even though each of the animals received five times the dose, on a molar basis, required to produce heart-cross-reactive antibody with the intact pep M5 molecule, none of the immunized animals developed heart-cross-reactive antibodies.

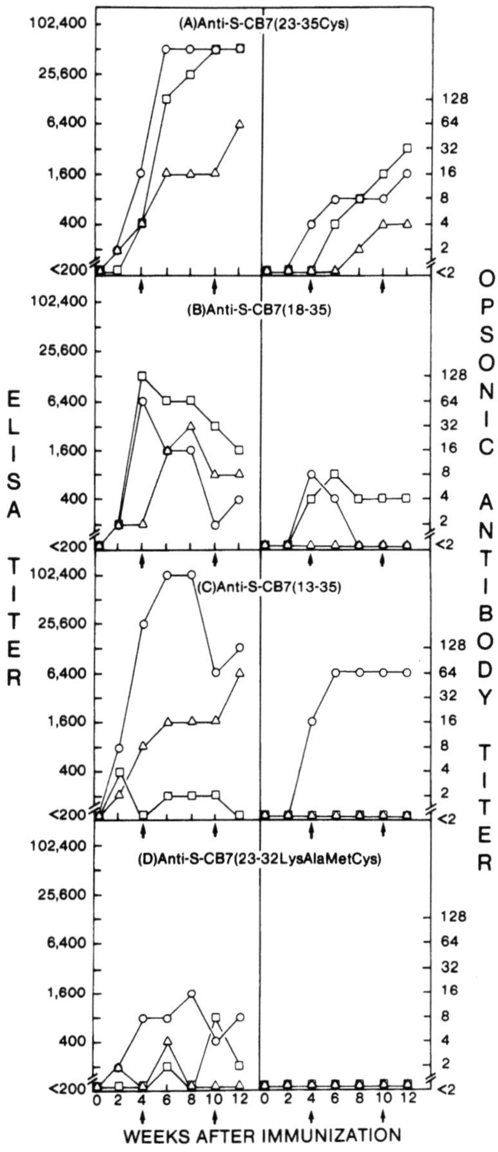

Fig. 5. Immune response of rabbits against tetanus toxoid-conjugated synthetic peptide fragments of type 24 streptococcal M protein as measured by ELISA against pep M24 (*left*) and by opsonic antibody assays (*right*). Sets of three rabbits (*triangles*, *squares*, *circles*) were immunized with 25 nmol tetanus toxoid-conjugated S-CB7(23-35) Cys(A); S-CB7(18-35)(B); S-CB7 (13-35)(C); or S-CB7(23-32 Lys-Ala-Met-Cys(D) emulsified in complete Freund's adjuvant. Booster injections of 25 nmol of the respective peptide conjugates in PBS were given as indicated by the *arrows*. In control experiments, none of the immune sera reacted with pep M5, pep M6, or pep M19 in ELISA, or opsonized heterologous serotypes 5, 6, or 19 streptococci, indicating the serotype specificity of the immune response. Reproduced with permission of Beachey et al. [32]

These studies should open the way to the development of streptococcal vaccines composed of small synthetic peptide regions of M protein that contain protective, but not tissue-cross-reactive antigenic determinants. The knowledge of the complete covalent structures of several serotypes of M protein should allow us to apply the principles reported by Hopp and Wood [34] on the prediction of which antigenic regions to isolate or synthesize based on the relative hydrophilicity of various peptide regions as determined by their amino acid sequences.

Table 2. Blastogenic responses of lymphocytes from rabbits immunized with S-CB7 or S-CB7(18-29) fragments of type 24 M protein[a]

Rabbit number	Immunizing antigen	Mean cpm ± standard error of lymphocytes cultured with:		
		Control	M5	M24
8026	S-CB7	98 ± 23	3743 ± 411	4721 ± 479
8027	S-CB7	181 ± 28	12684 ± 1454	829 ± 124
8028	S-CB7	156 ± 31	43391 ± 3094	36449 ± 5416
7919	S-CB7(18-29)	415 ± 27	11521 ± 3081	12038 ± 243
7921	S-CB7(18-29)	135 ± 31	17056 ± 3081	3575 ± 1265
8020	S-CB7(18-29)	705 ± 59	12487 ± 918	4916 ± 362
8007	CFA (control)	76 ± 102	64 ± 12	40 ± 2
8008	CFA (control)	31 ± 11	153 ± 25	83 ± 25

[a]CFA, complete Freund's Adjuvant. Control animals were injected with the same volume of complete Freund's adjuvant emulsified with 0.15 *M* NaCl without antigen. These data are from [23]. Heparinized (100 units/ml) peripheral blood was obtained from rabbits 2-6 weeks after immunization (see footnote, Table 1) by cardiac puncture. Mononuclear cells were isolated by Ficoll-Hypaque gradient centrifugation by the method of Boyum [10] and as previously described [11]. Lymphocytes were washed three times and resuspended in RPMI 1640 (Grant Island Biological Company, Grand Island, New York), supplemented with penicillin (100 units/ml), streptomycin (100 μg/ml), L-glutamine (2 m*M*), and HEPES buffer (25 m*M*). Lymphocytes (2×10^5) were incubated at 37°C with 50 μg per culture of each antigen tested in 96-well microculture plates (Falcon Plastics, 3040, Oxnard, California) in a total volume of 200 μl supplemented with 5% heat-inactivated fetal calf serum. Control cultures were incubated in the same volume of medium without antigen; 18 h before harvesting, 1 μCi thymidine ^3H (specific activity, 2 Ci/mmol, Research Products International Corporation, France) in 25 μl culture medium was added to each well. All cultures were harvested at 5 days with a multiple automated sample harvester and the cells assayed for radioactivity in a liquid scintillation counter.

Conclusion

It is now clear that the whole M protein molecule is not needed to immunize effectively against group A streptococcal infections. Chemically synthesized peptide fragments of carefully chosen regions of various M protein molecules should provide a vaccine that can be safely administered to humans without the fear of evoking host tissue-cross-reactive antibodies. There is some evidence to suggest that certain protective determinants of M protein may be shared among different serotypes. The identification and synthesis of such common protective determinants should provide the basis for the formulation of a broadly protective vaccine against many serotypes of rheumatogenic group A streptococci.

Acknowledgments. The research studies of the author are supported by Institutional Research Funds from the United States Veterans Administration and by NIH Research Grants AI-10085 and AI-13550. I thank my colleagues, Drs. Gene H. Stollerman, James B. Dale, Jerome M. Seyer, Andrew H. Kang, Louis Chedid, François Audibert, Michel Jolivet, Hélène Gras-Masse, and André Tarter for invaluable contributions over the years to the studies summarized in this report.

References

1. Stollerman GH (1975) Rheumatic fever and streptococcal infection. Grune and Stratton, New York
2. Kaplan MH (1963) J Immunol 90:595-606
3. Lancefield RC (1962) J Immunol 89:307-313
4. Beachey EH, Campbell GL, Ofek I (1972) Infect Immun 9:891-896
5. Beachey EH, Stollerman GH, Chiang EY, Chiang TM, Seyer JM, Kang JM (1977) J Exp Med 145:1479-1483
6. Beachey EH, Stollerman GH, Johnson RH, Ofek I, Bisno AL (1979) J Exp Med 150:862-877
7. Dale JB, Beachey EH (1982) J Exp Med 156:1165-1167
8. Phillips GN, Flicker PF, Cohen C, Manjula BN, Fischetti VA (1982) Proc Natl Acad Sci USA 78:4689-4693
9. Fox EN, Wittner MK (1969) Immunochemistry 6:11-24
10. Russel H, Facklam RR, Edwards LR (1975) Infect Immun 12:679-686
11. Fischetti VA, Gotschlich EC, Siviglia G, Zabriskie JB (1976) J Exp Med 144:32-53
12. Vosti KL, Williams WK (1978) Infect Immun 21:546-555
13. Beachey EH, Cunningham MW (1973) Infect Immun 8:19-24
14. Cunningham MW, Beachey EH (1975) J Immunol 115:1002-1006
15. Beachey EH, Seyer JM, Kang AH (1978) Proc Natl Acad Sci USA 75:3163-3167
16. Hasty DL, Beachey EH, Simpson WA, Dale JB (1982) J Exp Med 155:1010-1018
17. Fox EN, Wittner MK (1968) J Immunol 100:39-45
18. Wittner MK, Fox EN (1977) Infect Immun 15:104-108
19. Fischetti VA (1977) J Exp Med 146:1108-1123
20. Dale JB, Ofek I, Beachey EH (1980) J Exp Med 151:1026-1038
21. Beachey EH, Seyer JM (1982) In: Robbins JB, Hill JC, Sadoff JC (eds) Bacterial vaccines. Thieme-Stratton, New York, pp 401-410
22. Beachey EH, Seyer JM, Kang AH (1980) J Biol Chem 255:6284-6289
23. Beachey EH, Seyer JM, Dale JB, Simpson WA, Kang AH (1981) Nature 292: 457-459

24. Beachey EH, Seyer JM, Dale JB, Hasty DL (1983) J Biol Chem 258:13250-13257
25. Manjula BN, Fischetti VA (1980) J Immunol 124:261-267
26. Manjula BN, Fischetti VA (1980) J Exp Med 151:695-707
27. Fischetti VA, Manjula BN (1982) In: Robbins JB, Hills JC, Sadoff JC (eds) Bacterial vaccines. Thieme-Stratton, New York, pp 411-418
28. Manjula BN, Acharya AS, Mische SM, Fariwell T, Fischetti VA (1984) J Biol Chem 259:3686-3693
29. Hosein B, McCarty M, Fischetti VA (1979) Proc Natl Acad Sci USA 76:3765-3768
30. Merrifield RB (1963) J Am Chem Soc 85:2149-2155
31. Jolivet M, Audibert F, Beachey EH, Tarter A, Gras-Masse H, Chedid L (1984) Biochem Biophys Res Comm 117:359-366
32. Beachey EH, Tarter A, Seyer JM, Chedid L (1984) Proc Natl Acad Sci USA 81:2203-2207
33. Dale JB, Syer JM, Beachey EH (1983) J Exp Med 158:1727-1732
34. Hopp TP, Wood KR (1981) Proc Natl Acad Sci USA 78:3824-3828

Discussion

(pp. 193-218)

Binding to Connective Tissue

A rather extensive discussion was concerned with the specificity and relevance of microbial binding to fibronectin (and collagen and laminin); for example, inhibition of *Pseudomonas aeruginosa* binding to buccal epithelial cells by fibronectin of enterotoxogenic *E. coli* of human origin to the intestinal tract via fibronectin, since there is probably very little fibronectin in gut mucus and on epithelial cells. However, there is fibronectin exposed on epithelial cells or certain mucosal surfaces such as in the oral cavity. Findings suggest that *E. coli* strains (as well as *Streptococcus pyogenes*) which bind to fibronectin or laminin are noninvasive, but (e.g., uropathogenic *E. coli*) produce cytolytic toxins which can destroy epithelial cells and expose matrix proteins consisting of fibrinonectin, collagen, and laminin. In addition, laminin contains sugar sequences very similar to the ones P-fimbriae bind to which may be an important factor in the development of pyelonephritis. So what should be done is to grow organ cultures, lyse the cells, and expose the matrix to measure binding. Results with living streptococci do not differ from those obtained with heat-treated cells. With staphylococci, surface lipoteichoic acid cannot be involved and the proteins responsible for binding seem to be heat resistant. With regard to the binding domains on fibronectin, the middle portion of the molecule appears to be very sticky and bind to many charged and amphiphilic molecules as well as artificial surfaces. The insertion of the binding protein into staphylococcal cell walls is unknown and at present no mutant has been described which is unable to incorporate fibronectin receptor molecules in the cell wall.

Streptococcal M Protein, Fibrinogen

Streptococci are coated with fibrinogen. What are the consequences when they are exposed to plasmin, to thrombin, to streptococcal proteases, to streptokinase? Does it result in the unmasking of M epitopes? Does it allow complement to bind? Does it damage the bacterial cells in some way? What is the course of streptococcal infection in hypofibrinogenic mice, or in mice treated with drugs that would prevent the formation of plasmin? Will the proteases in localized infections help in spread? Experiments are under way to answer these questions. Plasmin, being a trypsin-like enzyme, might also remove M protein along with the fibrinogen. The complex between M protein and fibrinogen remains susceptible to thrombin digestion. Thrombin cleaves fibrinopeptide A from fibrinogen complexed to M protein or complexed to whole group A streptococci. Since macrophages have receptor sites on their surfaces that recognize the stub left on the fibrinogen molecule after cleavage of fibrinopeptide A, an interesting concept arises in that the resultant fibrin monomers may become an opsonin rather than an inhibitor of opsonization for mononuclear leukocytes and macrophages. Plasmin gives rise to fragments X, Y, D, and E of fibrinogen. M protein binds to each of these fragments except fragment E. Whether or not they block binding of complement to the surface of the organism remains to be tested.

Bayer-Symposium VIII
The Pathogenesis of Bacterial Infections, 221-234 (1985)

Molecular Analysis of Virulence Determinants of *Neisseria gonorrhoeae*

Th. F. Meyer, R. Haas, R. Halter, P. Nickel, J. Pohlner, A. Stern, J. Clarke, H. Delius, and M. So

Summary

Gonococcal virulence is thought to rely on multiple phenomena to which antigenic variation of surface proteins as well as the production of an extracellular protease specific for human IgA1 can be accounted. The expression of pilin and opacity (Op) protein in *Neisseria gonorrhoeae* can be switched on and off and a single cell apparently has a whole repertoire of genes to express many serologically distinguishable protein types. In order to investigate the molecular mechanisms associated with this surface variability, we have cloned the genes for pilin and Op expression in *Escherichia coli*. Using these genes as probes in DNA filter hybridizations, we revealed two complex gene systems which undergo genomic reorganizations and/or gene conversions which occur concomitant to changes in the expression of these surface proteins. To study the role of IgA proteases in bacterial pathogenesis, we cloned the IgA protease gene of *N. gonorrhoeae* MS11. This clone promotes expression and extracellular secretion of active enzyme in *E. coli* and other gram-negative bacterial species.

Introduction

Neisseria gonorrhoeae has developed efficient mechanisms to evade the immune surveillance of its host. Several gonococcal surface proteins are able to undergo dramatic changes in their immunologic and structural properties within few bacterial generations ([1-5]; Blake, this volume). This variability of gonococcal surface antigens is thought to allow the pathogen to adapt to the immune and infection status of the host organism. Furthermore, *N. gonorrhoeae* produces an extracellular protease which specifically cleaves human immunoglobulin A1 (IgA1) (for review see [6]). Although there is much speculation about a possible role of this enzyme in gonococcal virulence, its specific function in this process is still unknown. In order to improve our understanding of the implications of antigenic variation and immunoglobulin degradation for the gonococcal infection, we began to investigate these phenomena on a molecular level.

The Major Variable Surface Proteins of *N. gonorrhoeae*

Pilin, the subunit component of the pilus structure, and the opacity (Op) protein of the outer membrane represent the two most striking examples of gonococcal surface antigen variability. The expression of these proteins can be turned on and off and a single cell apparently has a large repertoire to produce many types of these proteins varying in size and antigenic properties [2, 7-10]. Changes in the expression of pilin and Op protein are reflected by distinct changes in the colony morphology of gonococci [2-4, 8, 11], and provide a convenient experimental system to monitor surface antigen variation of the bacterium. Four basic colony types (T1-T4) can be defined, representing the four possible combinations of the piliated or nonpiliated (P^+/P^-) and opaque or transparent (O^+/O^-) phenotypes of gonococci.

Gonococcal pili, which form fine hair-like structures on the cell surface, confer adhesion of the bacterium to the epithelium of the human mucosa ([12, 13]; Schoolnik and Rothbard, this volume). Pilus-mediated adhesion is the first critical event in the infection process by gonococci preceding invasion of the mucosal tissue ([14]; McGee and Robinson, this volume). Consistently, P^+ gonococci are much more infectious than P^- gonococci [8, 9]. The pili are composed of a protein subunit known as pilin. It consists of approximately 160 amino acids with strongly hydrophobic NH_2 terminal and a polar COOH terminal domain. The hydrophobic NH_2 terminus appears to be conserved among all gonococcal pilin types and is immunorecessive. In contrast, the polar pilin portion which is subject to antigenic variation is immunodominant.

The second variable surface protein, the Op protein, likewise seems to be involved in differential adhesion of gonococci to various cell types of the host [17-19]. Major parts of the protein are buried in the outer membrane and share common peptides, reminiscent of the constant region of pilin [1, 20, 21]. However, on the surface of intact gonococci, variant Op proteins appear to form classes of little antigenic relatedness. The strong association of Op protein with the outer membrane is reflected in its unusual temperature-modifiable mobility in SDS-polyacrylamide gels, which seems characteristic for the firm attachment of protein to lipopolysaccharide [22].

Using the well-characterized gonococcal strain MS11, we isolated various isogenic variants with different characteristics in pilin and/or Op protein expression. Several variants producing pilin of distinct antigenic properties or Op proteins of different sizes have been derived from a single parental line by in vitro culturing. Figure 1 shows outer membrane preparations of a few of our Op variants which express Op protein in the range between 29 and 35 kdaltons. These observations which have been made by other laboratories as well [2, 21, 23], raise a series of questions regarding the number of variant genes contained in the gonococcal genome and how their expression might be regulated. Approaching these questions by means of molecular cloning,

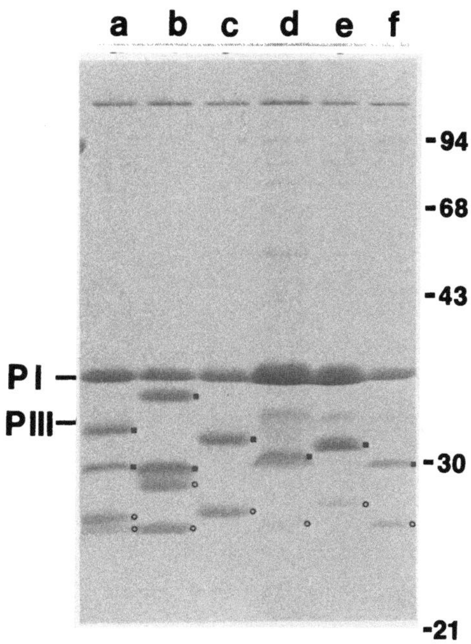

Fig. 1. Variability of OP protein in isogenic *N. gonorrhoeae*. Spontaneous isogenic variants of *N. gonorrhoeae* MS11 (*a* VO; *b* V1; *c* V18; *d* V28; *e* V32; and *f* V34) were isolated on culture plates. Outer membrane proteins from these variants were analyzed by SDS-gel electrophoresis. *Circles* and *squares* indicate the positions of partially and completely denaturated forms of Op protein, respectively. Variants V32 and V34 produce two Op proteins. Molecular weight markers are indicated at the right-hand side (kdaltons). The positions of outer membrane proteins I and III (PI and PIII) are indicated at the left-hand side

we detected a complex system of gene sequences which undergo rearrangements and conversions concomitant to variations in the expression of pilin and Op protein.

Analysis of Pilus Determinants

The strategy we used to clone the *N. gonorrhoeae* pilin gene in *E. coli* [24] was based on the assumption that both organisms are gram-negative and therefore likely share common transcription and translation signals required for the expression of genes. Consistently, we constructed a plasmid library of the chromosome of strain MS11 (P^+) and screened this library for expression of pilin with type-specific anti-pilin antibody. Fragments inserted in the plasmids of positive, pilin-producing colonies represented two different classes of pilin genes. Both classes expressed identical pilin and, consistently, shared a region of complete homology in the coding region. However, their border sequences differed in the arrangement of restriction sites. This indicated that they originated from different loci in the genome of *N. gonorrhoeae* MS11. These loci have been named *pil*E1 and *pil*E2 [6].

Using either of these clones as probes in DNA filter hybridizations with *N. gonorrhoeae* chromosomal DNA, we revealed a complex pattern of fragments which cross-hybridized to the pilin gene probe [24]. Further analysis indicated that at least five distinct gene loci exist which carry pilin genes or pilin-related gene sequences. An evaluation of the physical position of these pilin gene loci in the chromosome by hybridization analysis and cloning by chromosomal walking allowed us to link together some

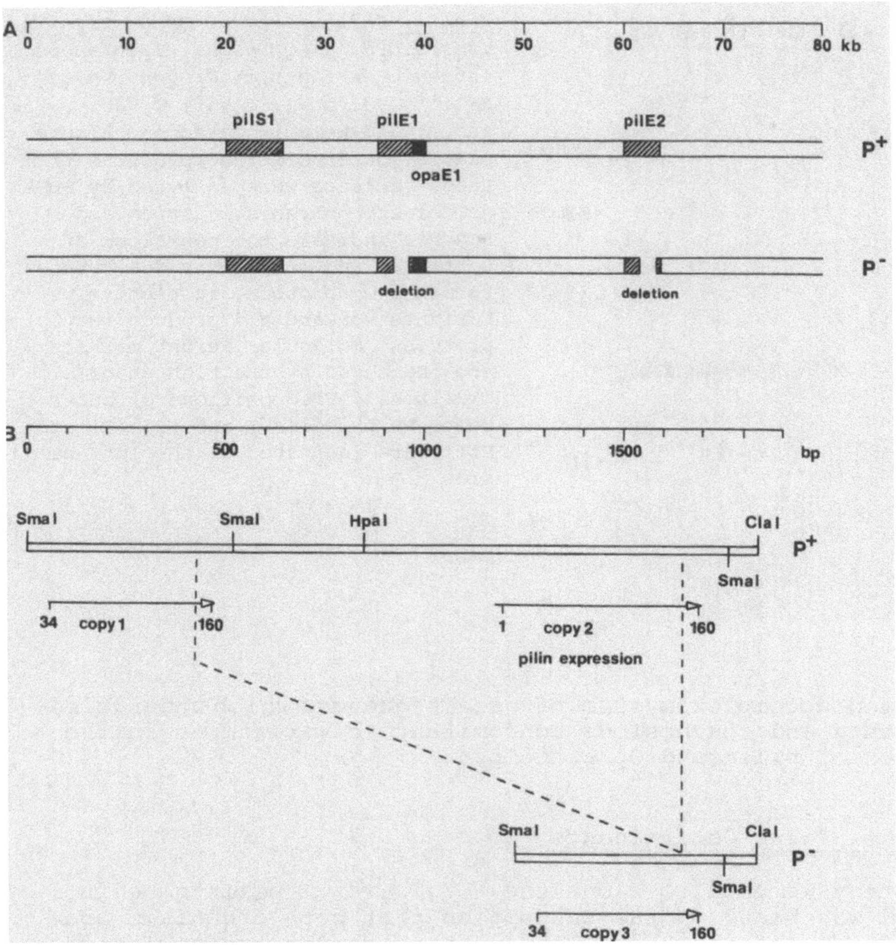

Fig. 2A,B. Organization of chromosomal gene loci for pilin and Op protein. (A) Arrangement of pilin and Op protein gene loci within an 80-kbase region of the *N. gonorrhoeae* MS11 genome. Location of two pilin expression loci (*pil*E1 and *pil*E2), a silent pilin gene locus (*pil*S1), and an expression site for Op protein (*opa*E1) near *pil*E1. The reading frames of pilin and Op sequences is from left to right in all gene loci. In the P^- state of MS11 (*lower part* of A), the pilin expression sites often carry deletions in the pilin structural gene. (B) Arrangement of pilin gene sequences within the locus *pil*E1. In the P^+ conformation of *pil*E1, two variant pilin gene sequences are arranged in tandem (copy 1 and copy 2). Only copy 2 expresses pilin whereas copy 1 misses expression signals as well as the sequence coding for the NH_2 terminal 33 amino acids of native pilin. Concomitant with the loss of pilin expression, deletion events (*lower part* of B) can occur. This particular type of deletion fuses together copies 1 and 2 and forms a novel variant pilin gene copy (copy 3) at the site of expression. Copy 3 is devoid of NH_2 terminal sequences and does not express pilin. Numbers drawn at individual gene copies indicate the positions of amino acids in native pilin (160 refers to the stop codon at the end of the pilin gene)

of these pilin gene loci in a linear map (Fig. 2A). In addition to the pilin expression loci *pil*E1 and *pil*E2, this part of the genome carries a pilus gene locus (*pil*S1) which does not express pilin when cloned in *E. coli*. Since *pil*S1 and all further (unmapped) pilus gene loci are missing certain restriction sites which are characteristic for a pilin expression site, we believe that *pil*E1 and *pil*E2 are the only gene loci in the MS11 genome which actively express pilin.

The hybridization pattern of pilin gene sequences obtained for the genome of P^- gonococci showed marked differences from that of isogenic P^+ gonococci [24]. A detailed analysis of the events that occurred upon loss of pilin expression indicated that deletions of different size classes had been introduced at one or both pilin expression sites (Fig. 2A,B). Such deletions always included parts of the pilin coding sequence. In contrast to the expression sites, for the silent gene loci we did not detect alterations in the hybridization analysis. Furthermore, when the cells spontaneously switched back to the piliated state, one or both pilin expression loci were refilled by pilin gene sequences from an as yet undefined source, giving rise to complete pilin structural genes regaining their properties to express pilin (M. So, personal communication).

A second type of recombination event involved in the regulation of pilin expression appeared to occur without involvement of dramatic genome alterations (M. So and T.F. Meyer, unpublished). Surprisingly, some of our isogenic P^- variants showed a hybridization pattern identical to that of the parental MS11 (P^+) variant. However, cloning of the expression copies from both variants and comparison at the nucleotide level showed significant heterologies inside as well as outside the coding sequences of the two pilin expression sites (S. Störzbach and T.F. Meyer, unpublished). It appears that reversions to the P^+ state in cells harboring such slight alterations in the pilin expression sites occur with frequencies much higher than reversions associated with the restoration of deleted expression sites.

Detailed restriction mapping, combined with DNA sequence analysis, allowed us to gain insight into the structural organization of silent loci and expression loci [6]. The coding sequences in *pil*E1 and *pil*E2 are surrounded by numerous direct and inverted repeats, some of which can be detected in the electron microscope (Fig. 3). In each of the expression loci, a second large open reading frame is located upstream of the coding genes. This open reading frame resembles a complete pilin gene, but is missing the first 100 nucleotides at its 5'-terminal portion (E. Billyard and M. So, unpublished). Comparing these two sequences at the nucleotide level shows a series of nucleotide substitutions as well as small deletions and insertions that do not alter the reading frame. One particular class of deletions associated with the switch to the P^- state leads to a recombination of these two variant sequences. As a result of this deletion, a novel variant pilin gene sequence is assembled in the expres-

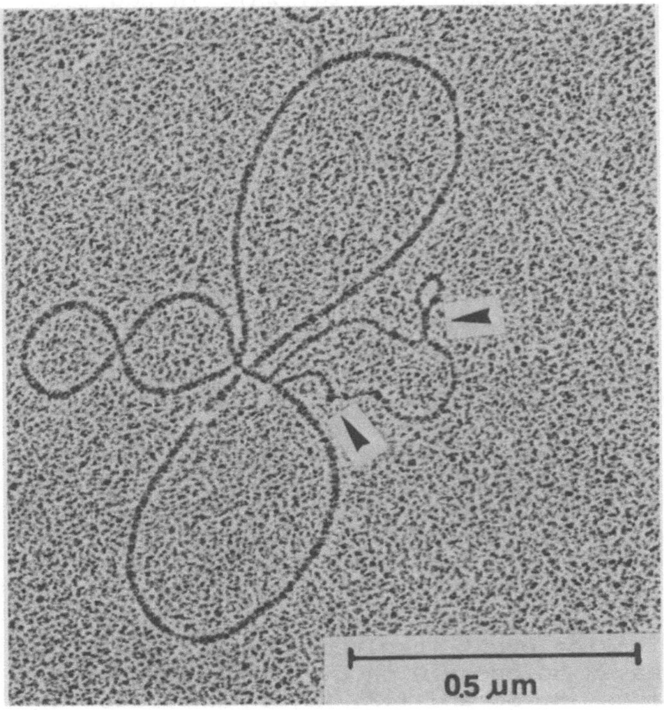

Fig. 3. Heteroduplex of cloned pilin gene loci *pil*E2 in the P^+ and P^- conformation as seen in the electron microscope. The site of pilin expression comprises a single-stranded region of 3.2 kbases in the P^+ strand of the heteroduplex. This DNA segment which is deleted in the P^- strand of the heteroduplex harbors the majority of the pilin structural gene and contains inverted sequences forming stable snapback structures in the single-stranded loop (*arrows*). The duplex is composed of one circular and one linear heterologous strand

sion locus. This new pilin sequence might be used as the basic frame for the expression of a variant pilin after the cell switches back to P^+.

Similar to the expression loci, the silent gene locus *pil*S1 harbors six characteristic pilin gene sequences (R. Haas, unpublished). These are slightly variant pilin sequences reminiscent of the central body of the pilin coding sequence in the expression locus which are missing defined 5' and 3' ends. They are arranged in tandem and interspersed by sequences that are not related to the pilin structural gene. We believe that these variant pilin gene sequences somehow participate in the formation of new expression genes. We do not know yet whether silent pilin loci just serve as pools for the reconstitution of novel variant pilin genes or whether they can be converted into expression sites themselves.

The Opacity Gene System

The strategy for cloning the gene coding for Op expression of *N. gonorrhoeae* MS11 in *E. coli* [25] was very similar to that used for the isolation of the gonococcal pilin gene. *E. coli* transformants were screened for expression of Op protein with rabbit antiserum raised against corresponding protein from *N. gonorrhoeae* MS11. The identity of the protein expressed in positive *E. coli* transformants with the Op protein from the parental MS11 strain was confirmed by digestion of the protein from both sources with *S. aureus* V8 protease and subsequent analysis of proteolytic fragments by electrophoresis.

The physical analysis of the cloned Op gene revealed an intriguing result. Next to the Op gene on the isolated fragment, we recognized one of the pilin expression loci, *pil*E1 [25]. Precise analysis showed that the Op expression site (*opa*E1) on the cloned fragment is located about 600 bp downstream of *pil* E1 and that it is transcribed in the same direction (see Fig. 2A). This was of considerable interest, since it was reported previously that in some cases of pilin variation there are simultaneous changes in the expression of Op protein [2]. Although both observations suggest a linked expression control which could provide reasonable advantage to the bacterium, the mechanism by which this could occur remains unknown.

When we probed chromosomal DNA of MS11 by filter hybridization with an Op subclone devoid of pilin gene sequences, the pattern was even more complex than that for the pilin genes [25]. At least 15 restriction fragments cross-hybridized under high stringency conditions. Interestingly, the pilin and the Op gene probes labeled different sets of bands in the filter hybridization, thus indicating that the two probes revealed unrelated gene families. It is therefore questionable if the gene systems for pilin and Op variation emerged from a common evolutionary origin.

In contrast to pilin variation, we detected no major DNA rearrangements when we hybridized the DNA from isogenic MS11 strains expressing variant Op protein (see Fig. 1) with our Op gene probe [25]. This result was obtained for several isogenic O^+ and O^- variants of strain MS11 with one exception. In the DNA of an Op variant (V28) expressing an Op protein slightly larger than the original Op protein (VO), we detected an additional Sal1 restriction site in the Op expression locus 1 (*opa*E1). In order to analyze this restriction site polymorphism in the DNAs of the MS11 variants VO and V28, we isolated an Op gene clone of variant V28 from the corresponding genomic locus. A detailed restriction analysis showed that the additional Sal1 site was located nearby or within the coding sequences of the Op gene. In addition, further restriction site alterations were found in this region of the variant gene. In Fig. 4 we show the results of a DNA sequence analysis of the heterologous area. Both sequences share common stretches and comprise a single open reading frame. The homology between the sequences is disturbed by numerous single and clustered nucleotide exchanges including a deletion

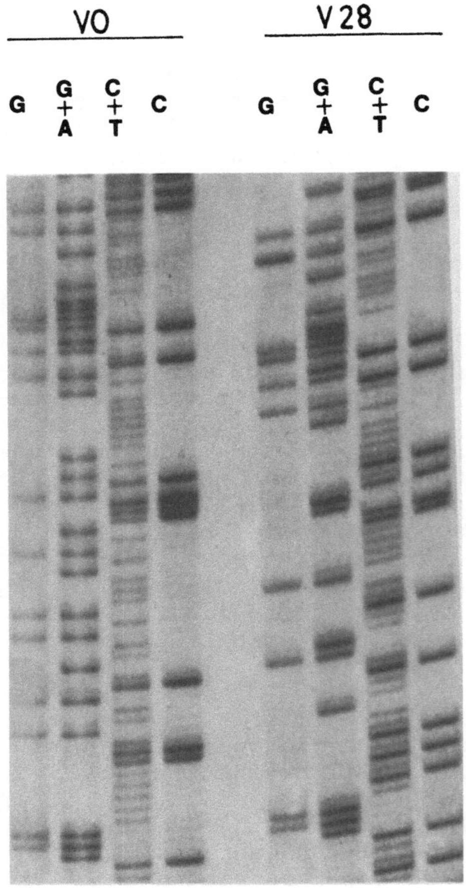

A

Fig. 4A,B. Comparison of two variant Op gene sequences. Corresponding expression loci (*opa*E1) of two variant MS11 strains (Vo and V28) were cloned in *E. coli* and shown to express altered Op proteins. DNA sequencing revealed heterologies in the coding region of both genes of which a short section is shown in the figure. (A) Maxam-Gilbert sequencing gel of VO and V28 Op segments. (B) Homologies between both sequences are indicated by *asterisks*. The reading frame of the Op genes is from left to right

```
  CTCGCTGTTATTTATAAGGCAGTCGTATTTTTTATACGCCCATGTATTTGTGTTATCGTTGTCCTTTTTGGACT   VO
  ** *******************  *******      * *  * **  * ***   ** * ** * ******
B CTTGCTGTTATTTATAAGGCAGCTGTATTTT------CTCAACCTTTTGTTCTTAGTCTTATTCTCTCTGGACT   V 28
```

(insertion) of six base pairs which does not affect the continuity of the reading frame.

In a similar approach, we compared a clone derived from an O^- MS11 variant which also failed to express Op protein in *E. coli* with our original O^+ clone [25]. The experiment was carried out by digestion of a heteroduplex between both cloned sequences by single-strand specific S1 nuclease. This enabled us to define an S1-sensitive site upstream of the putative Op coding sequence, an area we believe to harbor the promoter region of the Op gene. Therefore, minor rearrangements at the nucleotide level appear to play an important role in the regulation of Op gene expression. Whether deletion and insertion formation, as observed for the pilin genes, also can occur with the Op genes, cannot be excluded at this point. However, the sequence variations described here resemble those resulting from recombination events referred to as gene conversion.

The Gene of IgA Protease

While pilus and Op protein are cell-bound virulence factors of *N. gonorrhoeae*, IgA protease is extracellularly secreted by the bacterium [26]. It specifically degrades human IgA1 into intact Fab and Fc fragments, whereas other immunoglobulin allotypes, including IgA2, are not substrates [27, 28]. IgA proteases specific for human immunoglobulin are produced only by strictly human pathogens. Nonpathogenic species of the genus *Neisseria*, for example, and animal pathogens do not secrete the enzyme [6].

Owing to the possible involvement of IgA protease in pathogenesis, the molecular genetics of this enzyme became of substantial interest. The genes coding for IgA proteases of *N. gonorrhoeae* F62 and *H. influenzae* have been cloned in *E. coli* [29, 30]. The production and/or extracellular secretion of enzyme activity in these clones is relatively weak compared with the parental donor strains. In an effort to isolate an *E. coli* clone secreting reasonable amounts of *N. gonorrhoeae* MS11 IgA protease, we applied an enzymatic filter assay to detect IgA protease-secreting bacteria on an agar plate [31]. The assay is based on the degradation of radioactively labeled secretory IgA1 bound to a nitrocellulose filter via its secretory component. Since it is possible to introduce the majority of label into the Fab portion of the IgA1 antibody, a short incubation of the coated filter with IgA protease-producing colonies on an agar plate can remove a significant amount of radioactivity from the filter. Using this method, we were able to screen hundreds of *E. coli* transformants and to isolate a clone positive in secretion of IgA protease.

The original clone carried the IgA protease gene on a DNA fragment of 9.3 kbases [31]. This fragment could be shortened to 4.6 kbases by exonucleolytic digestion while still retaining the capacity to express and secrete IgA protease. Preliminary complementation studies of IgA protease gene fragments indicated that this minimal gene segment codes for a single independent gene product. This result was confirmed by linking this minimal gene segment to a temperature-inducible expression system (Fig. 5c,d). Upon induction, a protein of approximatly 180 kdaltons in size was produced in large quantities, indicating a contiguous open reading frame of about 4.5 kbases.

In a biochemical approach, we tried to identify the extracellular, enzymatically active IgA protease [31]. We therefore developed a procedure to purify IgA protease from culture supernatants of both *N. gonorrhoeae* MS11 and the *E. coli* hybrid clone. The procedure involved cation exchange chromatography as well as gel filtration. In all fractionation steps, a single protein of 105 kdaltons in SDS-polyacrylamide gels copurified with the activity of IgA protease. Since the same protein was obtained for both

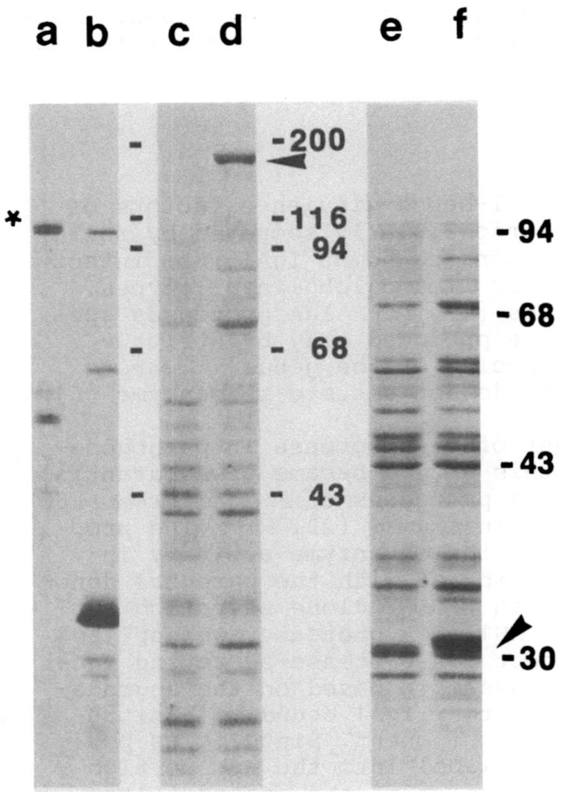

Fig. 5. Polyacrylamide gel electrophoresis of purified IgA protease and fusion proteins in total cell extracts. *Lanes a* and *b* represent IgA protease fractions purified from culture supernatants of *N. gonorrhoeae* MS11 and of the *E. coli* hybrid clone GC1 (pIP1), respectively. The protein band of 105 kdaltons present in both preparations was identified as the extracellular form of gonococcal IgA protease (*asterisk*). *Lanes c–f* represent total cell extracts of *E. coli* cells containing an expression system for protein fusions before (*c*, *e*) and after (*d*, *f*) induction. The proteins (*arrows*) of 175 kdaltons in *d* and of 31 kdaltons in *f* represent the gene products encoded by a major part of the IgA protease and the complete pilin gene, respectively. Both protein fusions carry at their NH_2 termini 10 kdaltons of unrelated protein in addition to gonococcal protein. Numbers refer to the size of protein markers (kdaltons)

preparations, we concluded that it represents the extracellular form of gonococcal IgA protease (Fig. 5a,b). An extra protein of 106 kdaltons which also copurified with the enzymatic activity in *N. gonorrhoeae* culture supernatants (Fig. 5a) was not expressed by the *E. coli* clone. Since the coding capacity of the cloned IgA protease gene exceeds the size of the recovered extracellular enzyme by about 65 kdaltons of protein, we assume that, in analogy to other secreted proteins, a considerable portion of the primary IgA protease gene product may be required for, and degraded during, the transport of the enzyme through the bacterial cell envelope.

Forthcoming Perspectives

We are using the means of gene technology to investigate the principles of antigenic variation and the expression of virulence factors of *N. gonorrhoeae*. The cloning of genes coding for pilin, Op protein, and IgA protease, and their use as labeled probes in hybridization experiments provide us with suitable tools to analyze the chromosomal organization of these genes and the mechanisms controlling their expression. For pilin and Op protein, a large number of structurally related gene copies exist, which apparently participate in the regulation of expression of variant types of these proteins. It appears that the variability of surface antigen expression involves at least two types of mechanisms: the formation of deletions and insertions at the expression loci, and the conversion of structural genes by variant gene sequences. Variant genes often differ by single and oligonucleotide exchanges as well as small insertions or deletions which maintain the reading frame of the coding sequences. We therefore believe that sophisticated mechanisms must have evolved to modulate the coding potential in distinct sections of the gene while maintaining the integrity of its reading frame and thereby the basic quality of its genetic information.

Unlike the gene systems for pilin and Op protein, the gene coding for IgA protease comprises a unique sequence in the genome of *N. gonorrhoeae*. This still does not exclude the possibility that IgA proteases are also subject to antigenic variation, although, perhaps to a lesser extent. In hybridization experiments, we found that the IgA protease genes of independent gonococcal isolates are very often structurally altered (R. Halter, unpublished). It is also known that different isolates can produce IgA proteases slightly differing in their cleavage specificity (M.H. Mulks, personal communication) and in the potential of their cloned genes to secrete active enzyme in *E. coli* [29, 31]. If one considers IgA protease as a serious factor in pathogenesis, the occasional variation of its antigenic properties could provide reasonable advantage to its function, but, since IgA protease is a soluble extracellular enzyme, an immune response directed against the enzyme does not directly affect the survival of the pathogen. This may have some bearing on the lesser complexity of the IgA protease gene system.

The cloning of *N. gonorrhoeae* virulence factors has significant potential for medical application. Pilin, as the cell component responsible for bacterial attachment to epithelial cells, represents a good candidate for the development of a vaccine for the prevention of gonorrhea ([15, 32]; G.K. Schoolnik, this volume). Despite the antigenic variability of pilin, this protein carries immunorecessive determinants which carry functions essential for the formation of the pilus structure and for hemagglutination and cell adhesion. If one removes the immunodominant portions from the pilin peptide chain, the residual common portion sequences become immunocompetent and also can be used as competitive inhibitors for pilin-specific adhesion in appropriate test systems ([15]; M. So, unpublished; G.K. Schoolnik, this volume). Since the cloning of the pilin gene provides access to its complete nucleotide sequence and variant sequences, this information provides a basis to design synthetic peptides representing common pilin determinants (M. So, unpublished). Such peptides can be used to elucidate essential functional domains of pilin and to stimulate specific immune responses against otherwise immunorecessive portions of pilin. Furthermore, the pilin gene can be used to construct genetic hybrids of the pilin gene and appropriate expression vectors (Fig. 5e,f). Such constructions produce stable fusion proteins of the constant portion of pilin and a carrier protein. These fusions combine the properties of synthetic peptides with the advantage of being synthesized in *E. coli* (H. Fiedler and T.F. Meyer, unpublished).

Another advantage of the expression of defined antigenic determinants in bacteria is their potential use in attenuated bacterial vaccination strains. To be successful, such strains may need to transport the antigenic material to the bacterial cell surface or, possibly, into the extracellular fluid. A reasonable candidate for the construction of a secretion system in gram-negative bacteria - we believe - is the gonococcal IgA protease. The gene we have isolated directs extracellular secretion of the enzyme in a number of gram-negative strains (S. Rahr and T.F. Meyer, unpublished). Our observation that IgA protease genes of independent gonococcal isolates show significant variations indicates that structural alterations in the enzyme do not necessarily affect its secretion. We therefore wonder if this gene can be manipulated in a manner that will allow the transport of antigenic determinants to the cell surface.

Acknowledgments. We wish to thank Dr. R.G. McKenzie and Dr. S. Rahr for critical comments and B. Werner for help in preparing the manuscript. These studies were supported by the National Science Foundation (PCM 823174), the Deutsche Forschungsgemeinschaft (Me 705/2-2), and the Bundesministerium für Forschung und Technologie (BCT 0364 1).

References

1. Blake MS, Gotschlich EC (1983) Gonococcal membrane proteins: speculation on their role in pathogenesis. Prog Allergy 33:298-313
2. Salit IE, Blake MS, Gotschlich EC (1980) Intra-strain heterogeneity of gonococcal pili is related to opacity colony variance. J Exp Med 151: 716-725
3. Swanson J (1978) Studies on gonococcus infection: XIV. Cell wall protein difference among colour/opacity colony variants of *Neisseria gonorrhoeae*. Infect Immun 21:292-302
4. Lambden PR, Heckels JE (1979) Outer membrane protein composition and colonial morphology of *Neisseria gonorrhoeae* strain P9. FEMS Microl Lett 5:263-265
5. Walstad DL, Guymon LF, Sparling PF (1977) Altered outer membrane protein in different colonial types of *Neisseria gonorrhoeae*. J Bacteriol 129: 1623-1627
6. Kornfeld SJ, Plaut AG (1981) Secretory immunity and the bacterial IgA proteases. Rev Infect Dis 3:521-534
7. Lambden PR, Robertson JN, Watt PJ (1980) Biological properties of two distinct pilus types produced by isogenic variance of *Neisseria gonorrhoeae* P9. J Bacteriol 141:393-396
8. Swanson J, Kraus SJ, Gotschlich EC (1971) Studies on gonococcus infection: I. Pili and zones of adhesion: their relationship to gonococcal growth patterns. J Exp Med 134:886-906
9. Kellog DS, Peacock WL, Deacon WE, Brown L, Pirkle CI (1963) *Neisseria gonorrhoeae*: I. Virulence genetically linked to colonal variation. J Bacteriol 85:1274-1279

10. Heckels JE (1981) Structural comparison of *Neisseria gonorrhoeae* outer membrane proteins. J Bacteriol 145:736-742
11. James JF, Swanson J (1978) Studies on gonococcus infection: XIII. Occurrence of colour/opacity colonial variants in clinical cultures. Infect Immun 19:332-340
12. Swanson J (1973) Studies on gonococcus infection: IV. Pili: their role in attachment of gonococci to tissue culture cells. J Exp Med 127:571-589
13. Buchanan TM (1977) Surface antigens: pili. In: Roberts RB (ed) The Gonococcus. Wiley, New York, pp 255-272
14. McGee ZA, Stephens DS, Hoffmann LH, Schlech III WF, Horn RG (1983) Mechanisms of mucosal invasion by pathogenic *Neisseria*. Reviews of Infectious Diseases 5, Suppl 4:708-714
15. Schoolnik GK, Tai JY, Gotschlich EC (1983) A pilus peptide vaccine for the prevention of gonorrhea. Prog Allergy 33:314-331
16. Meyer TF, Billyard E, Haas R, Störzbach S, So M (1984) Pilus genes of *Neisseria gonorrhoeae*: Chromosomal organization and DNA sequence. Proc Natl Acad Sci USA 81:6110-6114
17. Lambden PR, Heckels JE, James LT, Watt PJ (1979) Variations in surface protein composition associated with virulence properties in opacity types of *Neisseria gonorrhoeae*. Gen Microbiol 114:305-312
18. James JF, Lammel CJ, Draper DL, Brooks GF (1980) Attachment of *Neisseria gonorrhoeae* phenotype variants to eukaryotic cells and tissues. In: Danielson D, Normark S (eds) Genetics and immunobiology of pathogenic neisseria. University of Umea, Sweden, pp 213-216
19. Watt PJ, Ward ME (1981) Adherence of *Neisseria gonorrhoeae* and other *Neisseria* species to mammalian cells. In: Beachey E (ed) Bacterial adherence. Chapman and Hall, New York, pp 255-288
20. Swanson J (1980) ^{125}I-labeled peptide mapping of some heat-modifiable proteins of the gonococcal outer membrane. Infect Immun 28:54-64
21. Swanson J, Barrera O (1983) Immunological characteristics of gonococcal outer membrane protein II assessed by immunoprecipitation, immunoblotting, and coagglutination. J Exp Med 157:1405-1420
22. Russell RBR, Johnson KG, McDonald IJ (1975) Envelope proteins in *Neisseria*. Can J Microbiol 21:1519-1534
23. Lambden PR (1982) Biochemical comparison of pili from variants of *Neisseria gonorrhoeae* P9. J Gen Microbiol 128:2105-2111
24. Meyer TF, Mlawer N, So M (1982) Pilus expression in *Neisseria gonorrhoeae* involves chromosomal rearrangement. Cell 30:45-52
25. Stern A, Nickel P, Meyer TF, So M (1984) Opacity determinants of *Neisseria gonorrhoeae*: DNA sequence alterations associated with gene expression and chromosomal linkage to the gonococcal pilus gene. Cell 37:447-456
26. Plaut AG, Gilbert JV, Artenstein MS, Capra JD (1975) *Neisseria gonorrhoeae* and *Neisseria meningitidis*: Extracellular enzyme cleaves human immunoglobulin A, Science 190:1103-1105
27. Plaut AG, Gilbert JV, Wistar R Jr (1977) Loss of antibody activity in human immunoglobulin A exposed to extracellular immunoglobulin A proteases of *Neisseria gonorrhoeae* and *Streptococcus sanguis*. Infect Immun 17:130-135
28. Mulks HM, Kornfeld SJ, Plaut AG (1980) Specific proteolysis of human IgA by *Streptococcus pneumoniae* and *Haemophilus influenzae*. J Infect Dis 141:450-456
29. Koomey JM, Gill RE, Falkow S (1982) Genetic and biochemical analysis of gonococcal IgA1 protease: Cloning in *Escherichia coli* and construction of mutants of gonococci that fail to produce the activity. Proc Natl Acad Sci USA 79:7881-7885

30. Bricker J, Mulks MH, Plaut AG, Moxon ER, Wright A (1983) IgA1 proteases of *Haemophilus influenzae*: Cloning and characterization in *Escherichia coli* K-12. Proc Natl Acad Sci USA 80:2681-2685
31. Halter R, Pohlner J, Meyer TF (1984) IgA-protease of *Neisseria gonorrhoeae*: Isolation and characterization of the gene and its extracellular product. EMBO J 3:1595-1601
32. Brinton CC, Bryon J, Dillon JA, Guerina N, Jakobson LJ, Kraus S, Labik A, Lee S, Levence A, Lim S, McMichael J, Polen S, Rogers K, To ACC, To SCM (1978) Uses of pili in gonorrhoeae control: role of bacterial pili in disease, purification and properties of gonococcal pili, and progress in the development of a gonococcal pilus vaccine for gonorrhea. In: Brooks, Gotschlich, Holmes, Sawyer, Young (eds) Immunobiology of *Neisseria gonorrhoeae*. American Society for Microbiology, Washington, pp 155-178

Bayer-Symposium VIII
The Pathogenesis of Bacterial Infections, 235-245 (1985)

Clonal Polymorphism of Surface Antigens in a Relapsing Fever *Borrelia* Species

A. G. Barbour

Summary

Borrelia hermsii, the agent of relapsing fever, manifests an extensive antigenic repertoire during infection of a host. Abundant, trypsin-releasable proteins at the surface of the spirochete confer serotype specificity on each organism. These serotype-specific, or pI, proteins differ in apparent molecular weight, in structure as assessed by peptide mapping, and in activities with polyclonal and monoclonal antibodies. There is evidence for some conserved structure also; one of the monoclonal antibodies reacts with pI proteins from two or five serotypes examined. The biology of *B. hermsii* in both the mouse host and in synthetic medium, and the uniqueness of its surface proteins suggest that isogenic populations of *Borrelia* are polymorphic with respect to the pI proteins and that each pI protein represents a different allele.

Introduction

Most bacteriologists have observed sectored bacterial colonies on a culture plate. If one streaks a small portion of the phenotypically different sector onto a fresh plate, one usually discovers sectored colonies on the new plate as well. Always starting from an apparently pure inoculum, the researcher could repeat this maneuver several times in succession and always observe a predictable frequency of colonies that were either sectored or entirely the alternate phenotype. If growth conditions, such as medium constituents or temperature, are changed, the bacteriologist may find that the originally less frequent phenotype has become the predominant one. The environment can determine the representation of each trait.

Such reversible changes in state by bacteria are generally termed phase variation. Phase variation is most commonly noted to be between two different phenotypes on solid medium and, therefore, could also be called colony-type dimorphism. Visually distinctive examples of such dimorphisms are the choices between light and dark colonies of the bioluminescent marine bacterium, *Vibrio harveyi* [17, 24] and between pigmented and nonpigmented colonies of *Serratia marcescens* [10].

Some pathogenic bacteria are also dimorphic with respect to phenotypes easily discernible on culture plates or with antisera. In many cases, the morphological or serologic phenotypes have been identified or correlated with virulence factors or major surface antigens. One such phase variation, and the one whose mechanism of switching is best understood at a molecular level, involves the H flagellar antigen alleles of *Salmonella typhimurium* [20, 30, 32]. Other examples of phase variation among pathogenic bacteria are the colony morphologies of *Bordetella pertussis* [18], type 1 pili of *Escherichia coli* [9, 13], and, acting independently [35], the pili [19, 28] and colony opacities [34] of *Neisseria gonorrhoeae*.

While there are many examples of dimorphisms, instances of clonal polymorphisms [31], i.e., the presence of more than two alleles in a population derived from a single cell, have been less frequently observed in species of bacteria and other unicellular organisms. A situation where such polymorphisms have been found was, as Beale predicted, "...in microbes parasitic on a higher organism in which the host defense mechanisms involve the production of specific antibodies" [7]. Two of the more striking examples of pathogens which "developed" polymorphisms in their antigens as a response to host antibodies are salivarian trypanosomes and relapsing fever *Borrelia* species.

Salivarian trypanosomes, the agents of sleeping sickness in humans and other mammals, are protozoa. Populations of trypanosomes in the host manifest sequential changes in their surface antigens, thus avoiding final immune clearance. The extensive antigenic repertoire in trypanosomes is generated through gene duplications and genome rearrangements [8, 16, 25, 36].

Our knowledge of the mechanism of antigenic variation in *Borrelia* is comparatively meager, although it has been recognized for half a century that spirochetes recovered during the first fever relapse differed antigenically both from the original infecting serotype and from the borreliae isolated from subsequent relapses [11, 14, 23, 27, 29]. More recently, however, Stoenner and colleagues at the Rocky Mountain Laboratories reported the the isolation from the progeny of a single *Borrelia hermsii* organism at least 24 different serotypes [33]. The frequency of spontaneous appearance of new serotypes in populations growing in mice was estimated to be 10^{-3}-10^{-4} per cell per generation [33]. Although any of the 24 serotypes (25 including an additional isolate, 7 × 16, that reacted with two antisera) may occur during the first relapse of spirochetemia in mice, a few serotypes predominate [4, 33] (Fig. 1).

This collection of isogenic serotypes provided a resource for our studies of the variable antigens of *B. hermsii* [4, 5] and of in vitro variation [3]. The variable antigens are abundant proteins of the spirochete's outer membrane. For the most part, the variable proteins, hereafter called pI proteins, are antigenically and structurally distinct from each other. However, there is evidence of structure that is shared between some pI proteins.

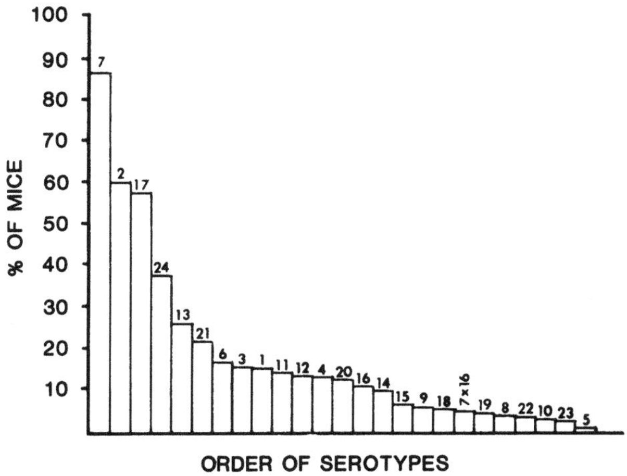

Fig. 1. Distribution of serotypes of *B. hermsii* HS1 among 230 mice undergoing first relapses. Each of serotypes 1-24 were inoculated into groups of mice. On the sixth and seventh days after inoculation, blood samples from the mice were examined with an IFA as to their borrelial populations. Detailed procedures and results are given in references [3] and [33]. The means of the percentages for each of the 24 serotypes are given. Serotype 7 was the most frequent serotype; 87% of mice undergoing relapse had detectable concentrations of this serotype; 7 × 16 was a new serotype that reacted with both anti-serotype 7 and anti-serotype 16 sera

Materials and Methods

Organisms and Culture Conditions

The origin of the HS1 strain (ATCC 35209) of *B. hermsii* and the isolation of 24 numbered serotypes of this strain from mice have been described previously [33]. The lettered serotypes, C and Y, were isolated during in vitro cultivation of HS1. Serotype C (culture) was found in culture tubes after several passages of serotype 7; antigenically identical organisms were also recovered from multipassaged populations of serotypes 1, 3, 14, and 21 [4, 33]. Serotype Y was isolated from a population of serotype 21 organisms that had been passed in medium containing rabbit antiserum to serotype C [3].

The borreliae were cultivated in mice and broth medium essentially as described previously [5]. Exceptions were an X-irradiation dosage per mouse of 650 rad instead of 900 rad and the use of BSK II medium [2] for the broth cultivations. Cultures were harvested, assessed as to homogeneity of serotype, and stored frozen as described previously [4, 5].

Production of Hybridomas

For the majority of hybridomas reported here, the mouse immunization schedule was as follows: frozen suspensions of spirochetes were thawed, centrifuged, and resuspended in phosphate-buffered saline, pH 7.4, with 5 m*M* $MgCl_2$ (PBS/Mg). BALB/c mice (6 weeks old; Rocky Mountain Laboratories substrain) were each inoculated intraperitoneally with approximately 10^8 borreliae on day 0. On day three, after peak spirochetemia followed by immune-mediated clearance of the spirochetes had occurred, the mice were begun on oral tetracycline hydrochloride (0.5 mg per milliliter drinking water) to prevent emergence of new serotypes [33]. The antibiotic was continued until day 13. On day 21, the mice were inoculated intravenously with the same inoculum and the same serotype of borreliae as on day 0. On day 24, the mice were killed and their spleens were removed. The remaining steps in the production of hybridomas through fusions of the spleen cells with derivatives of NS1 myeloma cells have been described [4]. The hybridomas were usually cloned by limiting dilution, but in some cases cloning was done in semisolid medium by the method of Davis et al. [12].

In the alternative immunization protocol, a spirochete suspension in PBS/Mg was emulsified in Freund's complete adjuvant and injected intraperitoneally into mice on day 0. The spirochete inocula were approximately 10^8 per mouse. The mice were boosted with live organisms on day 21 and killed on day 24 as described.

The supernatant fluids of the hybridomas were screened by indirect immunofluorescence assay (IFA) [6] and also by a solid-phase radioimmunoassay [6]. In a modification of the method for use with whole cells, 10 µl of a suspension of spirochetes in PBS/Mg (approximately 10^9 cells/ml) was applied to 6.4-mm diameter discs of Whatman 540 filter paper. The discs were dried at 42°C, fixed for 30 min in methanol, dried again, and stored at 4°C. In the assay itself, the discs were placed in microtiter plate wells, blocked with a solution of bovine albumin, incubated with hybridoma supernatant, washed, and probed for bound immunoglobulin G with radioiodinated protein A, as described previously [6].

Protease Treatment of Spirochetes

Spirochetes were thawed, washed three times with PBS/Mg, and resuspended in this buffer at a concentration of approximately 2×10^9 cells/ml. In a Microfuge tube, the cell suspensions were incubated with trypsin (50 µg/ml; Sigma Chemical Company, St. Louis, Missouri), Pronase (2.5 µg/ml; Calbiochem-Behring Corporation, La Jolla, California), or no protease. After incubation of the cells with enzyme for 30 min at room temperature, proteolysis was stopped by the addition of phenylmethylsulfonylfluoride (1 mg/ml, final concentration; Sigma). Four volumes PBS/Mg were added to the tube, and the suspension was centrifuged for 4 min in a Microfuge (Beckman Instruments, Incorporated, Fullerton, California). After removal of the supernatant, the pellet was suspended in sample buffer for polyacrylamide gel electrophoresis (PAGE).

PAGE and Western Blotting

Whole cell lysates of the spirochetes were subjected to PAGE under conditions previously described [4]. An exception was the use in some gels of a separating gel containing an acrylamide: bisacrylamide ratio of 30:0.1 instead of 30:0.8. In all gels, the pH of the separating gel buffer was 8.6. The Western blot procedure was also essentially that previously described [6]. In the present study, however, the solvent for the blocking step, the antibody and protein A incubations, and the washes was 50 m*M* Tris (pH 7.5)-150 m*M* NaCl-5 m*M* EDTA-0.05% Tween 20 (TSE/Tween). Hybridoma supernatants were diluted 1:10.

Results and Discussion

A Coomassie blue-stained PAGE gel of serotypes C, Y, 21, 7, and 14 is shown in Fig. 2. The apparent subunit molecular weights of the variable pI proteins of the five serotypes were 21, 23, 36, 38, and 39 $\times 10^3$, respectively, when compared with the migrations of the molecular weight standards. The other major protein in the lysates had an apparent molecular weight of 41 $\times 10^3$ in each of the serotypes. This protein has been designated the pII protein [4]. The electrophoretic migrations of the pI proteins relative to the pII protein and also to each other vary with the pH of the separating gel buffer [4] and also the amount of cross-linking of acrylamide in the gel. The apparent molecular weights of the lettered, in vitro-derived serotypes were considerably smaller than those of the numbered, mouse-derived serotypes. There were also minor differences between serotypes in the lower molecular weight proteins. For instance, serotype 7 and 14 lysates had proteins of approximately 15 000 molecular weight that were not seen in the lysates of the other three serotypes.

Past studies showed that polyclonal and monoclonal antibodies which are serotype-specific as assessed by immunofluorescence bind only to the homologous pI proteins in Western blots [4]. The monoclonal antibodies employed in these previous studies were IgM molecules appearing during the early phase of clearance of the infecting spirochetes. We have since raised IgG monoclonal antibodies by boosting the mice with a second dose of the homologous serotype three weeks after the initial infection. Tetracycline administration prevented relapses with other serotypes between the two immunizations. The patterns of reactivities of four of the monoclonal antibodies obtained as a result of this immunization protocol are shown in Fig. 3. The results of both IFA and Western blot assays are given. In the IFA, a 3+ (out of a possible 3) reaction was seen only when a monoclonal antibody was incubated with the serotype against which it was raised. In all cases of hybridomas derived from "natural" infections, i.e., those in which an initial spirochetemia was produced by intraperitoneal injection of live organisms without an adjuvant, monoclonal antibodies which were serotype specific by IFA bound to the homologous, but not heterologous pI proteins in Western blots. These reactions are exemplified by monoclonal antibodies H4825, H9326, and H9245 (Fig. 3).

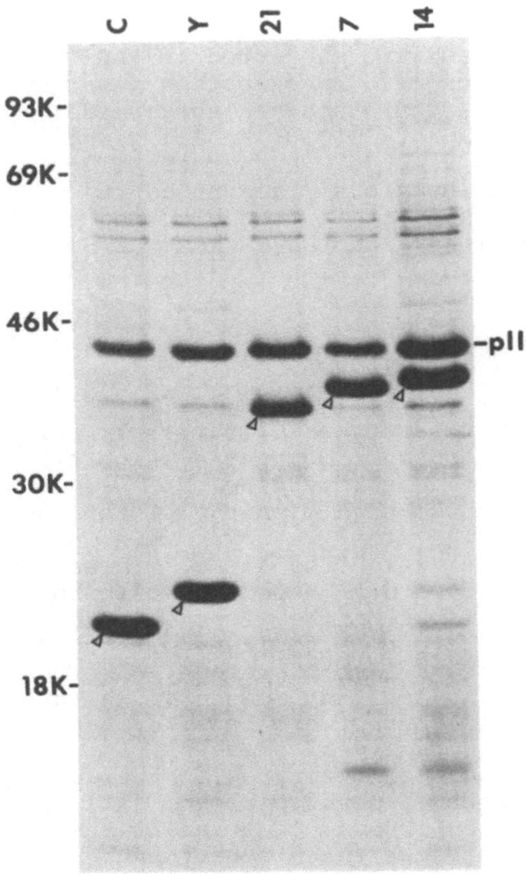

Fig. 2. Coomassie blue-stained PAGE gels of *B. hermsii* HS1 serotypes C, Y, 21, 7, and 14. The location of the variable pI protein in each serotype is indicated by the *open triangles*. The pII proteins have the same apparent molecular weight in each serotype. The acrylamide concentration in the separating gel was 15% (acrylamide:bisacrylamide 30:0.1). The molecular weight standards, the migrations of which are shown at the left, are phosphorylase B (93 000), bovine albumin (69 000), ovalbumin (46 000), carbonic anhydrase (30 000), and β-lactoglobulin (18 000)

During the course of screening, we found a few antibodies that reacted weakly by IFA with all serotypes examined. An example of one of these monoclonal antibodies is H9826 (see Fig. 3). This antibody was found by Western blot to react with a protein with the same electrophoretic migration as the invariable pII proteins. Subsequent studies have shown that the pII proteins are associated with the axial filaments (periplasmic flagellae) of the spirochetes (A.G. Barbour, R. Heiland, S.F. Hayes, manuscript in preparation). I assume the drying and methanol fixation of the spirochetes allowed access of H9826 to the axial filaments within the cell and thus resulted in the observed immunofluorescence. There is no evidence for a surface exposure of pII proteins in situ [4, 5].

The PAGE protein profiles and the reactivities of the serotype-specific antibodies in the Western blots indicated that a change in serotype is synonymous with a change in pI protein and that a borrelia's uniqueness in a crowd of its siblings is determined by its pI protein. Further indication of the critical role of these proteins in antigenic variation came from determinations

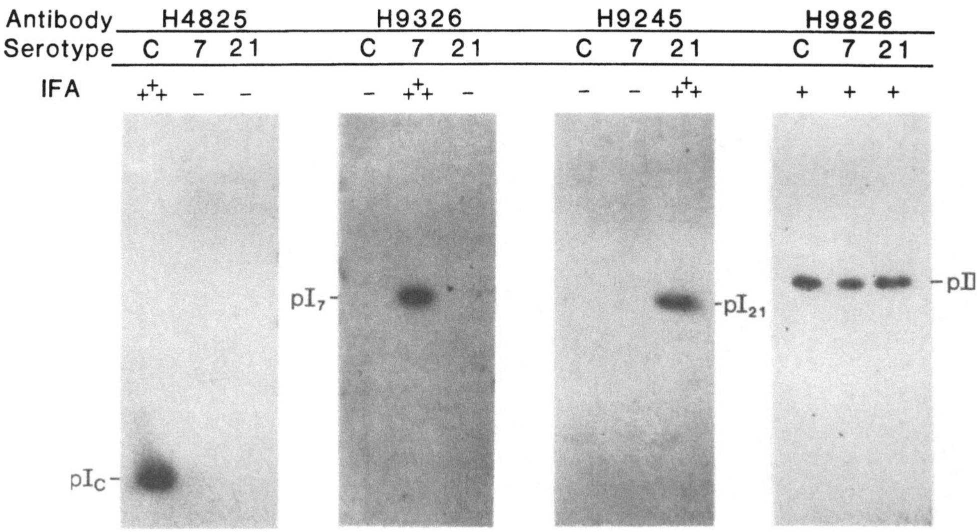

Fig. 3. Western blot (WB) and IFA reactions of four anti-borrelial IgG monoclonal antibodies. Antibodies H4825, H9326, H9245, and H9826 were examined by IFA for binding with methanol-fixed spirochetes of *B. hermsii* HS1 serotypes C, 7, and 21, and by WB for reactivies with serotype C, 7, and 21 components separated by PAGE. The IFA reactions were graded on a 0-3 scale. The location of pI_C, pI_7, pI_{21}, and pII proteins in the blots are shown. The acrylamide concentration was 10% (acrylamide:bisacrylamide 30:0.8)

of the location of the pI proteins in the cell. A simple-minded view of the relapse phenomenon is that the borreliae change their "coats" between fever peaks. Thus, a candidate variable antigen should have evidence of being on the surface of the cell. That this is a characteristic of the pI proteins was indicated by the preferential radiolabeling of these proteins with iodine under surface-specific labeling conditions [4, 5]. Additional evidence was provided by experiments in which intact spirochetes were exposed to the proteases trypsin and Pronase. The result of an experiment with serotype 21 is shown in Fig. 4. Both trypsin and Pronase effectively removed pI_{21} from the gel. While trypsin apparently did not affect other proteins, Pronase's cleavage of a higher molecular weight protein yielded a smaller fragment that was still associated with the cellular fraction in the pellet. Similar results were obtained with serotype 7 (data not shown). The association of the epitope recognized by the serotype 21-specific monoclonal antibody H10121 and the abundant protein cleaved by the proteases is shown by the Western blot on the right-hand side of Fig. 4.

Accepting at this point the probability that the pI proteins solely provide for serotype specificity, we arrive at the important question of how one pI protein is replaced by another. As discussed in a past report, there are several possible mechanisms by which this event could happen [5]. The hypothesis

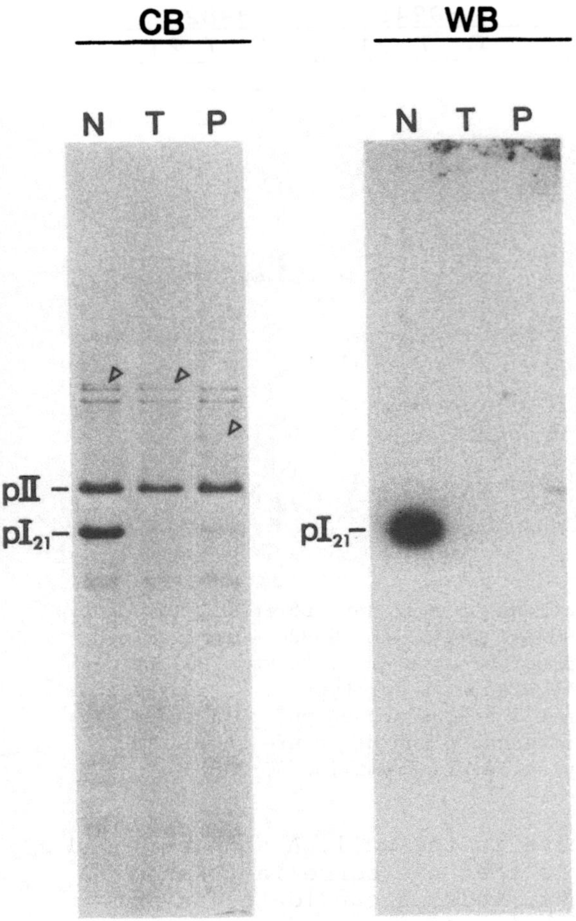

Fig. 4

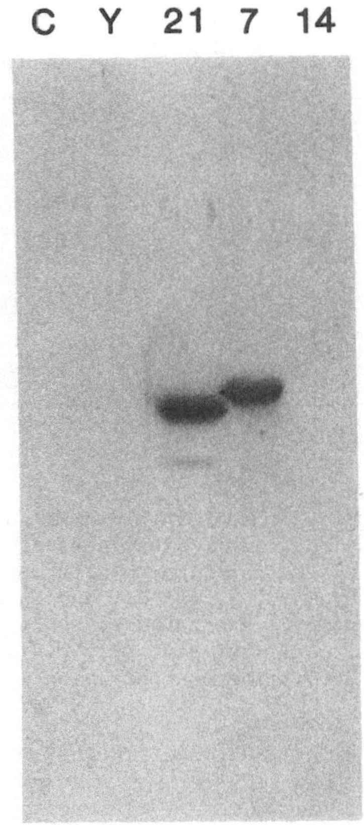

Fig. 5

Fig. 4. PAGE and Western blot (WB) analyses of protease-treated cells of *B. hermsii* HS1 serotype 21. Intact spirochetes were incubated with trypsin (T), Pronase (P), or no protease (N). Following removal of the protease and any released peptides, the cells were pelleted and subjected to PAGE and WB. The Coomassie blue (CB)-stained proteins are shown on the left. The *open triangles* indicate a protein which is present in untreated and trypsin-treated cells, but apparently cleaved to a smaller fragment by Pronase. In the WB (right), the cellular components were reacted with the serotype 21-specific monoclonal antibody H10121. The acrylamide concentration was 15% (acrylamide:bisacrylamide 30:0.1)

Fig. 5. Western blot reactions of monoclonal antibody H12135 with components of *B. hermsii* HS1 serotypes C, Y, 21, 7, and 14. The antibody bound only to the pI proteins of serotypes 21 and 7. There is also a minor band below the major band (pI_{21}) in the serotype 21 lysate. The acrylamide concentration was 12.5% (acrylamide:bisacrylamide 30:0.8)

spectrum runs from simple point mutations in a single gene to site-specific recombinations to a "cassette" model. The latter mechanism occurs with yeast mating types [15] and with trypanosomal variant antigens [16, 25, 36]. There is effectively a different gene for each protein, and only one gene (the "cassette") is expressed (in the "player") at a time.

Our previous studies, which employed both one- and two-dimensional peptide mapping procedures, showed that there were structural differences between the pI proteins of serotypes C, 7, and 21 [5]. This finding was not very surprising to us, knowing the near exclusiveness of antibody reactivities for these proteins. These results indicated to us that antigenic variation would probably not be explained by evoking one or a few mutations during the serotypic changeover. Rather, the evidence suggests that either there is a different gene for each protein or there are extensive rearrangements of whole or portions of genes at one or a few loci. However, even assuming that there is a different gene for each pI protein, we had no reason not to expect to find some relatedness between the different pI genes or their products. Indeed, this would be the case if variant genes arose through gene duplications and divergent genes shared conserved regions. Regions of homology have been documented in variant antigen genes of *T. brucei* [1, 21, 26].

Antibody H12135, which is the product of a hybridoma derived from a mouse immunized with serotype 7 borreliae in complete Freund's adjuvant, revealed that there are epitopes common to serotypes 7 and 21. I found that this monoclonal antibody reacted with both serotypes 7 and 21 by IFA. Similar results were obtained with Western blots: H12135 bound to both pI_7 and pI_{21} (Fig. 5). In contrast, there were no detectable cross-reactivities with serotypes C, Y, or 14 by this assay. The immunization protocol cannot be considered one that mimicked a "natural" infection, but, because of differences in processing of the antigens, it may have improved the chances for isolating antibodies that recognized cross-reactive epitopes in pI_7 and pI_{21}. Whether the epitopes themselves are determined by the primary structure of the protein remains to be determined, but amino acid sequencing has revealed that between the pI_7 and pI_{21} proteins there are some homologous stretches of amino acid sequence (P.A. Barstad, J. Coligan, A.G. Barbour, submitted for publication).

It may be presumptuous to apply the terms "polymorphism" and "allele" to a prokaryote which is undoubtedly haploid. Nevertheless, when confronted with the diversity of gene products that are clonally expressed in an otherwise isogenic population of borreliae, one might at this point appropriately use terminology originally relating to population genetics of higher organisms.

Acknowledgments. I thank Sandy Tessier and Merry Schrumpf for expert technical assistance, Joe Meier and Paul Barstad for advice, Susan Smaus for preparation of the manuscript, Bob Evans and Chuck Taylor for photographic assistance, Herb Stoenner for teaching me borrelial lore, and John Swanson for encouragement.

References

1. Barbet F, McGuire TC (1978) Cross reacting determinants in variant-specific surface antigens of Africa trypanosomes. Proc Natl Acad Sci USA 75:1989-1993
2. Barbour AG (1984) Isolation and cultivation of Lyme disease spirochetes. Yale J Biol Med 57:521-525
3. Barbour AG, Stoenner HG (1984) Antigenic variation of *Borrelia hermsii*. In: Herskowitz I, Simon M (eds) Genome rearrangement. Liss, New York (UCLA Symposia on Molecular and Cellular Biology, New Series, vol 20)
4. Barbour AG, Tessier SL, Stoenner HG (1982) Variable major proteins of *Borrelia hermsii*. J Exp Med 156:1312-1324
5. Barbour AG, Barrera O, Judd R (1983) Structural analysis of the variable major proteins of *Borrelia hermsii*. J Exp Med 158:2127-2140
6. Barbour AG, Tessier SL, Todd WJ (1983) Lyme disease spirochetes and ixodid tick spirochetes share a common surface antigenic determinant defined by a monoclonal antibody. Infect Immun 41:795-804
7. Beale GH (1961) Antigenic variation in unicellular organisms. Ann Rev Microbiol 15:263-296
8. Borst P, Cross GAM (1982) Molecular basis for trypanosome antigenic variation. Cell 29:291-303
9. Brinton CC (1959) Non-flagellar appendages of bacteria. Nature 183: 782-786
10. Bunting MI (1940) A description of some color variants produced by *Serratia marcescens*, strain 274. J Bacteriol 40:57-68
11. Coffey EM, Eveland WC (1967) Experimental relapsing fever initiated by *Borrelia hermsii*: II. Sequential appearance of major serotypes in the rat. J Infect Dis 117:29-34
12. Davis JM, Pennington JE, Kubler AM, Conscience JF (1982) A simple, single step technique for selecting and cloning hybridomas for the production of monoclonal antibodies. J Immunol Methods 50:161-171
13. Eisenstein BI (1981) Phase variation of type 1 fimbriae in *Escherichia coli*. Science 214:337-339
14. Geigy R, Burgdorfer W (1951) Unterschiedliches Verhalten verschiedener Stämme von *Spirochaeta duttoni* in der weißen Maus. Acta Trop (Basel) 8: 151-154
15. Hicks JB, Strathern JN, Herskowitz I (1977) The cassette model of mating type interconversion. In: Bukhar A, Shapiro J, Adhya S (eds) DNA insertion elements, plasmids, and episomes. Cold Spring Harbor, New York, pp 457-462
16. Hoeijmakers JHJ, Frasch ACC, Bernards A, Borst P, Cross GAM (1980) Novel expression-linked copies of the genes for variant surface antigens in trypanosomes. Nature 284:78-80
17. Keynan A, Hastings JW (1961) The isolation and characterization of dark mutants of luminescent bacteria. Biol Bull (Woods Hole, Mass) 121:375
18. Lacey BW (1960) Antigenic modulation of *Bordetella pertussis*. J Hyg (Lond) 58:57-93
19. Lambden PR, Robertson JN, Watt PJ (1980) Biological properties of two distinct pilus types produced by isogenic variants of *Neisseria gonorrhoeae* P9. J Bacteriol 141:393-396
20. Lederberg J, Iino T (1956) Phase variation in Salmonella. Genetics 41: 743-757
21. Majumber HK, Boothroyd JC, Weber H (1981) Homologous 3'-terminal regions of mRNAs for surface antigens of different antigenic variants of *Trypanosoma brucei*. Nucleic Acids Res 9:4745-4753

22. Matthysses G, Michiels F, Hamers R, Pays E, Steinert M (1981) Two variant surface glycoproteins of *Trypanosoma brucei* have a conserved C-terminus. Nature 293:230-233
23. Meleney HE (1928) Relapse phenomena of *Spironema recurrentis*. J Exp Med 48:65-82
24. Nealson KH, Hastings JW (1979) Bacterial bioluminescence: its control and ecological significance. Microbiol Rev 43:496-518
25. Pays E, Van Meirvenne N, Le Ray D, Steinert M (1981) Gene duplication and transposition linked to antigenic variation in *Trypanosoma brucei*. Proc Natl Acad Sci USA 78:2673-2677
26. Rice-Ficht AC, Chen KK, Donelson JE (1981) Sequence homologies near the C-termini of the variable surface glycoproteins of *Trypanosoma brucei*. Nature 294:53-57
27. Russell H (1936) Observations of immunity in relapsing fever and trypanosomiasis. Trans R Soc Trop Med Hyg 30:179-190
28. Salit IE, Blake M, Gotschlich EC (1980) Intra-strain heterogeneity of gonococcal pili is related to opacity colony variance. J Exp Med 151: 716-725
29. Schuhardt VT, Wilkerson M (1951) Relapse phenomena in rats infected with single spirochetes (*Borrelia recurrentis* var. *turicatae*). J Bacteriol 62:215-219
30. Silverman M, Zieg J, Hilmen M, Simon M (1979) Phase variation in *Salmonella*: genetic analysis of a recombinational switch. Proc Natl Acad Sci USA 76:391-395
31. Simon MI, Silverman M (1984) Recombinational regulation of gene expression in bacteria. Ann Rev Genet 18
32. Stocker BAD (1949) Measurements of rate of mutation of flagellar antigenic phase in *Salmonella typhimurium*. J Hyg (Lond) 47:398-413
33. Stoenner HG, Dodd T, Larsen C (1982) Antigenic variation of *Borrelia hermsii*. J Exp Med 156:1297-1311
34. Swanson J (1978) Studies on gonococcus infection: XII. Colony color opacity variants of gonococci. Infect Immun 19:320-331
35. Swanson J, Barrera O (1983) Gonococcal pilus subunit size heterogeneity correlates with transitions in colony piliation phenotype, not with changes in colony opacity. J Exp Med 158:1459-1472
36. Williams RO, Young JR, Majiwa PAO (1979) Genomic rearrangements correlated with antigenic variation in *Trypanosoma brucei*. Nature 282:847-849

Discussion

(pp. 221-245)

Variations in the pilus-type expression which occur in the progenies of a given organism are often associated with changes in the ligand receptor interaction. This appears to be true also for the opacity proteins (protein II) which influence the attachment of the organism to mucosal surfaces. Such alterations in the expression of proteins can be detected in culture, as demonstrated by Heckels by the isolation of isogenic pilus variants, as well as in the infected host. Considering the possible role of this surface protein variability, it seems that the organism requires different surface components at different stages in the pathogenic process.

An intriguing observation which was made during the culturing of gonococcal strains is that clinical isolates and even isogenic variants of laboratory strains vary their colonial morphologies with different frequencies. The ability to create new surface proteins with variant characteristics within a short period of growth may not be intrinsically related to virulence, but rather provides the organism with the opportunity of greater adaptability. Changes in the colonial morphology can be observed of the order of 10^{-7} to 10^{-2}.

On the molecular level, deletions and insertions could be observed in the expression sites of the pilus gene. There are also switching events in the pilus system which are not associated with major rearrangements. Such minor changes are also found for variations in the opacity genes. Apparently, these latter recombination events (gene conversions) occur with higher frequencies than deletions and insertions. Thus, the differences in the frequencies of gonococcal surface variability may rely on the differences of the molecular mechanisms involved in the variation.

Antigenic variation in *Borrelia* shows formal similarities with that of trypanosomes. This organism seems to express its surface proteins in a pronounced order. The question was raised if the surface proteins of *Borrelia* have functional properties, for example porin-like functions, besides their obvious involvement in antigenic masquerade.

Bayer-Symposium VIII
The Pathogenesis of Bacterial Infections, 247-256 (1985)

The Role of the Cell Surface Components of *Pseudomonas aeruginosa* in Virulence

R. E. W. Hancock

Summary

A variety of roles in virulence, both direct and indirect, can be ascribed to the outer membrane components of *Pseudomonas aeruginosa*. These include the endotoxic nature of *Pseudomonas* lipopolysaccharide (LPS) owing to a lipid A region which cross-reacts antigenically with other gram-negative lipid As. In addition, LPS composition has a direct influence on serum susceptibility of *P. aeruginosa*. A variety of outer membrane proteins are mitogenic for murine B lymphocytes and immunogenic in both animals and humans. Presumably, these properties could be involved in modulation of virulence. A major role in the virulence of *P. aeruginosa* in antibiotic-treated humans is afforded by the low outer membrane permeability and consequent intrinsic antibiotic resistance of this organism. Some of these properties have now been manipulated to provide new methods of anti-pseudomonal therapy.

Introduction

In the past few years, considerable attention has been focused on the role of extracellular products and excreted cellular components as virulence determinants for gram-negative bacteria. For example, Young [33] summarized work describing no fewer than 15 different excreted products implicated as virulence factors in *Pseudomonas aeruginosa* pathogenicity. However, if we take the broadest definition of pathogenicity, that is, the ability of a bacterium to grow in a host and produce sufficient quantities of toxic or harmful products to cause damage to the host, it becomes clear that many different cellular components can be defined as virulence factors. In particular, cell surface (outer membrane) components are important since they are involved in primary interactions with the host immune system and have also been implicated in resistance to the serum bactericidal response, to phagocytosis, and to antibiotics (which could be considered the major handicap to the growth of a gram-negative bacterium in a human host). In this paper, I will expand on this concept with specific reference to our own research on *P. aeruginosa*.

In the past 30 years, *P. aeruginosa* has emerged as a primary opportunistic pathogen in immunocompromised patients. It is now recognized as one of the three major causative agents of gram-negative septicemia in North America [34]. In patients who develop *P. aeruginosa* bacteremia, the onset of disease can be rapid and often leads to death [34]. *Pseudomonas* is also the major pathogen associated with chronic and fatal lung disease in patients with cystic fibrosis. In these clinical situations, two factors are of major importance, the failure of the host immune system to counteract the bacterial infection (which may be caused, in part, by the fact that some of these patients are immunocompromised) and the poor success of antimicrobial chemotherapy. In each case, the cell surface (outer) membrane is of major importance.

P. aeruginosa, being a gram-negative bacterium, has two cell envelope membranes separated by a single layer of peptidoglycan [26]. The outer membrane is an asymmetric bilayer containing phospholipids on the inner leaflet of the outer membrane and lipopolysaccharide (LPS) as the major lipidic molecule of the outer (cell surface) monolayer. LPS is an amphiphilic molecule containing a hydrophobic region (lipid A, also known as endotoxin) which has five or six fatty acids linked to diglucosamine phosphate. Covalently attached to this is the rough oligosaccharide core containing in its proximal portion an unusual sugar, 2-keto-3-deoxyoctanate (KDO), as well as a variety of heptose and hexose residues [26]. The rough oligosaccharide core may be substituted with a variable number of repeated trisaccharide to pentasaccharide units called the O-antigen [26].

In addition to LPS and phospholipids, the *P. aeruginosa* outer membrane contains between five and nine polypeptides (depending on growth conditions) which are present in high copy number (10^4–5×10^5 copies per cell) and thus are called major outer membrane proteins. Three of these major proteins, F, D1, and P, have been shown to form hydrophilic channels of defined size through the outer membrane [1, 2, 11] and thus bear the common name porins. In addition, protein F as well as the outer membrane lipoproteins H2 and I, are strongly noncovalently bound to the underlying peptidoglycan [13] and may have structural roles. Protein H1 has been implicated in the development of resistance to polycationic antibiotics and chelators in media containing low concentrations of divalent cations [24]. This paper will focus upon the role of specific outer membrane components of *P. aeruginosa*, namely LPS and porin protein F, as virulence determinants, using this broad definition of virulence.

Lipopolysaccharide

Increasing attention has been focused on the LPS of *P. aeruginosa* in recent years (see [32] for review). However, although the composition has been partially defined, the structure of some portions of the LPS, especially the rough core and lipid A portions, is poorly understood. There are a number of reasons for this, including the high molecular weight and substantial variety of constituents of LPS [32], the complexity and lack of available standards for some of these constituents [32], the heterogeneity within given populations of LPS [7, 32], and the fact that many of the more common analytic procedures cause degradation and loss of some of the components of LPS [7, 32]. Three recent developments may have a major impact on LPS analyses: the development of an LPS isolation procedure which allows recovery of about five times as much LPS from *P. aeruginosa* strains as previously used methods [7], the developing use of nuclear magnetic resonance as a nondegradative method for analyzing sugar compositions [17, 31] and preliminary studies of monoclonal antibodies as specific probes for assisting the analysis of LPS composition [18, 21]. Since this work is in its early stages, the discussion below will consider LPS as a simple tripartite structure (lipid A, rough core, O-side chain).

Antigenicity: Common and Unique Determinants

LPS from *P. aeruginosa*, like other bacterial LPS, has a variety of interesting biologic properties, including mitogenicity towards mouse B lymphocytes [27], pyrogenicity in rabbits, tumor-nectrotizing activity, endotoxicity, interferon-inducing activity, adjuvanticity [29], and strong immunogenicity [27]. With the exception of this latter trait, most of these properties are thought to be caused by the lipid A portion of the LPS [27, 29]. Because lipid A from *P. aeruginosa* has similar biologic properties to the lipid A of *E. coli*, *Salmonella*, and other bacteria [3], we investigated the antigenic similarities between the lipid A moieties of these organisms. To do this, we obtained monoclonal antibodies specific for the lipid A of *E. coli* [22]. These monoclonal antibodies were isolated by Centocor Corporation, Pennsylvania, after the fusion of myeloma cells with the B lymphocytes of mice injected with intact *E. coli* J5 cells. Two of these antibodies, 5E4 and 8A1, reacted with purified lipid A from *Salmonella minnesota* and *P. aeruginosa*; in addition, they cross-reacted with outer membrane and LPS preparations from 36 *P. aeruginosa* strains and 22 other gram-negative bacteria from the families *Vibrionaceae*, *Enterobacteriaceae*, *Rhizobiaceae*, and *Pseudomonadaceae*, but not with the cell walls of three gram-negative bacteria. One of the monoclonal antibodies, 8A1, interacted on Western blots with a similar fast migrating band corresponding to the rough LPS (rough core plus lipid A) from strains of *E. coli*, *Salmonella typhimurium*, *Klebsiella pneumoniae*, *Salmonella minnesota* (Fig. 1), and with strains representing all 17 serotypes of *P. aeruginosa* [23].

This extensive cross-reactivity of the lipid A-specific monoclonal antibodies explains, in part, the protective effects of antisera to *E. coli* J5 organisms against bacteremia caused by other gram-negative bacteria including *P. aeruginosa* [4]. The strong conservation of these antigenic determinants throughout gram-negative bacteria suggests that lipid A has an important role in these bacteria and may indicate a common evolutionary lipid A molecule.

In contrast, we have shown that monoclonal antibodies against the LPS rough core of our wild-type *P. aeruginosa* strain interact only with LPS strains representing 4-6 of the 17 serotypes [15, 21], suggesting that the rough core of *P. aeruginosa* is heterogeneous. A monoclonal antibody against the O-antigen of serotype 5 LPS is relatively specific for this LPS, in agreement with the

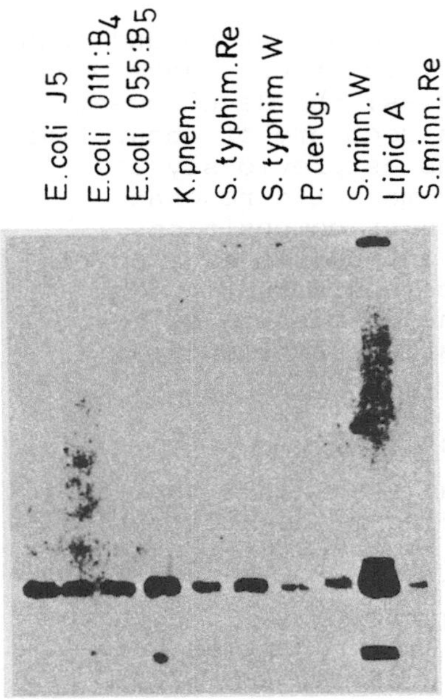

Fig. 1. Reactivity of a monoclonal antibody to lipid A with various lipopolysaccharides (LPS) and lipid A. Purified LPSs were separated by SDS-polyacrylamide gel electrophoresis and then transferred to nitrocellulose by the Western blotting procedure. They were than interacted with monoclonal antibody 8A1 followed by ^{125}I-labeled protein A and autoradiography to reveal the position of the monoclonal antibody-reactive material. The LPSs used were derived from the strains indicated above the respective lanes. The lipid A was derived from *S. minnesota*. The band stained in all preparations is equivalent to rough LPS (i.e., rough core plus lipid A), except, of course, in the lipid A lane

concept that LPS O-antigen heterogeneity is the basis for serotyping in *P. aeruginosa* [32].

Rough, LPS-Altered Strains Associated with Disease

The overwhelming majority of *E. coli* and *Salmonella* strains isolated from human infections are O-serotypable, suggesting that they possess an O-antigen attached to the lipid A-rough core regions of their LPS. Such strains are called smooth strains owing to their characteristic colony morphology. When LPS is isolated from such strains and separated according to molecular size on SDS-polyacrylamide gel, extreme heterogeneity is observed in the length of the O-side chain (i.e., number of repeating trisaccharide units); however, a large number of LPS molecules contain less than four repeating units and somewhere between 5% and 62% of the LPS is rough, i.e., lacking O-side chains (e.g., [9]). Despite this, the rough cores of the LPS are masked as judged by the resistance of these smooth strains to phages which use this portion of the LPS as their receptor.

P. aeruginosa also shows substantial LPS heterogeneity, although a larger amount of rough LPS, estimated as between 75% (A. Kropinski, personal communication) and 90% [15, 32] of the total LPS, is present. We studied a series of *P. aeruginosa* strains isolated from patients with cystic fibrosis [15]. Many of these strains were not serotypable and exhibited two patterns; failure to agglutinate with any typing sera, or polyagglutinability with more than one typing serum. We were able to demonstrate that these abnormal typing patterns, occurring in up to 60% of cystic fibrosis isolates [35], correlated with deficiencies in the amounts of O-antigen in the LPS of these strains [15]. Admittedly, such strains exist in a unique ecological niche (the lungs of patients with cystic fibrosis), but these observations have several important implications. First, they call into question the broad application of O-antigen-based antisera for serotyping *P. aeruginosa* [35]. Second, they tend to suggest that immunotherapy using the recent LPS-based vaccines will not be successful in some disease situations. Third, they demonstrate that there is no obligate association between possession of an O-antigen and ability to persist in a host. While other studies have suggested this for intracellular pathogens like *Yersinia pestis* [8] and *Neisseria* [30], this has not been widely recognized among organisms which do not protect themselves by internalization in host cells. Significantly, *P. aeruginosa* infections can persist in the lungs of cystic fibrosis patients for more than 10 years and are the primary infections associated with terminal lung disease in these patients [21].

Role in Serum Resistance

Using these rough strains from the lungs of patients with cystic fibrosis as well as rough, LPS-altered, phage-resistant derivatives of our laboratory wild-type *P. aeruginosa* strain PAO1, we were able to demonstrate a dramatic enhancement in susceptibility to killing by normal human serum of these rough strains when compared with smooth strains, including both patient isolates and strain PAO1. Indeed, smooth strains were able to grow in concentrations of serum exceeding 40% (vol/vol), whereas rough strains were killed by 2% serum [15]. Similar observations have been made in other organisms [28] and it has been proposed that this result reflects blocking of some components by the O-side chains of LPS. Alternatively, I recently proposed [10] that differences in the relative affinities of smooth and rough LPS for Mg^{2+} can explain these phenomena, given evidence that complement attacks an LPS divalent cation binding site on the surface of the outer membrane. In any case, the high susceptibility to serum of the rough *P. aeruginosa* strains from the lungs of cystic fibrosis patients may help explain why these strains are apparently non-invasive and cystic fibrosis patients rarely, if ever, succumb to *P. aeruginosa* bacteremia.

Outer Membrane Proteins

Mitogenic Response

Unlike LPS, none of the *P. aeruginosa* outer membrane proteins appears to be toxic for mice. For example, injection of 5 mg/kg protein F into mice causes no lethality and no obvious clinical symptoms (E.C.A. Mouat and R.E.W. Hancock, unpublished work). Outer membrane proteins are, however, like LPS [5] capable of interacting with host cells, namely B lymphocytes. Proteins F, H2, and I in picomole amounts were each capable of stimulating resting murine B lymphocytes to proliferate [5]. This capability was not diminished in C3H/Hej mice which did not interact with *P. aeruginosa* LPS [5]. T cells were not mitogenically stimulated by these proteins. Interestingly, two of these proteins are outer membrane lipoproteins and their mitogenic effects can be compared to that of Braun's outer membrane lipoprotein of *E. coli* [19]. The significance of these observations has not, as yet, been elucidated.

Antigenicity

We have demonstrated that outer membrane proteins E, F, H2, and I are strongly antigenically conserved in *P. aeruginosa* strains by using polyclonal rabbit antisera and the Western immunoblotting technique [22]. In addition, we have demonstrated, using monoclonal antibodies, the conservation, among 16 clinical isolates and the 17 serotypes of *P. aeruginosa*, of single antigenic sites on proteins H2 and F [13, 21]. In the case of the two protein F antigenic sites recognized by two separate classes of monoclonal antibodies, indirect immunofluorescence studies have shown that both of these common antigenic sites are surface located; in contrast, the epitope of protein H2 recognized by monoclonal antibody MA1-6 is buried in smooth *P. aeruginosa* strains, but exposed in rough LPS O-antigen-deficient mutants [21]. One of the monoclonal antibodies against protein F, MA4-4, protects mice against subsequent lethal challenge by a virulent *P. aeruginosa* strain PA103 (Hancock and Mouat, manuscript submitted).

These data pose a major question; given the existence of conserved, surface-exposed antigenic sites on protein F of *P. aeruginosa* strains, why are the *P. aeruginosa* strains not rapidly cleared? One possible answer might be that *P. aeruginosa* protein F is weakly immunogenic in vivo or that these antigenic sites are masked. In agreement with this, we have been able to isolate insertion sequence mutants of *P. aeruginosa* strain PAO1 in which these antigenic sites are masked in whole cells, but not in membrane preparations (Angus and Hancock, unpublished work). Furthermore, the sera of four cystic fibrosis patients which were collected shortly after their first episode of *P. aeruginosa* lung infection, had antibody titers against outer membrane proteins that did not differ from those of uninfected patients (although multiply infected patients had extremely high antibody titers to these proteins [16]). Also, four patients with bacteremic *P. aeruginosa* infections did not have antibodies against protein F. In contrast, the sera of rats infected for only seven days with *P. aeruginosa* using the agar bead model demonstrated antibodies against protein F [18]. Thus, while protein F clearly has the potential to be immunogenic in vivo, as demonstrated by our studies using chronically infected rats [18] and cystic fibrosis patients [16], it is uncertain as yet whether antibodies to protein F contribute to clearance of *P. aeruginosa* or whether they are produced too late or in too small quantities to influence these infections.

Restricted Outer Membrane Permeability as a Virulence Factor

The outer membrane shields gram-negative cells against many toxic agents and potentially harmful enzymes in the host. For example, intact *P. aeruginosa* cells are resistant to bile salts, proteases, lysozyme, and phospholipases ([10]; unpublished work). In addition, *P. aeruginosa* demonstrates substantial resistance to antibiotics and disinfectants. This provides an explanation for its rise in prominence as a pathogen over the past 30-40 years.

Treatment of patients with antibiotics would tend to select, over time, for more resistant microorganisms. Significantly, *P. aeruginosa* infections are often hospital-acquired complications of other underlying diseases [34]. The high intrinsic resistance of *P. aeruginosa* to germicidal agents would favor its persistence in hospital environments.

The primary reason for the high intrinsic resistance of *P. aeruginosa* to most commonly used antibiotics is the low permeability of its outer membrane [10, 25]. This low outer membrane permeability appears to be due to the low efficiency in pore formation across the outer membrane of protein F, the major porin of *P. aeruginosa* [25]. We have estimated that despite the larger channel size of porin protein F pores (which are threefold greater in area than *E. coli* porin pores), that only 1 in 400 of the 100 000 trimers in the outer membrane forms active functional pores. The resultant decrease in the rate of permeation across the outer membrane decreases the exposure of the interior of the cell to antibiotics and increases the efficiency of other defense systems (e.g., the low level of constitutive β-lactamase in the periplasm of *P. aeruginosa*). Interestingly, it could be argued that the large channel size of *P. aeruginosa* porin protein F 2.3 nm diameter [1]) is itself significant in pathogenesis. Thus, one could consider a scheme whereby the excreted proteases of *P. aeruginosa* digested host proteins into large peptides. These large peptides could be taken up through protein F channels and serve as substrates for peptidases located on the periplasmic surface of the cytoplasmic membrane [20]. In agreement with this, proteolytic *P. aeruginosa* strains grow more rapidly on burnt skin extracts than nonproteolytic strains [6]. Similarly, one might argue that large channels would enhance the uptake of hydrophobic compounds produced as a result of the action of the excreted lipases of *P. aeruginosa*.

Conclusions and Perspectives

With the exception of the lipid A (endotoxin) portion of LPS, it is hard to argue that outer membrane components are classical virulence factors. However, in the broadest definition of virulence, outer membrane components contribute significantly to the ability of *P. aeruginosa* to grow in a host. Thus, since outer membrane proteins and LPS are present on the surface of *P. aeruginosa*, they are the major structures which interact with the host immune system and consequently help determine the outcome of the infection. In addition, the low permeability of the *P. aeruginosa* outer membrane to extrinsic agents like antibiotics and disinfectants, and to host factors like serum (for smooth strains only), lysozyme, proteases, lipases, and bile salts, etc., can be a major factor in determining the virulence of *P. aeruginosa* during bacteremic infections. Having identified two major contributions of the outer membrane to the course of *P. aeruginosa* infections, we have begun to design therapeutic strategies against this organism. One of these strategies involves the use of monoclonal antibodies against protein F as passive vaccines (see the section on antigenicity of outer membrane proteins) in an attempt to bolster the host immune system. A second strategy consists of our recent finding that a group of diverse compounds, which we have given the group name "permeabilizers", will increase the permeability of the outer membrane of *P. aeruginosa* to β-lactams, lysozyme, and hydrophobic compounds [12]. Since low outer membrane permeability is a significant impediment to antimicrobial therapy, we hope that one of these permeabilizer compounds, given together with an antibiotic, will provide a more successful method of therapy.

Acknowledgments. My research in these areas has been supported generously by the Canadian Cystic Fibrosis Foundation, Medical Research Council of Canada, and British Columbia Health Care Research Foundation.

References

1. Benz R, Hancock REW (1981) Properties of the large ion-permeable pores formed by protein F of *Pseudomonas aeruginosa* in lipid bilayer membranes. Biochim Biophys Acta 646:298-308
2. Benz R, Gimple M, Poole K, Hancock REW (1983) An anion-selective channel from the *Pseudomonas aeruginosa* outer membrane. Biochim Biophys Acta 730:387-390
3. Bradley SG (1979) Cellular and molecular mechanisms of action of bacterial endotoxins. Annu Rev Microbiol 33:67-94
4. Braude AI, Ziegler EJ, McCutchan JA (1978) Antiserum treatment of gram-negative bacteremia. Schweiz Med Wochenschr 108:1872-1876
5. Chen YU, Hancock REW, Mishell RI (1980) Mitogenic effects of purified outer membrane proteins from *Pseudomonas aeruginosa*. Infect Immun 28:178-184
6. Cicmanec JF, Holder IA (1979) Growth of *Pseudomonas aeruginosa* in normal and burned skin extract: Role of extracellular proteases. Infect Immun 25:477-483
7. Darveau RP, Hancock REW (1983) Procedure for the isolation of bacterial lipopolysaccharide from both smooth and rough *Pseudomonas aeruginosa* and *Salmonella typhimurium* strains. J Bacteriol 155:831-838
8. Darveau RP, Chernetzky WT, Hurlbert RE, Hancock REW (1983) Effect of growth temperature, 47 megadalton plasmid and calcium deficiency on the outer membrane protein, porin, and lipopolysaccharide composition of *Yersinia pestis* EV76. Infect Immun 42:1092-1101
9. Goldman RC, Leive L (1980) Heterogeneity of antigenic-side-chain length in lipopolysaccharide from *Escherichia coli* O111 and *Salmonella typhimurium* LT2. Eur J Biochem 107:145-153
10. Hancock REW (1984) Alterations in outer membrane permeability. Annu Rev Microbiol 38:237-264
11. Hancock REW, Carey AM (1980) Protein D1 — a glucose-inducible, pore-forming protein from the outer membrane of *Pseudomonas aeruginosa*. FEMS Microbiol Lett 8:105-109
12. Hancock REW, Wong PGW (1984) Compounds which increase the permeability of the *Pseudomonas aeruginosa* outer membrane. Antimicrob Agents Chemother 26:48-52
13. Hancock REW, Irvin RT, Costerton JW, Carey AM (1981) *Pseudomonas aeruginosa* outer membrane: peptidoglycan associated proteins. J Bacteriol 145:628-631
14. Hancock REW, Wieczorek AA, Mutharia LM, Poole K (1982) Monoclonal antibodies against *Pseudomonas aeruginosa* outer membrane antigens: isolation and characterization. Infect Immun 37:166-171

15. Hancock REW, Mutaria LM, Chan L, Darveau RP, Speert DP, Pier GB (1983) *Pseudomonas aeruginosa* isolates from patients with cystic fibrosis: A class of serum sensitive, nontypable strains deficient in lipopolysaccharide O side chains. Infect Immun 42:170-177
16. Hancock REW, Speert DP, Mouat ECA (1984) Quantitation and identification of antibodies to outer membrane proteins of *Pseudomonas aeruginosa* in sera of patients with cystic fibrosis. J Infect Dis 149:220-226
17. Knivel YA, Vinogradov EV, Shashkov AS, Dmitriev BA, Kochetkov NK, Stanislavsky ES, Mashilova GM (1982) Somatic antigens of *Pseudomonas aeruginosa*. The structure of O-specific polysaccharide chains of P. aeruginosa O:3a,b and O:3a,d lipopolysaccharides. Eur J Biochem 128:81-90
18. Lam JS, Mutharia LM, Hancock REW, Hoiby N, Lam K, Balk L, Costerton JW (1983) Immunogenicity of *Pseudomonas aeruginosa* outer membrane antigens examined by crossed immunoelectrophoresis. Infect Immun 42:88-98
19. Melchers F, Braun V, Galanos C (1975) The lipoprotein of the outer membrane of *Escherichia coli:* A B-lymphocyte mitogen. J Exp Med 142:473-482
20. Miller RV, Becker JM (1978) Peptide utilization in *Pseudomonas aeruginosa*: evidence for membrane associated peptidases. J Bacteriol 133:165-171
21. Mutharia LM, Hancock REW (1983) Surface localization of *Pseudomonas aeruginosa* outer membrane porin protein F by using monoclonal antibodies. Infect Immun 42:1027-1033
22. Mutharia LM, Nicas TI, Hancock REW (1982) Outer membrane proteins of *Pseudomonas aeruginosa* serotyping strains. J Infect Dis 146:770-779
23. Mutharia LM, Crockford G, Bogard WC, Hancock REW (1984) Monoclonal antibodies specific for *Escherichia coli* J-5 lipopolysaccharide: Cross-reaction with other gram-negative bacterial species. Infect Immun 45:631-636
24. Nicas TI, Hancock REW (1980) Outer membrane protein H1 of *Pseudomonas aeruginosa*: Involvement in adaptive and mutational resistance to ethylenediamineteraacetate, polymyxin B, and gentamicin. J Bacteriol 143: 872-878
25. Nicas TI, Hancock REW (1983) *Pseudomonas aeruginosa* outer membrane permeability: Isolation of a protein F-deficient mutant. J Bacteriol 153: 281-285
26. Nikaido H, Nakae T (1979) The outer membrane of gram-negative bacteria. Adv Microb Physiol 19:163-250
27. Pier GB, Markham RB, Eardley D (1981) Correlation of the biological response of C3H/Hej mice to endotoxin with the chemical and structural properties of the lipopolysaccharides from *Pseudomonas aeruginosa* and *Escherichia coli*. J Immunol 127:184-191
28. Rowley D (1968) Sensitivity of rough gram-negative bacteria to the bactericidal action of serum. J Bacteriol 95:1647-1652
29. Tanamoto K, Homma JY (1982) Essential regions of the lipopolysaccharide of *Pseudomonas aeruginosa* responsible for pyrogenicity and activation of the proclotting enzyme of horseshoe crabs. Comparison with antitumor, interferon-inducing and adjuvant activities. J Biochem 91:741-746
30. Tsai CM, Frasch CE (1982) A sensitive silver stain for detecting lipopolysaccharide in polyacrylamide gels. Anal Biochem 119:115-119
31. Wilkinson SG (1981) ^{31}P N.m.r. evidence for the presence of triphosphate residues in the lipopolysaccharides from *Pseudomonas aeruginosa*. Biochem J 199:833-835
32. Wilkinson SG (1983) Composition and structure of lipopolysaccharides from *Pseudomonas aeruginosa*. Rev Infect Dis 5 Suppl:S941-S949
33. Young LS (1980) The role of exotoxins in the pathogenesis of *Pseudomonas aeruginosa* infections. J Infect Dis 142:626-630

34. Young LS, Stevens P, Kaijser B (1982) Gram-negative pathogens in septacaemic infections. Scand J Infect Dis [Suppl] 31:78-94
35. Zierdt CH, Williams RL (1975) Serotyping of *Pseudomonas aeruginosa* isolates from patients with cystic fibrosis of the pancreas. J Clin Microbiol 1:521-526

Bayer-Symposium VIII
The Pathogenesis of Bacterial Infections, 257-266 (1985)

Extracellular Factors in the Virulence of *Pseudomonas aeruginosa*

B. H. Iglewski and T. I. Nicas

Summary

Investigators have studied the effects of purified extracellular products of *Pseudomonas aeruginosa* in a variety of animals or utilized active or passive immunization against a given product in order to elucidate the role of a given product in the pathogenesis of *P. aeruginosa* infections [31, 33]. Both of these approaches require that the product be available in purified form and assume that purification has not altered it in any biologically important respect. Furthermore, both approaches ignore potential interplay of different bacterial products which would occur during infection. Alternatively, others have compared different strains of *P. aeruginosa* possessing various combinations of potential virulence properties in animal models in an effort to correlate a suspected product with virulence [31, 33]. Such studies are complicated by the fact that independently isolated strains of *P. aeruginosa* are quite heterogeneous and may differ in many respects.

A genetic approach to *P. aeruginosa* virulence has been used which circumvents many of the problems inherent in earlier studies. Mutants specifically deficient in toxin A, exoenzyme S, elastase, or alkaline protease have been isolated and characterized both in vitro (see Table 3) and in vivo (see Tables 4 and 5). The results of these studies indicate that virulence of *P. aeruginosa* is multifactorial. Furthermore, these studies indicate that the relative contribution of a given extracellular product to virulence of *P. aeruginosa* can differ, depending on the type of infection. Thus, toxin A and alkaline protease were shown to be major virulence factors in *P. aeruginosa* infections of the mouse cornea, but to be relatively less important than exoenzyme S in infections of burned mice. Similarly, elastolytic activity appears to be required for maximum virulence of *P. aeruginosa* in burned mouse infections, but it is not involved in the pathogenesis of mouse eye infections by *P. aeruginosa*.

Introduction

The pathogenesis of *Pseudomonas aeruginosa* infections is poorly understood. This organism causes a number of different kinds of disease. These range through acute localized infections (*Pseudomonas* keratitis), chronic localized infections (lung infections in cystic fibrosis patients), to acute systemic infections in patients with burns or certain neoplasias [30]. Just as *P. aeruginosa* causes multiple disease syndromes, its virulence appears to be multifactorial. A large number of bacterial products have been identified which have the potential to contribute to the virulence of *P. aeruginosa* [10, 18, 31]. Determining the relative contribution of each of these bacterial products to the virulence of *P. aeruginosa* and the role of each in the pathogenesis of the various different *P. aeruginosa* infections represents a sizeable challenge. This paper summarizes recent studies utilizing a genetic approach to determine the relative contribution of four extracellular proteins to virulence of *P. aeruginosa* in *Pseudomonas* keratitis and burn wound sepsis. The four proteins studied include two with ADP-ribosyl transferase activity (toxin A and exoenzyme S) and two proteases (alkaline protease and elastase).

Toxin A

The most toxic extracellular protein produced by *P. aeruginosa* is toxin A (LD_{50} = 0.2 µg per 22-g mouse [18]). The toxicity of toxin A is due to its ability to catalyze the transfer of the adenosine 5'-diphosphate ribosyl (ADPR) moiety of nicotinamide adenide dinucleotide (NAD) onto the diphthamide residue of eukaryotic elongation factor 2 (EF-2) [13]. The resultant ADPR-EF-2 complex is inactive in protein synthesis. When EF-2 becomes rate limiting, protein synthesis ceases and the intoxicated cell dies. This reaction catalyzed by toxin A is identical to that catalyzed by the fragment A moiety of diphtheria toxin [3, 31]. Also like diphtheria toxin, *Pseudomonas* toxin A is released by bacteria as a proenzyme which is toxic to cultured cells and animals, but is devoid of ADPR transferase activity [28]. The intact toxin A has a molecular weight of 66 000 and contains four disulfide bridges [16]. Its enzymatic activity can be potentiated by fragmenting the molecule enzymatically (by proteolysis), or chemically, or by treating toxin A with reducing and denaturing agents such as dithiothreitol (DTT) and urea. The latter treatment does not detectably alter the size of toxin A. The toxin A molecule is composed of at least two functionally important domains, one which interacts and binds to a specific, but as yet uncharacterized, receptor on the surface of susceptible cells and a second domain containing the enzymatic sites involved in NAD binding, cleavage, and the ADPR transferase activity [16, 28]. Recently, the toxin A gene has been cloned in *E. coli* and sequenced [7]. Analysis of the sequences suggests that the enzymatically active site is located at the COOH terminus of the toxin A molecule whereas the opposite is true for diphtheria toxin, in which the enzymatically active site resides near the NH_2 terminus.

The structural gene encoding toxin A is located at approximately 85' on the chromosome of strain PAO [8]. This gene is widely disseminated among *P. aeruginosa* strains as approximately 90% of all clinical isolates produce detectable toxin A [1]. Recent hybridization studies utilizing the cloned toxin A gene as a probe indicate an even greater percentage of *P. aeruginosa* strains contain the toxin A structural gene [29]. Regulation of the toxin A structural gene is poorly understood. However, genes distally located from the structural gene appear to be involved in the regulation of toxin A. Thus, a mutation resulting in a specific toxin A deficiency (*tox*-2) has been mapped at 39' on the chromosome of strain PAO [6]. The nature of the regulation exerted by this gene is as yet unknown. It is known, however, that toxin A is not produced constitutively by tox+ strains of *P. aeruginosa*, but rather toxin A yields are influenced by the carbon source and iron concentration of the growth medium as well as the degree of aeration and growth temperature [2, 18]. The general properties of toxin A are summarized in Table 1.

Table 1. Comparison of *Pseudomonas aeruginosa* toxin A and exoenzyme S

Property	Toxin A	Exoenzyme S
Molecular weight	66 000	53 000
Size of enzymatically active fragments (kdaltons)	25-45K	20-49K
Enzymatic activity	ADPR-transferase	ADPR-transferase
Substrate	EF-2	Multiple proteins not EF-2
Effect of urea-DTT	Potentiates activity	Destroys activity
Location of structural gene	85' on chromosome	Unknown
Incidence of production (%)	90	>40
LD_{50} (mice) (µg)	0.2	>1.0

Exoenzyme S

A second *P. aeruginosa* extracellular protein with ADPR transferase activity is exoenzyme S. Whereas the substrate for toxin A is EF-2, exoenzyme S does not modify EF-2, but rather transfers ADPR to a number of as yet unidentified proteins present in eukaryotic cell extracts. Exoenzyme S differs from toxin A in a number of other properties (see Table 1). Thus, treatment of exoenzyme S with urea-DTT destroys its enzymatic activity, and these two proteins are immunologically distinct [14]. On the other hand, exoenzyme S, like toxin A, exists in at least two forms. The larger exoenzyme S protein (molecular weight 53 000) is devoid of enzymatic activity whereas smaller peptides (20 000-49 000) are enzymatically active. Detergents are required in order to purify all of the different exoenzyme S proteins and therefore it is not surprising that these purified exoenzyme S proteins are relatively nontoxic (Iglewski and Lile 1984, unpublished work).

The structural gene encoding exoenzyme S has not yet been located. However, initial studies indicated that approximately 40% of all clinical isolates of *P. aeruginosa* produce exoenzyme S [26]. These studies detected exoenzyme S by virtue of its ADPR transferase activity. More recently, we have developed specific antisera against exoenzyme S which recognize the enzymatically inactive as well as the enzymatically active forms of S. A number of strains formerly thought to be exoenzyme S-negative react with this antiserum and can be shown to produce the 53 000 molecular weight exoenzyme S protein (Lile and Iglewski 1984, unpublished work). It therefore seems likely that the incidence of exoenzyme S production is much higher than formerly reported.

P. aeruginosa Proteases: Elastase and Alkaline Protease

Most strains (90%) of *P. aeruginosa* produce two proteases: elastase and alkaline protease. These proteases have been purified and characterized in a number of laboratories [10, 33]. Their basic properties are summarized in Table 2. Elastase is thought to be synthesized as a cell-associated proenzyme which is activated as it is secreted by limited proteolysis, either by itself or by alkaline protease [15]. The purified extracellular elastase has a molecular weight of 39 000, a pK_i of 5.9, and a pH optimum of 7-8. Each elastase molecule contains one atom of zinc,

Table 2. Comparison of *Pseudomonas aeruginosa* elastase and alkaline protease

Property	Elastase	Alkaline protease
Molecular weight	39 000	48 000
pK_i	5.9	4.1
pH optimum	7-8	8-9
Specific activity (casein)(mPU/mg)	50	5
Location of structural gene	75' on chromosome	Unknown
Incidence of production (%)	90	90
LD_{50} (mice)(μg)	125	200

and elastase activity is inhibited by metal chelators, heavy metal ions, and reducing agents. Phosphoramidon and plasma α-2-macroglobulin also inhibit elastase activity [10, 33]. Alkaline protease has a molecular weight of 48 000, a pK_i of 4.1, and a pH optimum of 8-9. It is approximately tenfold less active in degrading casein than is elastase. Calcium or cobalt are required for maximum activity of alkaline protease and its enzymatic activity is inhibited by chelators [10, 33]. Elastase has a specificity for bulky and hydrophobic amino acids at the amino side of the splitting point [19]. It is of interest that elastase degrades elastin and human IgG [5] and that it inactivates complement components (C1, C3, C5, C8, and C9) and human α-1-proteinase inhibitor [33]. The specificity of alkaline protease is broad and is determined by the amino acid residues distant from the splitting point. Alkaline protease does not degrade elastin and does not specifically degrade IgG [5]. The elastase structural gene is located at approximately 75' on the chromosome of strain PAO [12]. The structural gene for alkaline protease has yet to be located.

Contribution of Toxin A, Exoenzyme S, Elastase, and Alkaline Protease to Virulence of *P. aeruginosa*: A Genetic Approach

A genetic approach to determine the contribution to virulence of a potential virulence factor was described by Holmes [9]. Mutants (from a virulent strain) which are altered with respect to the factor desired are isolated. Because potent mutagenic agents may be required, these mutants must then be extensively characterized in vitro and compared with the parental strain in order to establish that they are not altered in any property other than the one desired. The virulence of appropriate mutants is then compared with that of the parental strain in selected animal models. We have used this genetic approach to determine the contribution of toxin A, exoenzyme S, elastase, and alkaline protease to virulence of *P. aeruginosa* [11, 20, 22]. Three parental strains were chosen for these studies, PA103, PAO, and 388. The phenotypes of these parental strains are shown in Table 3. Strain PA103 was chosen because it produces large amounts of toxin A (about 30 μg/ml) and low but significant levels of alkaline protease (1.0 μg/ml), but no elastase or exoenzyme S activity, although exoenzyme S protein (molecular weight 53 000) is produced. Following mutagenesis with *N*-methyl-*N*'-nitro-*N*-nitrosoguanidine, a specific toxin A mutant (PA103-29) was identified using an immunologic assay. This mutant was deficient in the production of toxin A (0.2% parental levels), but it was otherwise identical to the parental strain PA103 [24]. Following mutagenesis with methanesulfonic acid ethyl ester, a mutant (PA103-AP1) specifically deficient in alkaline protease was isolated [11]. It was identical to the parental strain PA103 except for its alkaline protease deficiency (see Table 3).

A second parental strain, PAO, was chosen because it produces toxin A, exoenzyme S protein (molecular weight 53 000), but no exoenzyme S enzyme activity, and it produces both alkaline protease and elastase. Two different types of toxin A mutants were isolated following mutagenesis with NTG. When an immunologic

Table 3. Characterization of *Pseudomonas aeruginosa* strains and mutants

Strain	Toxin A	Exoenzyme S	Elastase	Alkaline protease
PA103(parent)	+++	+[b]	-	+
PA103-29	- (0.2%)	+[b]	-	+
PA103-AP1	+++	+[b]	-	- (0.1%)
PAO(parent)	+	+[b]	+++	+
PAO-T1	- (0)	+[b]	+++	+
PAO-PR1	CRM[a]	+[b]	+++	+
PAO-E64	+	+[b]	CRM[d]	+
388(parent)	-	+++[c]	+	+
388 *exs*1::Tn*1*	-	- (0)	+	+

[a]Enzymatically inactive, antigenically cross-reactive protein.
[b]Exoenzyme S protein (molecular weight 53 000), no exoenzyme S activity.
[c]Exoenzyme S activity.
[d]Enzymatically altered (nonelastolytic) cross-reactive protein.

assay was employed, a toxin A-deficient mutant (PAO-T1) was isolated [22]. When a toxicity assay was used, a mutant (PAO-PR1), which produces inactive toxin A protein (cross-reactive material, CRM) was identified [4]. A specific elastase mutant (PAO-E64) was also isolated from PAO by an elastolysis assay. Mutant PAO-E64 produces parental levels of elastase antigen which is greatly reduced in elastase activity (CRM type mutant) [23].

A third parental strain (388) was chosen because it produces no detectable toxin A, but it does produce large amounts of both forms of exoenzyme S (molecular weight 53 000 and 49 000). This strain also produces both elastase and alkaline protease. Using a temperature-sensitive derivative of plasmid RP1, a Tn*1*-induced mutant (388 *exs*1::Tn*1*) was found which had no detectable exoenzyme S activity or antigen in culture supernatants or in cell lysates. Except for its exoenzyme S deficiency and its resistance to carbenicillin (specified by Tn*1*), this mutant was identical to its parental strain [20]. The relevant phenotypes of these mutants are shown in Table 3.

Virulence of Extracellular Product Mutants in a Mouse Eye Model

We have utilized a mouse eye model and a number of the mutants described to investigate the relative contribution of toxin A, alkaline protease, and elastase to *P. aeruginosa* infections of the cornea [11, 22]. The progression of infection was determined by culturing the eyes every other day and by examination of the eyes with a ×50 stereoscopic microscope. The extent of damage was quantitated according to a corneal damage index (CDI) where a score of 0 is normal and 4.0 indicates a perforated cornea [11]. Two parental strains were examined in this model, strain PA103 and PAO. Infection of the mouse cornea with strain PA103 resulted in a more severe infection (average CDI = 3.2) than occurred with strain PAO (CDI = 1.5). However, both of these strains were able to establish an infection which resulted in permanent damage at an inoculum of 10^6. In contrast, three different toxin A mutants, PA103-29, PAO-T1, and PAO-PR1, were each less virulent than the parental strains from which they were derived. The mutants PAO-T1 and PAO-PR1 caused no permanent damage (CDI = 0) whereas the mutant PA103-29 caused some permanent damage (CDI = 1.3) or 40% of the damage caused by its parental strain PA103. In addition, the three toxin A mutants were cleared more rapidly from the mouse eyes then were their parental strains [22]; Cryz and Iglewski 1984, unpublished work). The alkaline protease mutant PA103-AP1 was virtually avirulent in this eye model (CDI = 0.1). Further, mutant PA103-Ap1 was deficient in establishing infections and 60% of eyes infected with this mutant were sterile after only two days whereas 100% of the eyes infected with the parental strain PA103 were culture-positive after four days [11]. In contrast to the decreased virulence of the toxin A and alkaline protease mutants in this eye model, the elastase mutant (PAO-E64) was as virulent as its parent strain PAO [22] (Table 4). These data indicate that both toxin A and alkaline protease

Table 4. Virulence of *Pseudomonas aeruginosa* mutants in a mouse eye model

Strain	Mutant phenotype	% Parent	Reference
PA103	Parent	(100)	[22]
PA103-29	Toxin A	40	[22]
PA103-AP1	Alkaline protease	0-3	[11]
PAO	Parent	(100)	[22]
PAO-E64	Elastase CRM	100	[22]
PAO-T1	Toxin A	0	[22]
PAO-PR1	Toxin A CRM	0	S.J. Cryz and B.H. Iglewski (1984, unpublished work)

contribute to the virulence of *P. aeruginosa* in this mouse eye model and that both of these extracellular products are required for maintenance of these infections and for maximum damage. In contrast, elastolytic activity is not a required virulence factor in these eye infections.

Virulence of Extracellular Product Mutants in a Burned Mouse Infection Model

An experimental burned infection model has been described in which *P. aeruginosa* spread from the initial site of infection (subcutaneous at the burn site) [27]. The virulence of the mutants described in Table 3 were compared with that of their parental strains in this burned infection model (Table 5). As in the mouse eye infection model, there was considerable difference in the virulence of the three different parental strains ($LD_{50} = 3 \times 10^1 - 1 \times 10^4$). All of the mutants tested were less virulent than their respective parental strain. In the case of the toxin A mutants, the alkaline protease mutant, and the elastase mutant, the difference in virulence compared with their parental strains was less than 100-fold [21, 25]. On the other hand, the exoenzyme S-deficient mutant (388 *exs*1::Tn*1*) was at least 2000-fold less virulent than its exoenzyme S-producing parental strain 388 [20]. The marked decrease in virulence of the exoenzyme S-deficient mutant was not due merely to the presence of the transposon (Tn*1*) since a second Tn*1*-induced mutant (a leucine auxotroph) which produced parental levels of exoenzyme S was as virulent as its parental strain 388 ($LD_{50} = 3 \times 10^1$) [20]. These data (Table 5) indicate that, while each of the extracellular products examined

Table 5. Virulence of *Pseudomonas aeruginosa* mutants in a burned mouse model

Strain	Mutant phenotype	LD_{50}	Reference
PA103	Parent	7.1×10^3	[25]
PA103-29	Toxin A	3.0×10^5	[21]
PA103-AP1	Alkaline protease	1.2×10^5	[21]
PAO	Parent	1.3×10^4	[21]
PAO-T1	Toxin A	5.6×10^4	[21]
PAO-E64	Elastase CRM	9.2×10^4	[21]
388	Parent	3.0×10^1	[21]
388 *exs*1::Tn*1*	Exoenzyme S	1.6×10^5	[20]

(toxin A, exoenzyme S, alkaline protease, and elastase) contributes to the virulence of *P. aeruginosa* in this burned mouse infection model, exoenzyme S appears to have the greatest effect. This finding underscores the contribution of this type of experimental approach, since exoenzyme S purified by our current methods has been nontoxic, and there was previously little evidence to indicate that exoenzyme S contributed to the pathogenesis of *P. aeruginosa* infections.

Acknowledgments. This work was supported in part by grant DAMD 17-83-G-9556 from the United States Army and AI 14671 from the National Institute of Allergy and Infectious Disease. T.I.N. was supported by a fellowship from the Natural Sciences and Engineering Research Council of Canada.

References

1. Bjorn MJ, Vasil ML, Sadoff JC, Iglewski BH (1977) Incidence of exotoxin production by *Pseudomonas* species. Infect Immun 16:362-366
2. Bjorn MJ, Iglewski BH, Ives SK, Sadoff JC, Vasil ML (1978) Effect of iron on yields of exotoxin A in cultures of *Pseudomonas aeruginosa* PA-103. Infect Immun 19:785-791
3. Collier RJ (1975) Diphtheria toxin: Mode of action and structure. Bacteriol Rev 39:54-85
4. Cryz SJ, Friedman RL, Iglewski BH (1980) Isolation and characterization of a *Pseudomonas aeruginosa* mutant producing a nontoxic, immunologically cross-reactive toxin A protein. Proc Natl Acad Sci USA 77:7199-7203
5. Doring G, Oberneser HJ, Bozenhart K (1981) Extracellular toxins of *P. aeruginosa*: II. Effect of two proteases on human immunoglobulins IgG, IgM, and secretory IgA. Zentralbl Bakteriol Mikrobiol Hyg 249:89-93
6. Gray GL, Vasil ML (1981) Isolation and genetic characterization of toxin deficient mutants of *Pseudomonas aeruginosa* PAO. J Bacteriol 147:275-281
7. Gray GL, Smith DH, Baldridge JS, Harkins RN, Vasil ML, Ellson Y, Heynecker HL (1984) Cloning, nucleotide sequencing, and expression in *E. coli* of the exotoxin A structural gene of *Pseudomonas aeruginosa*. Proc Natl Acad Sci USA 81:2645-2649
8. Hanne LF, Howe TR, Iglewski BH (1983) Locus of the *Pseudomonas aeruginosa* toxin A gene. J Bacteriol 154:383-386
9. Holmes RK (1975) Genetic aspects of toxinogenesis in bacteria. In: Schlessinger D (ed) Microbiology — 1975. American Society for Microbiology, Washington, pp 296-301
10. Homma JY (1980) Role of exoenzymes and exotoxin in the pathogenicity of *Pseudomonas aeruginosa* and the development of a new vaccine. Jap J Exp Med 50:149-165
11. Howe TR, Iglewski BH (1984) Alkaline protease deficient mutants of *Pseudomonas aeruginosa*: Isolation and characterization in vitro and in a mouse eye model. Infect Immun 43:1058-1063
12. Howe TR, Wretlind B, Iglewski BH (1983) Comparison of two methods of genetic exchange in determination of the genetic locus of structural gene for *Pseudomonas aeruginosa* elastase. J Bacteriol 156:58-61
13. Iglewski BH, Kabat D (1975) NAD-dependent inhibition of protein synthesis by *Pseudomonas aeruginosa* exotoxin A, Proc Natl Acad Sci USA 72:2284-2288
14. Iglewski BH, Sadoff JC, Bjorn MJ, Maxwell ES (1978) *Pseudomonas aeruginosa* exoenzyme S: An adenosine diphosphate ribosyltransferase distinct from toxin A. Proc Natl Acad Sci USA 75:3211-3215

15. Jensen SE, Pecyz IT, Stemke GW, Campbell JN (1980) Demonstration of a cell-associated, inactive precursor of an extracellular protease of *Pseudomonas aeruginosa*. J Bacteriol 144:844-847
16. Leppla SH, Martin OC, Muel LA (1978) The exotoxin of *P. aeruginosa*: A proenzyme having an unusual mode of activation. Biochem Biophys Res Commun 81:532-538
17. Lory S, Collier RJ (1980) Expression of enzymatical activity of exoenzyme A from *Pseudomonas aeruginosa*. Infect Immun 28:494-501
18. Liu PV (1974) Extracellular toxins of *Pseudomonas aeruginosa*. J Infect Dis 130:S94-S99
19. Morihara K (1964) Production of elastase and proteinase by *Pseudomonas aeruginosa*. J Bacteriol 84:745-757
20. Nicas TI, Iglewski BH (1984a) Isolation and characterization of transposon induced mutants of *Pseudomonas aeruginosa* deficient in exoenzyme S. Infect Immun 45:470-474
21. Nicas TI, Iglewski BH (1984b) The contribution of exoproducts to virulence of *Pseudomonas aeruginosa*. Can J Microbiol 31:103-108
22. Ohman DE, Burns RP, Iglewski BH (1980a) Corneal infections of mice with toxin A and elastase mutants of *Pseudomonas aeruginosa*. J Infect Dis 142:547-555
23. Ohman DE, Cryz SJ, Iglewski BH (1980b) Isolation and characterization of a *Pseudomonas aeruginosa* PAO mutant that produces altered elastase. J Bacteriol 142:836-842
24. Ohman DE, Sadoff JC, Iglewski BH (1980c) Toxin A deficient mutants of *Pseudomonas aeruginosa* PA103: Isolation and characterization. Infect Immun 28:899-908
25. Pavloskis OR, Edman DC, Leppla SH, Wretlind B, Lewis L, Martin KE (1981) Protection against experimental *Pseudomonas aeruginosa* infection in mice by active immunization with exotoxin A. Infect Immun 24:181-187
26. Sokol PA, Iglewski BH, Hagar TH, Sadoff JC, Cross AS, McManus A, Farber BF, Iglewski WJ (1981) Production of exoenzyme S by clinical isolates of *Pseudomonas aeruginosa*. Infect Immun 34:147-153
27. Stieritz DD, Holder IA (1975) Experimental studies on the pathogenesis of infections due to *Pseudomonas aeruginosa*: Description of a burned mouse model. J Infect Dis 131:699
28. Vasil ML, Kabat D, Iglewski BH (1977) Structure activity relationships of an exotoxin of *Pseudomonas aeruginosa*. Infect Immun 16:353-361
29. Vasil ML, Gray GL, Grant C (1984) Molecular analysis of the exotoxin A gene of *Pseudomonas* species. Abstracts of the Annual Meeting of the American Society for Microbiology, p 62
30. Wood RE (1976) *Pseudomonas*: The compromised host. Hosp Pract 11:91-100
31. Woods DE, Iglewski BH (1983) Toxins of *Pseudomonas aeruginosa*: New Perspectives. Rev Infect Dis 5:S715-S721
32. Woods DE, Cryz SJ, Friedman RL, Iglewski BH (1982) Contribution of toxin A and elastase to virulence of *Pseudomonas aeruginosa* in chronic lung infections in rats. Infect Immun 36:1223-1228
33. Wretlind B, Pavloskis OR (1984) *Pseudomonas aeruginosa* proteases and their role in *Pseudomonas* infections. Rev Infect Dis 5:S998-S1004

Discussion

(pp. 247-266)

Pseudomonas aeruginosa infections of cystic fibrosis patients may last for years, despite their high sensitivity to carbenicillin and serum. Strains may contain a rough lipopolysaccharide and may be mucoid. Both phenotypes can be obtained by selection for phage resistance in the laboratory and may also be caused by phage in the lung. Despite high titers of antibodies against *Pseudomonas*, these antibodies apparently do not reach the bacteria in the lung. Antibodies to outer membrane proteins can function as opsonins, but it is unknown whether they have protective activity under these circumstances. Antibodies against lipopolysaccharide are also present in the serum of patients with long-lasting infections, but it is unknown whether they contribute in any sense to the outcome of the infection. The same conclusion can be drawn for the exoproteases released from *Pseudomonas* with a potential activity against immunoglobulins. As far as it is known, exoenzyme is not identical with leukocidin. The reported incidence of production for leukocidins by clinical isolates is around 4%.

Bayer-Symposium VIII
The Pathogenesis of Bacterial Infections, 268-279 (1985)

Damage to the Host by Channel-Forming Bacterial Toxins

S. Bhakdi, W. Seeger, N. Suttorp, and J. Tranum-Jensen

Summary

The perturbation of membrane by complement, staphylococcal α-toxin, and streptolysin-O are three examples of bilayer damage by channel formers. In all cases, primarily water-soluble proteins self-associate on the membrane to form channel-structured oligomers. Hydrophobic surfaces become exposed that permit these channels to insert into and become stably embedded within the bilayer. Secondary events can follow that will augment the primary damage induced through pore formation. Staphylococcal α-toxin activates the arachidonic acid cascade, possibly by serving as nonphysiologic calcium bypass channels. Membrane-bound streptolysin-O binds host antibody and thus induces self-attack of cells by the autologous complement system. Such secondary processes are probably responsible for major pathophysiologic effects elicited by channel-forming toxins in host tissues.

Introductory Overview

Formation of aqueous transmembrane channels is being increasingly recognized as a major mechanism through which target membranes can be damaged by alien proteins. The first clear documentation of this principle was made in the complement field, where it was found that self-association of the terminal five serum complement components into channel-forming C5b-9 protein complexes inserting into the target bilayer constituted the molecular principle underlying the phenomenon of immune cytolysis [4, 5, 16]. Subsequently, it was found that membrane damage by channel formers occurred in many other instances. The present discussion will focus on two prototypes of channel formers which we have been studying, i.e., staphylococcal α-toxin and streptolysin-O. Both of these bacterial exotoxins represent important pathogenic factors and their study has furthered our understanding of the mechanisms responsible for their deleterious effects in the host organism.

Certain features appear common to all channel formers. The proteins are produced as water-soluble polypeptides, but they undergo an irreversible transition from a hydrophilic to an amphiphilic state after binding and insertion into the target bilayer. In their final, membrane-bound form, they thus assume properties characteristic of integral membrane proteins. This is possible because of exposure of lipid-binding, apolar surfaces on the molecules that firmly anchor them to the lipid matrix. Membrane insertion and channel formation is invariably the consequence of self-association (oligomerization) of the protein monomers on and in the lipid bilayer. Lipids and proteins of the membrane targets, although sometimes involved in the initial binding of native toxin molecules to the cell surface, probably never themselves significantly contribute to formation of the channel structures per se.

The initial binding of the channel formers to the membrane surface requires specific "binder" or "acceptor" molecules in some cases, but may require none in others. Examples of the former category of molecules are the C9 complement component, and the sulfhydryl-activated bacterial exotoxins such as streptolysin-O. C9 binds to membrane-bound C5b-8 "precursor" terminal complexes, whereas the sulfhydryl-activated toxins bind to membrane cholesterol. These proteins will not bind to membranes lacking the respective binder molecules. Examples of membrane insertion of proteins without the apparent requirement for specific binders are given in the case of precursor C5b6/C5b-7 complement complexes and staphylococcal α-toxin. These proteins bind to protein-free liposomes and specific lipidic binders have not been unequivocally identified. When specific binders are present, membrane attachment is generally very effective, even at low protein molarity. In contrast, binding of proteins directly to the bilayer in the absence of a high-affinity acceptor is generally of low efficacy. For this reason, the presence of relatively high concentrations of the latter category of channel formers as opposed to the former is usually required to generate the channels and induce cytolysis.

The protein channels may constitute a homogeneous population of structures (e.g., staphylococcal α-toxin hexamers), or they may exhibit marked heterogeneity owing to the presence of varying numbers of monomeric subunits harbored in a given polymer. Examples of the latter are the channels formed by C9, which is the major channel-forming subunit of the C5b-9 complement complex, and by the sulfhydryl-activated toxins such as streptolysin-O. The process of oligomerization directly leads to exposure of lipid-binding surfaces on the proteins probably owing to changes in their conformation. The molecular basis for this unique hydrophilic-amphiphilic transition has not yet been elucidated for any single channel former. However, structural studies at a molecular genetic level are now under way and considerable progress in this field should be made in the near future. Although the native proteins are sensitive to proteolytic degradation, membrane-bound channel structures are generally indestructible by proteases at neutral pH. In the organism, phagocytosis may therefore be the only means for removal of these stably membrane-bound structures.

Antigenic determinants are always exposed on the channel oligomers and specific antibodies bind to the proteins in detergent solutions as well as on the membranes. The channels can usually be isolated quite easily from target membranes after their solubilization with detergents, and can then be used for raising specific antibodies.

The primary function of channel formers is to perturb membrane integrity by generating aqueous transmembrane pores. This process of protein insertion and pore formation can in turn trigger important secondary pathophysiologic events, examples of which will be discussed in the second part of this paper. Such secondary processes probably play major roles in eliciting the final tissue reactions in the host organism.

Molecular Properties of Staphylococcal α-Toxin and Streptolysin-O

Staphylococcal α-Toxin

Staphylococcal α-toxin is produced by most pathogenic strains of staphylococci and is considered one of the major factors of staphylococcal pathogenicity [17]. The toxin is secreted as a hydrophilic, 3.3 *S* monomer of M_r 34 000 [6] with an isoelectric point of approximately 8.5. Upon contact with an appropriate target membrane, the monomers self-associate to form small channels that appear to represent a homogeneous population of 11-12 *S* hexamers ($M_r = 200\,000$; [6]). The latter bind lipid and detergent. They generate circumscribed functional "holes" in the membrane of resealed erythrocyte ghosts whose effective diameter appears to be approximately 2 nm [15]. In the electron microscope, the channels indeed display a central pore of these dimensions (Fig. 1). The external diameter of the hexamers measures 8.5-10 nm as determined on the extramembranous portion of the cylinder.

Fig. 1. (A) Negatively stained fragment of rabbit erythrocyte lysed with staphylococcal α-toxin. Numerous 10 nm ring-shaped structures are seen over the membrane (*arrows*). (B) Isolated toxin hexamers in detergent solution. (C) Lecithin liposomes carrying reincorporated α-toxin hexamers. The hexamers are seen as stubs along the edge of the liposomal membrane and as rings over the membrane (*arrows*). Characteristically, liposomes that escape incorporation of the toxin are impermeable to the stain. (D) Negatively stained erythrocyte membrane lysed by streptolysin-O, showing numerous 25-100 nm long and approximately 7.5 nm broad, curved rods of 13-16 nm inner radius of curvature. Most rods are approximately semicircular, often joined in pairs at their ends. Dense accumulations of stain are seen at the concave side of the rods. When these do not form closed profiles, the stain deposit is partly bordered by a "free" edge of the erythrocyte membrane (*arrows*). (E) Negative staining of isolated streptolysin-O oligomers, showing numerous curved rod structures identical to those found on toxin-treated membranes. (F) Purified streptolysin-O complexes reincorporated into cholesterol-free lecithin liposomes. The toxin oligomers form holes in the liposomes (*unlabeled arrows*); *p* indicates a lesion seen in profile. *Scale bars* indicate 100 nm in all frames. Sodium silicotungstate was used as negative stain in B-F. Uranylacetate was used in A. Reproduced from reference [5] with permission of The Royal Society, London

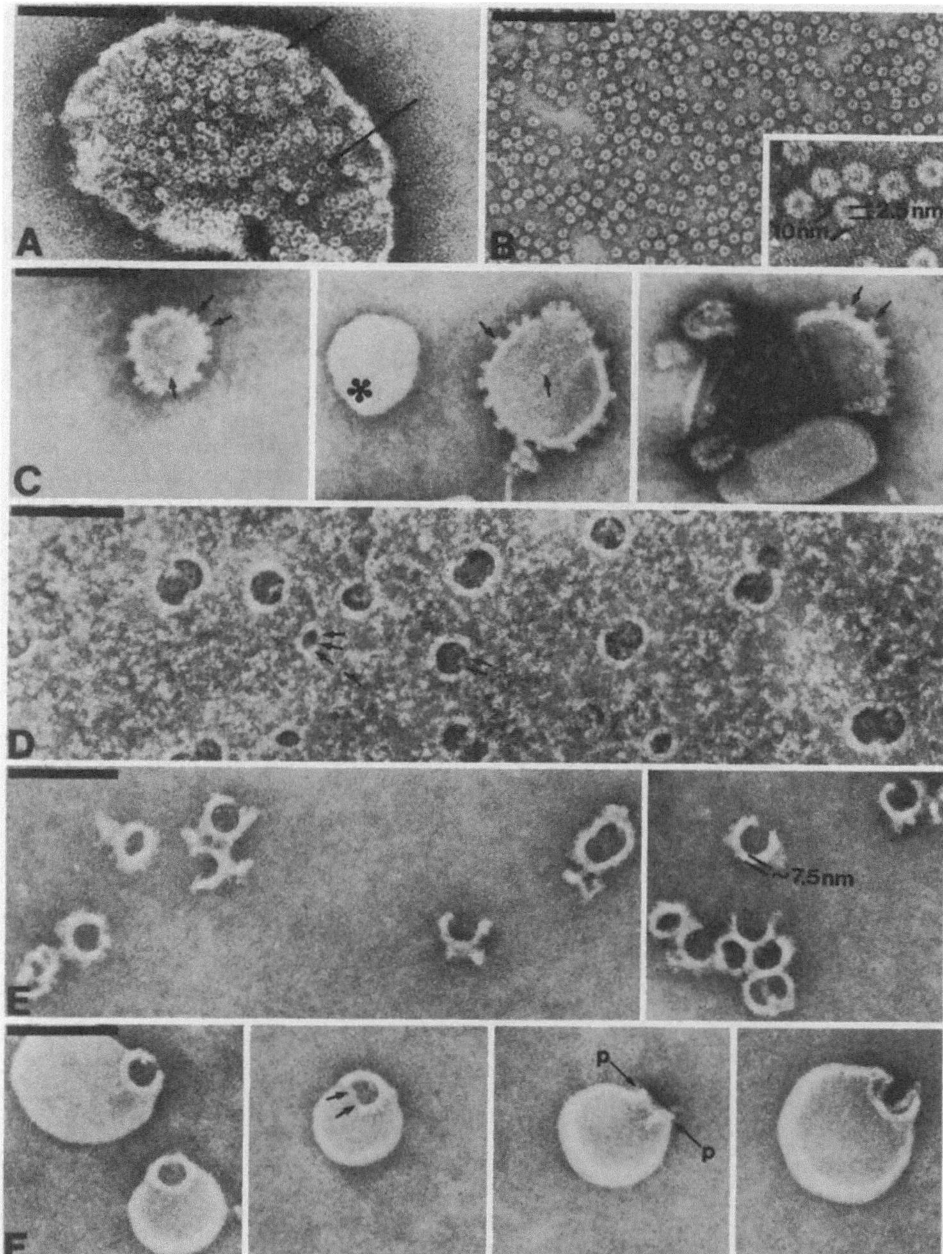
A
B
2.5 nm
10 nm
C
D
E
7.5 nm
F
p
p

Triggering of the hexamerization process is not recognizably dependent on the presence of a biochemically defined membrane binding site [14, 17]. Spontaneous hexamer formation occurs in the absence of a lipid bilayer when purified toxin is exposed to specific heating conditions [2] or to deoxycholate detergent [6]. Hexamers also form when toxin molecules come into contact with human plasma low density lipoprotein, probably through nonspecific triggering of the oligomerization process by lipid contained in the lipoprotein particle [7]. As with all other channel formers, toxin oligomers are hemolytically inactive, probably owing to their low solubility in water. Binding and hexamer formation of the toxin on lipoprotein thus causes toxin inactivation and may represent a significant nonimmune defense mechanism of the host toward this toxin.

The efficacy of toxin binding to cell membrane is low: at toxin concentrations of 3×10^{-8}–10^{-6} *M* (1-30 μg/ml), less than 5% of toxin offered to a surplus of cells becomes membrane bound. We believe that this is due to the absence of specific membrane binders for the toxin. As toxin levels are raised, overall binding will increase to reach, quite abruptly, levels of 50%-70% of total toxin offered to the cells (Fig. 2). This binding behavior clearly shows that binding of the toxin to cells does not exhibit characteristics of a simple ligand-receptor interaction [8]. It further indicates that cooperative processes operate to augment toxin binding as its concentration is raised.

Since specific binders are absent, the initial diffusion of the toxin to the cell surface can probably be influenced by a number of quite nonspecific factors, including surface charge. It is probably for this reason that different cell species display a

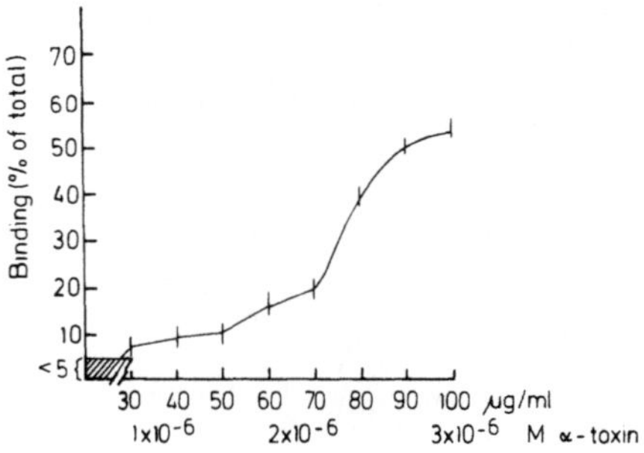

Fig. 2. Binding of staphylococcal α-toxin to erythrocytes estimated by hemolytic titrations; 0.1 ml human or rabbit cell suspensions (10^8 cells) received toxin at the final concentrations indicated. After incubation at 37°C for 60 min, the cell supernatants were titrated for hemolytic activity. The degree of toxin binding to membranes was calculated from titer loss and expressed as binding in percentage of total toxin in a given sample. Similar results were obtained for both human and rabbit erythrocytes. Binding to rabbit cells was below the limit of detection (less than 5%) at toxin concentrations below 20-30 μg/ml

very wide variation in overall sensitivity toward cytolytic toxin action. For example, it has long been known that human erythrocytes are lysed at toxin concentrations that are approximately 100-fold higher than those required to lyse rabbit erythrocytes [17]. Doubts regarding the true biologic relevance of the toxin in the human organism have therefore occasionally been voiced. However, we have noted a marked pH dependence in sensitivity of human red cells toward lytic toxin action. At pH 5-5.5, these cells are lysed by toxin levels approximately fivefold lower than those required at neutral pH. We have suggested that this phenomenon derives from neutralization of negative charges on the membrane surface which otherwise restrict diffusion of the toxin molecules to the lipidic surface through binding of the positively charged toxin (pI 8.5). The enhancement of toxic potential at low pH has obvious implications for the pathogenetic role of α-toxin in humans. Thus, pH reduction due to inflammatory processes probably allows the toxin to exert its cytotoxic action on human cells at far lower concentrations than hitherto assumed. This could be taken as an indirect argument for a true pathophysiologic role of the toxin in staphylococcal disease.

Streptolysin-O

This toxin is a secreted product of group A β-hemolytic streptococci and represents the prototype of sulfhydryl-activated bacterial cytolysins [1, 19]. At least 14 other bacterial exotoxins belong to this group and share the following properties. All are reversibly inactivated by atmospheric oxygen. The initial binding of toxin is to membrane cholesterol, and membrane damage can thus be produced in a very wide variety of mammalian cells. In contrast, bacterial membranes which lack cholesterol are not attacked by the toxins. All toxins of this class consist of a single polypeptide chain with individual molecular weights in the range 40-80 000. In many cases, cytolysis has been shown to be accompanied by the occurrence of circular and semicircular structures on the target membrane [3, 13].

We have recently isolated streptolysin-O from bacterial culture supernatants and identified two hemolytically active forms [9]. Native toxin has $M_r = 69\ 000$ and an isoelectric point of approximately 6.1. During purification procedures, it can be proteolytically cleaved to yield a hemolytic 57 000 daltons polypeptide with an isoelectric point of approximately 7.4. Both toxin forms bind to erythrocyte membranes, yielding the characteristic channel structures. Oligomers of streptolysin-O exhibit marked heterogeneity, and a broad array of structures ranging from C-shaped curved rods to fully closed rings is observed (see Fig. 1). These toxin complexes insert into the membrane to generate very large, 30- to 35-nm defects in the bilayer. Functional studies also reveal the existence of large hydrophilic pores across such membranes [11]. The channels can be particularly well visualized following their reincorporation into bilayers of pure egg lecithin (see Fig. 1). When C-shaped oligomers become membrane incorporated, the ensuing channels appear lined only in part by protein (see Fig. 1). Facing the concave sides of the protein channel, a sharp edge of lipid appears to line the residual part of the channel. Insertion of frankly "incomplete" channels consisting of C-shaped oligomers thus already appears to create transmembrane pores, probably because lipid is repelled by the hydrophilic concave sides of the membrane-inserted complexes. It will be of great interest eventually to determine the state of molecular packing and orientation of lipids in these membrane regions.

The fact that isolated and extensively delipidated toxin oligomers can reassociate with pure lecithin serves to underline the fact that cholesterol, although important in triggering the oligomerization process, does not itself significantly contribute to the structure of the channels. Once exposed, the apolar regions of the protein complexes also exhibit no recognizable specificity with regard to the type of lipid that can be bound [10].

Initial estimates yield volumes of streptolysin-O oligomers ranging from approximately 2000 to 6000 nm^3, corresponding to a range in mass of $1.5\text{-}5.0 \times 10^6$ daltons. This corresponds to a heterogeneous population of complexes containing a range of 25-80 molecules of native toxin. Hemolytic titrations indeed indicate that the presence of 70-125 toxin monomers per cell suffice to generate one functional lesion per cell [9]. It is clear that such titrations can only give an indication of the true number of lesions required to lyse a cell. They clearly suggest, however, that very few toxin oligomers (perhaps only one) formed on a membrane will induce hemolysis.

Secondary Effects Elicited by Staphylococcal α-Toxin and Streptolysin-O

Staphylococcal α-Toxin: Stimulation of the Arachidonic Acid Cascade

As already discussed, the efficacy of toxin binding to the target cell membrane is generally low, and the pore size of the toxin hexamers is comparatively small. It is therefore conceivable that nucleated target cells will be able to cope with and repair the membrane damage inflicted by the action of toxin doses occurring in vivo. In order to examine whether subcytolytic toxin concentrations might elicit detectable pathophysiologic tissue reactions, studies were undertaken in the isolated rabbit lung model as well as with cultured endothelial cells. The results obtained in both experimental systems lead us to conclude that subcytolytic toxin doses can effectively activate the arachidonic acid cascade in target cells.

In the first model, isolated rabbit lungs were ventilated and recirculatingly perfused with buffer. Injection of 0.5-5.0 µg toxin elicited a steep, dose-dependent pressure increase in the pulmonary artery. The pressor response was paralleled by the release of the arachidonic acid (AA) metabolites thromboxane B2 and 6-keto-prostaglandin $F_1\alpha$ into the perfusion fluid. They were blocked by inhibitors of thromboxane synthetase (imidazole), cyclooxygenase (indomethacin), phospholipase (mepacrine) as well as by substances interfering with intracellular Ca-calmodulin function (TMB 8, trifluoperazine). The toxin induced selective release of K (in contrast to the Ca ionophore A 23187), but not of LDH into the perfusion fluid [18].

In further studies, it became apparent that the observed release of AA metabolites was dependent on influx of calcium ions from the extracellular to the intracellular space. Thus, calcium depletion of the intravascular space by recirculation with calcium-free, EGTA-containing buffer did not suppress the toxin-dependent K release, but did abrogate the pressor response and the release of AA metabolites. This indicated that, although toxin became cell bound and transiently created small channels, no activation of the AA cascade occurred. When calcium ions were reintroduced into the circulation without application of a second toxin stimulus, marked pressor responses were registered, paralleled by release of the AA metabolites. We inferred from these findings that the reintroduced calcium ions traversed the toxin-treated cell membranes, probably via the toxin channels, to activate the AA cascade.

In order to corroborate these findings, experiments were conducted in a second model of confluent monolayers of pig pulmonary artery endothelial cells. Again, α-toxin dose-dependently stimulated release of radiolabeled AA and PG-12 production. Following an initial lag period (10 min), a rapid formation of 6-keto-PG $F_{1\alpha}$ similar to that of the Ca ionophore A 23187 was observed. The effect was abolished by preincubation of the toxin with neutralizing antibodies. The toxin response was strictly dose dependent on extracellular caclium, but not on magnesium. It was completely blocked in the absence of calcium and was promptly restored by subsequent readdition of Ca. Following toxin treatment, it was moreover found that the endothelial cells showed a significant (over fourfold) increase of transmembrane flux of Ca^{45}. Inhibition of cyclooxygenase and interference with intracellular Ca-calmodulin function again dose-dependently blocked the observed release of AA and 6-keto-PG $F_{1\alpha}$ formation [20].

These experiments thus show that staphylococcal α-toxin stimulates the AA cascade with subsequent formation of cyclooxygenase products in the vascular bed of isolated lungs as well as in cultured pulmonary endothelial cells. The data are compatible with the hypothesis that this triggering of the AA cascade occurs because of transmembrane Ca flux, possibly taking place through toxin pores (Fig. 3). It is apparent that similar processes occurring in infected tissues may well be responsible for many of the pathophysiologic effects (including inflammatory processes) encountered in staphylococcal disease.

Streptolysin-O: Autologous Complement Activation on Host Membranes

Complement activation does not occur on autologous cells and tissues under normal circumstances owing to the presence of several regulatory membrane factors, and to the absence of complement-activating autoantibodies. Complement activation on an autologous cell surface needs to be avoided since it could not only lead to generation of the biologically active polypeptides

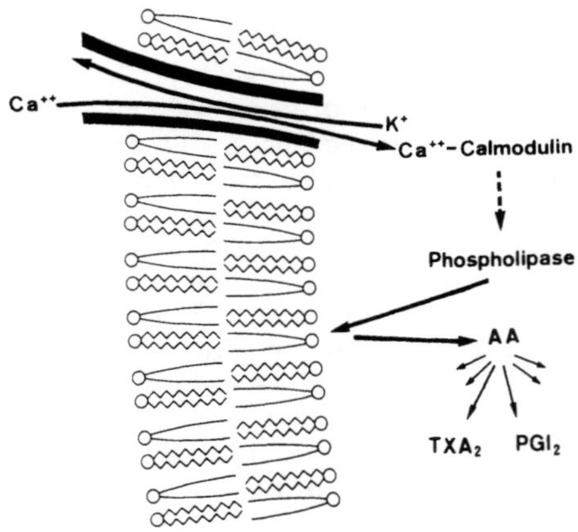

Fig. 3. Proposed mechanism for activation of the arachidonic acid cascade in nucleated cells by staphylococcal α-toxin. A toxin pore serves as a nonphysiologic calcium channel. Incoming calcium, possibly after binding to calmodulin, activates phospholipases with subsequent cleavage of arachidonic acid and formation of tissue-specific arachidonic acid metabolites

C3a/C5a, but also to the binding of C3b that will act as an opsonin, and of the terminal C5b-9 complex that will directly inflict damage to the membrane.

Through its entry into the host membrane, streptolysin-O becomes a stable, membrane-bound focus for triggering of the autologous complement system in the host. This occurs as a consequence of binding of host anti-streptolysin-O antibodies to the membranes. The activated complement system overruns all regulatory membrane factors and C5b-9 terminal complexes are generated on the autologous membranes (Fig. 4). A unique situation thus arises in which a soluble bacterial product, through its entry into the host membrane, induces self-attack by a major host defense system. The consequences in vivo may be central to the understanding of the pathogenetic mechanisms operative in streptococcal disease. When occurring in the immediate vicinity of the invading bacteria, these self-attack events probably perpetuate tissue destruction and inflammatory processes. The extraordinary stability of streptolysin-O polymers in their membrane-bound form could serve to prolong the duration of these deleterious reactions, and phagocytic removal of the afflicted tissue may represent the only possibility of interrupting the vicious circle of events. At the same time, deviation of the complement system away from the bacteria may indirectly support their invasion and persistence in the host tissues.

There may be other important consequences. If toxin is able to be transported to distant organs (e.g., the kidney), its deposition at predisposed sites could provide a later focus for autologous complement activation. It is tempting to speculate that such a process may be at least partly responsible for the pathogenesis of certain poststreptococcal diseases such as acute glomerulonephritis.

Staphylococcal α-toxin, although also a channel former, does not induce similar self-attack of cells by complement. This divergence probably is due to structural and immunologic features of

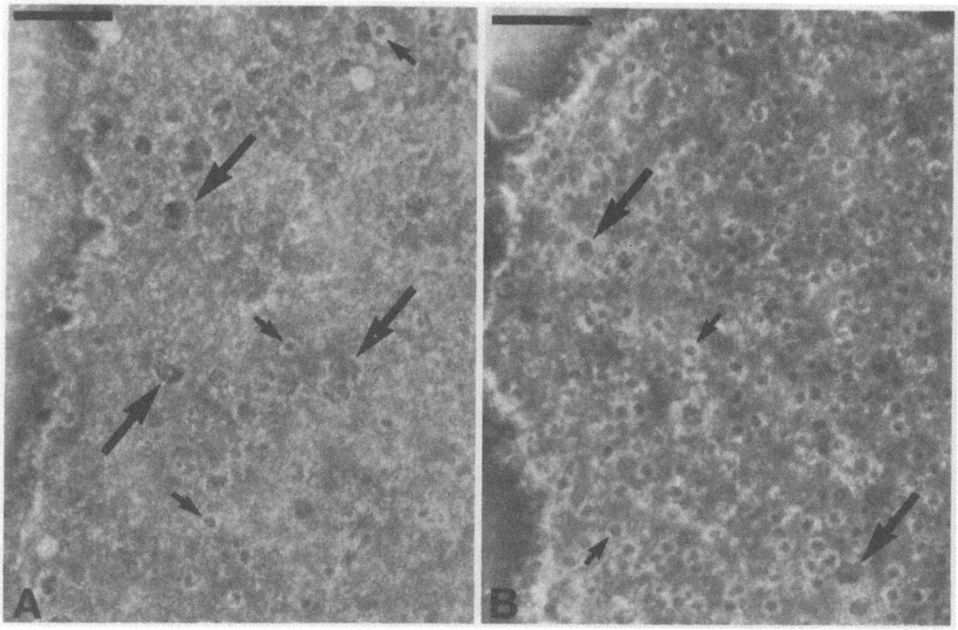

Fig. 4. Human erythrocyte membranes, lysed with streptolysin-O, washed, and posttreated with fresh autologous serum. Streptolysin-O lesions are labeled by *bold arrows*. "Classical" complement lesions are labeled by *medium-sized arrows*. Binding of host anti-SLO antibodies to toxin-damaged membranes causes activation and self-attack of autologous cells by the complement system with formation of terminal C5b-9 complexes. *Scale bars* indicate 100 nm. Sodium silicotungstate negative staining

the streptolysin-O molecule that specifically bestow strong complement-activating capacity upon the immune complexes formed with human antibody.

Concluding Remarks

Membrane damage by channel formers is still a relatively new concept in microbiology and it is clear that many interesting aspects now await investigation. The intrinsically interesting and central problem of how water-soluble proteins enter membranes is flanked by equally intriguing questions regarding the biologic effects of these proteins in the host organism. The pathophysiologic reactions elicited by staphylococcal α-toxin and streptolysin-O discussed in this paper represent but two of a multitude of secondary processes that probably may occur, depending on the nature of the toxin and the site of attack. It appears possible that relatively simple explanations will eventually be found to account for many of the diverse cellular effects known to be induced by staphylococcal α-toxin [17], streptolysin-O [1], and other channel formers.

Acknowledgments. We thank Margit Pohl and Marion Muhly for outstanding technical assistance. These investigations were supported by the Deutsche Forschungsgemeinschaft (Bh 2/1-3,4,5 and SFB 47).

References

1. Alouf JE (1980) Streptococcal toxins. Pharmacol Ther 11:661-717
2. Arbuthnott JP, Freer JH, Bernheimer AW (1967) Physical states of staphylococcal α-toxin. J Bacteriol 94:1170-1177
3. Bernheimer AW (1974) Interactions between membranes and cytolytic bacterial toxins. Biochim Biophys Acta 344:27-50
4. Bhakdi S, Tranum-Jensen J (1983) Membrane damage by complement. Biochim Biophys Acta 737:343-373
5. Bhakdi S, Tranum-Jensen J (1984) Mechanism of complement cytolysis and the concept of channel-forming proteins. Philos Trans R Soc Lond [Series B] 306:311-324
6. Bhakdi S, Füssle R, Tranum-Jensen J (1981) Staphylococcal α-toxin: Oligomerisation of hydrophilic monomers to form amphiphilic hexamers induced upon contact with deoxycholate detergent micelles. Proc Natl Acad Sci USA 78:5475-5479
7. Bhakdi S, Tranum-Jensen J, Utermann G, Füssle R (1983) Binding and partial inactivation of *S. aureus* α-toxin by human plasma low density lipoprotein. J Biol Chem 258:5899-5904
8. Bhakdi S, Muhly M, Füssle R (1984a) Membrane damage by staphylococcal α-toxin: Correlation between toxin-binding and hemolytic activity. Infect Immun 46:318-323
9. Bhakdi S, Roth M, Sziegoleit A, Tranum-Jensen J (1984b) Streptolysin-O: Isolation and identification of two hemolytic forms. Infect Immun 46: 394-400
10. Bhakdi S, Tranum-Jensen J, Sziegoleit A (1984c) Structure of streptolysin-O in target erythrocyte membranes. FEMS Symposium Proc 24:173-180
11. Buckingham L, Duncan JL (1983) Approximate dimensions of membrane lesions produced by streptolysin-S and streptolysin-O. Biochim Biophys Acta 729: 115-122
12. Duncan JL (1974) Characteristics of streptolysin-O hemolysis: Kinetics of hemoglobin and ^{86}rubidium release. Infect Immun 9:1022-1027
13. Duncan JL, Schlegel R (1975) Effect of streptolysin-O on erythrocyte membranes, liposomes, and lipid dispersions – a protein cholesterol interaction. J Cell Biol 67:160-173
14. Freer JH, Arbuthnott JP, Bernheimer AW (1968) Interaction of staphylococcal α-toxin with artificial and natural membranes. J Bacteriol 95: 1153-1168
15. Füssle R, Bhakdi S, Sziegoleit A, Tranum-Jensen J, Kranz T, Wellensiek HJ (1981) On the mechanism of membrane damage by *S. aureus* α-toxin. J Cell Biol 91:83-94
16. Mayer MM (1978) Complement, past and present. Harvey Lect 72:139-175
17. McCartney C, Arbuthnott JP (1978) Mode of action of membrane-damaging toxins produced by staphylococci. In: Bacterial toxins and cell membranes. Jeljaszewicz J, Wadström T (eds) Academic, New York, pp 89-122
18. Seeger W, Bauer M, Bhakdi S (1984) Staphylococcal α-toxin elicits hypertension in isolated rabbit lungs: Evidence for thromboxane formation and the role of extracellular calcium. J Clin Invest 74:849-858

19. Smyth CJ, Duncan JL (1978) Thiol-activated (oxygen-labile) cytolysins. In: Bacterial toxins and cell membranes. Jeljaszewicz J, Wadström T (eds) Academic, New York, pp 129-183
20. Suttorp N, Seeger W, Dewein E, Bhakdi S, Roka L (1985) Staphylococcal α-toxin stimulates synthesis of prostacyclin by cultured endothelial cells from pig pulmonary arteries. Am J Physiol 248:C127-C135

Discussion

(pp. 268-279)

Regarding the diameter of channels formed by complement, the data obtained with the black lipid membrane system yielded results comparable to those obtained by marker release studies. In both experiments, maximal channel diameters were estimated to be of the order of 5-7 nm. There is no evidence to indicate that the channel extends only halfway through the lipid bilayer, or that lipids are actually blocking the channel on one side of the bilayer. However, this possibility may be considered whenever a membrane target is thicker than 5 nm.

The freeze-fracture electron microscopy data indicate that the channel is truly transmembrane in its orientation since holes on the inner lipid monolayers are always observed complementary to the C5b-9 cylinders that are extracted together with the E-face (external monolayer). It is impossible to conclude that the holes on the inner monolayer are identical in dimensions to the internal diameter of the C5b-9 cylinder. However, the marker release studies showing escape of large molecules (diameter up to 7 nm) indeed suggest that the defect on the inner monolayer must be of comparable size.

Streptolysin-O will only bind to and attack cell membranes containing cholesterol. This forms the basis for the specificity of its action and explains why self-destruction of streptococci, spheroplasts, or L-phase variants is avoided. Concern regarding the specificity of the blockers used to inhibit the AA cascade induced by staphylococcal α-toxin was answered in the sense that all blockers used up to now support the conclusion that the Ca influx into cells mediated by the toxin is the cause of the observed effects. The model was moreover based on direct measurements of Ca influx into endothelial cells, and on the mimicking action of Ca ionophores.

Bayer-Symposium VIII
The Pathogenesis of Bacterial Infections, 281-291 (1985)

Virulence Promotion by Mixed Bacterial Infections

D. Mayrand

Summary

Virulence promotion by mixed bacterial populations has three underlying features: bacterial interactions, expression of virulence factors, and host-bacteria interactions. This paper describes examples of two of these features in relation to some bacteria that are associated with periodontal diseases. However, specific forms of periodontal disease, along with other clinical manifestations of mixed bacterial infections are still inexplicable. In view of the dynamic nature of these infections, further model testing as well as better definition of in situ relevant pathogenic properties are needed to understand the basic mechanisms in the initiation and subsequent development of such polymicrobial infections.

> Nothing is harder, yet nothing is more necessary, than to speak of certain things whose existence is neither demonstrable nor probable. The very fact that serious and conscientious men treat them as existing things brings them a step closer to existence and to the possibility of being born.
>
> Hermann Hesse, *Das Glasperlenspiel*

The very idea of mixed bacterial infections is a fairly new concept which can explain various infectious diseases, some of which have been known for centuries. For the sake of clarity, let us first define this type of infection. Generally speaking, a mixed bacterial infection is any infection which is caused by at least two bacterial entities. In practice, most cases of mixed infections involve multiple species of bacteria, of which 60%-70% are anaerobes [9, 31]. This definition by itself can partly explain why such infections have only recently been studied.

Improved sampling techniques, along with improved culture and identification methods, have helped to demonstrate the anaerobic component in mixed infections. Experimental models have also helped, in specific cases, to explain the disease process [2] and to devise ways to counteract the infection [4, 6, 7, 39].

Yet, as you probably know, the mechanisms by which mixtures of bacteria initiate and sustain infections in clinical situations and in experimental animals have only been studied in detail in the last 25 years. Still, in some cases, we have not been able: (a) to determine the bacterial species required to initiate and maintain the infectious process; (b) to explain the interbacterial relationships that exist in such infections; and (c) to define the virulence factors and the mechanisms of virulence promotion. Why? The explanation in part resides in three inherent characteristics of mixed infections:

1. The organisms can be recovered not only from a clinical infection, but also as part of the normal complex flora residing at that site. It is thus sometimes difficult to implicate specific bacteria as a cause of disease on the basis of culture alone.
2. As individuals, the members of such infections are only minimally virulent under most conditions.
3. Predisposing factors may play an important role in the initiation of such diseases. Indeed, a change, say in environmental conditions, may enable particular members of the ecosystem to become more prominent and/or to express some of their potential pathogenic features.

Another aspect, common to studies of mixed infections, relates to the fact that the organisms that could be of importance in mixed bacterial infections usually do not fulfill Koch's postulates. This is particularly true of various forms of human destructive periodontal disease. In order to circumvent this problem, a number of criteria for an etiologic role of a microorganism have been put forward by Socransky [28] as an alternative to Koch's postulates. These criteria include: (a) association with disease; (b) elimination of the microorganisms; and (c) host response to the presence of a specific organism. Other slightly less important criteria include animal pathogenicity testing, the presence of virulence factors, and mechanisms of pathogenicity.

But, even if we take into account those criteria, various clinical manifestations of mixed infections still remain inexplicable. Some types of periodontal disease can illustrate this point: the first criterion in recognizing a pathogen is its association with a specific clinical entity. However, in contrast to the more acute versions of mixed infections, most forms of periodontal disease may be considered as chronic diseases. This does not necessarily mean that these diseases proceed at a regular or constant rate. On the contrary, it now seems that periodontal diseases are characterized by bursts of activity interspersed with periods of remission or even repair [28, 30]. Thus, a key problem here is to be able to detect bacterial species of importance in periods of activity. This is, of course, complicated by the fact that the sites surrounding the lesions are also heavily colonized and that probable pathogens such as *Bacteroides gingivalis*, *Bacteroides intermedius*, *Fusobacterium nucleatum*, *Actinobacillus actinomycetemcomitans*, and species of *Eubacterium* are always isolated together with other bacteria for which a role in the disease process cannot be excluded.

Despite the complex nature of these infections and our lack of understanding of them, a number of studies have shown that virulence can be enhanced by mixed bacterial infections. Examples include a natural infection, sheep foot rot [22], and experimental infection models such as the well-known intra-abdominal infections in rats [21] or mice [19], and liver abscess infections in mice [11]. A number of experimental mixed infections involving bacteria of oral origin have also been studied. These last experimental observations are summarized in Table 1.

Looking at the results of these studies, one can conclude that:
1. Except for one study [36], all experiments dealt with mixtures of anaerobes and facultative organisms.
2. Most of the studies, if not all, showed a synergistic effect, e.g., individual bacterial species or isolates did not induce an infection whereas mixtures of two or more bacteria did produce the effects.
3. Most of these mixed infections have one common bacterial species: a black-pigmented *Bacteroides*.

Table 1. Experimental mixed infections involving oral bacteria

Model	Number of bacteria and type	Interactions	References
Fusospirochetal infection	>15 (Anaerobe/ facultative)	Synergy?	[23]
Mixed infection	2 (Anaerobe/ facultative)	Synergy (hyaluronidase)	[20]
Mixed infection	2-4 (Anaerobe/ facultative)	Synergy (nutritional dependency)	[16, 29]
Mixed infection	3 (Anaerobe)	Synergy (nutritional dependency)	[36]
Purulent infection	2-4 (Anaerobe/ facultative)	Synergy?	[33]
Mixed infection	2 (Anaerobe/ facultative)	Synergy (nutritional dependency)	[17]
Apical periodontitis	2-8 (Anaerobe/ facultative)	Synergy?	[8]
Mixed infection	4 (Anaerobe/ facultative)	Synergy	[10]

In some cases, the results obtained from these experimental infections in guinea pigs correlated very nicely, at least in terms of the bacterial species present, with results found in ligature-induced periodontitis in monkeys [15, 27] and with human clinical studies which showed the association of certain species of black-pigmented *Bacteroides* with specific clinical entities [24, 32, 37, 38, 40].

The genus *Bacteroides* as a whole and, more particularly, members of the black-pigmented *Bacteroides* thus seem to be good candidates to participate in mixed infections. Why? One reason is that these species cannot be considered as true pathogens in the sense that they do not fulfill Koch's postulates. Evidence at hand points to this conclusion (see Table 1), although some isolates of these species have been shown to induce abscesses in guinea pigs or mice and have to be considered as true pathogens [4, 13, 35].

In order to understand the whole process of a mixed infection, we first have to study the basic features exhibited by individual members of mixed bacterial infections that are part of virulence promotion. These features include bacterial interactions, virulence factors, and host-bacteria interactions. Some examples of each of these in a specific environment, the oral cavity, will be given. Three species have been chosen: *B. gingivalis*, *B. intermedius*, and *Capnocytophaga* species. The two *Bacteroides* species have definitively been associated with specific forms of periodontal diseases whereas *Capnocytophaga* species have not. It should be remembered that some of these factors can be significant in other situations and environments.

Other speakers at this Symposium have already given examples of physical relationships which can exist between two bacteria or between the host and one bacterium. Oral bacteria can also exhibit such properties via surface components (Table 2). Possible nutritional interrelations or food chains may also exist between two microorganisms in dental plaque. In this case, a sugar, for example, can be transformed by one bacterium into another compound (an organic acid) which in its turn can be utilized by a second bacterial species (Fig. 1). The result of these nutritional relationships can either be beneficial (*Streptococcus* >*Veillonella*) or detrimental (*Capnocytophaga* >*B. gingivalis*) to the host. One should also note that the growth factors indicated are bacterially derived and similar or equivalent factors can be provided by the host.

The second feature to be considered is the virulence factors of each of the bacterial species which are necessary to initiate and sustain a mixed infection. It should be evident that we do not have a clear picture of these factors for every bacterial species associated with specific oral diseases because we are still unable to specify which species are important in the whole disease process. The only thing we can do now is to determine the virulence factors of some of the bacteria: the ones associated with the actual clinical symptoms and bacteria which are generally thought to be somewhat important in the disease process. We can divide the characteristics that may play a role in

Table 2. Attributes of colonization and survival[a]

Item	*B. gingivalis*	*B. intermedius*	*Capnocytophaga*
Surface components in attachment			
Pili	+	+	?
Long fibers	+	+	*C. sputigena* +
Capsule	+	+	*C. sputigena* +
Vesicles	+	+	*C. sputigena* +
Lipopoly-saccharide	+	+	+
Growth-stimulatory factors			
Bacteria-derived	Naphthaquinone	Naphthaquinone	?
Bacteria-derived	Succinate	Succinate	?

[a]Modified from Slots and Genco [26]. Additional references: Grenier and Mayrand [10]; Mouton and Mayrand (unpublished work).

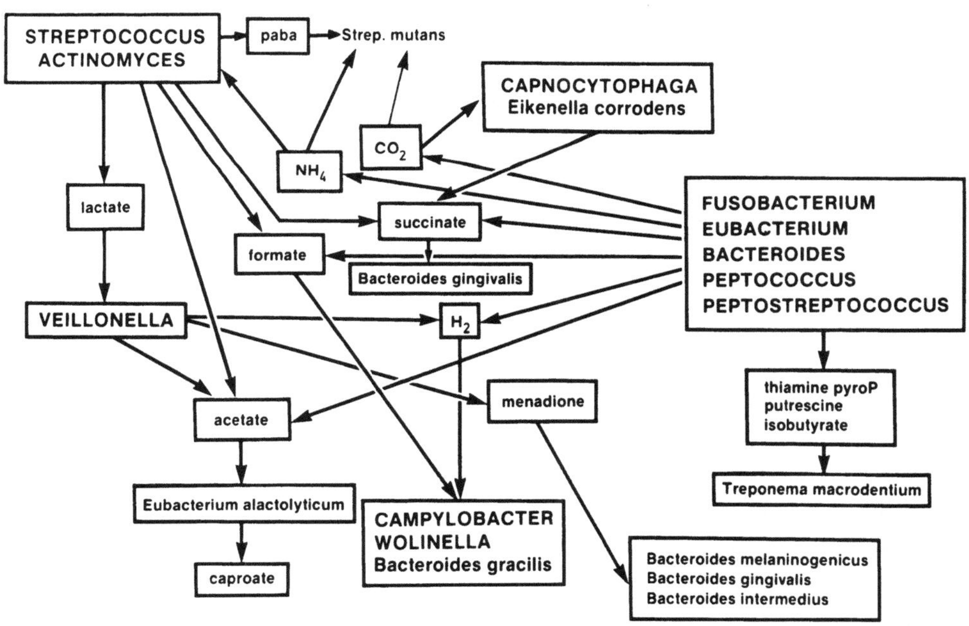

Fig. 1. Possible nutritional relationships between oral bacteria

virulence into three categories: (a) those important in colonization (already seen in Table 2); (b) those important in evading host defense systems; and (c) products with potential to destroy host tissues.

Oral bacteria possess a number of properties which facilitate bacterial evasion from or even destruction of host defense systems (Table 3). These include inhibition of PMN functions, resistance to complement-mediated killing, immunoglobulin proteases, etc. Recently, Sundqvist and co-workers [34] showed that one particular *B. gingivalis* strain could degrade in vivo protein C3 of the complement system. Most of these properties could at least lead to a local paralysis of the host defense system, thus enabling bacteria to advance the front of the lesion.

Table 3. Attributes of evasion or destruction of host defense systems[a]

Item	*B. gingivalis*	*B. intermedius*	*Capnocytophaga*
Inhibition of polymorphonuclear leukocytes			
Leukotoxin	-	-	-
Chemotaxis inhibitors	+	+	+
Decreased phagocytosis and intracellular killing	+	+	?
Resistance to complement-mediated killing	+	+	?
C3 (complement) degradation	+	-	?
Lymphocyte alterations	?	?	+
Endotoxicity	Weak	Weak	Weak to moderate
Immunoglobulin proteases			
IgA	+	+	+
IgG	+	+	+
Fibrinolysin	Strong	Weak	-
Superoxide dismutase	+	+	+

[a] Modified from Slots and Genco [26]. Additional references: Sundqvist et al. [34]; Grenier and Mayrand (unpublished work).

Finally (Table 4), these bacteria, and particularly *B. gingivalis*, exhibit a vast array of enzymatic activities and produce potent toxic factors which have the potential to destroy various types of host tissues [12, 25]. Since the particular habitat of these bacteria is the gingival sulcus or pocket, butyric acid, collagenase, trypsin-like enzyme, hyaluronidase, and various bone-resorbing factors should be considered as significant entities.

Table 4. Attributes of tissue destruction[a]

Item	*B. gingivalis*	*B. intermedius*	*Capnocytophaga*
Abscess former	Strong	Moderate	-
Enzymes			
Degradation of proteinase inhibitors	+	-	?
Collagenase	+	-	-
Trypsin-like	+	-	-/+
Gelatinase	Strong	Moderate	-
Aminopeptidases	+/-	-	+
Phospholipase A	+	+	?
Alkaline phosphatase	+	+	+
Acid phosphatase	+	+	+
Hyaluronidase	+	-	-
Toxic factors			
Epitheliotoxin	+	+	+
Fibroblast growth inhibitors	+	+	+
Endotoxicity	Weak	Weak	Weak to moderate
Lipopolysaccharide-induced bone resorption	+	+	+
Other bone-resorbing factors	?	?	?
Volatile sulfur compounds	+	+	?
Butyric and propionic acids	+	-	-
Indole	+	+	-
Ammonia	+	+	-

[a]Modified from Slots and Genco [26]. Additional references: Carlsson et al. [5]; Mayrand et al. [18]; Grenier and Mayrand [10]; Grenier and Mayrand (unpublished work).

The third feature, bacteria-host interactions, implies, in a sense, that the host, in response to a bacterial invasion, can in some instances, via inflammmation processes and various lymphokines, aggravate its own condition. Various types of periodontal disease show such interactions which are not protective for the host and thus lead to tissue destruction [1]. However, very little is actually known about these interactions between the host cells and the various bacterial components and excreted products and how the bacteria can profit from them.

Now that we have seen the basic features of some bacterial species which take part in mixed infections, the next and last item that I want to address is the question of mechanisms of virulence promotion. Unfortunately, it is very difficult at this point to describe such mechanisms. At best, we only can imagine the mechanistic events which will lead to a recognized mixed infection.

We can envision three basic types of mechanism which could explain virulence promotion by mixed bacterial populations. These I call the "addition" model, the "cascade" model, and the "sequential" model. Of course, we can also imagine a number of combinations of these basic types (Fig. 2). These rather simplistic models may in part explain different types of mixed infection; first, from the point of view of time of appearance of clinical symptoms and second, from the mechanistic events which take place.

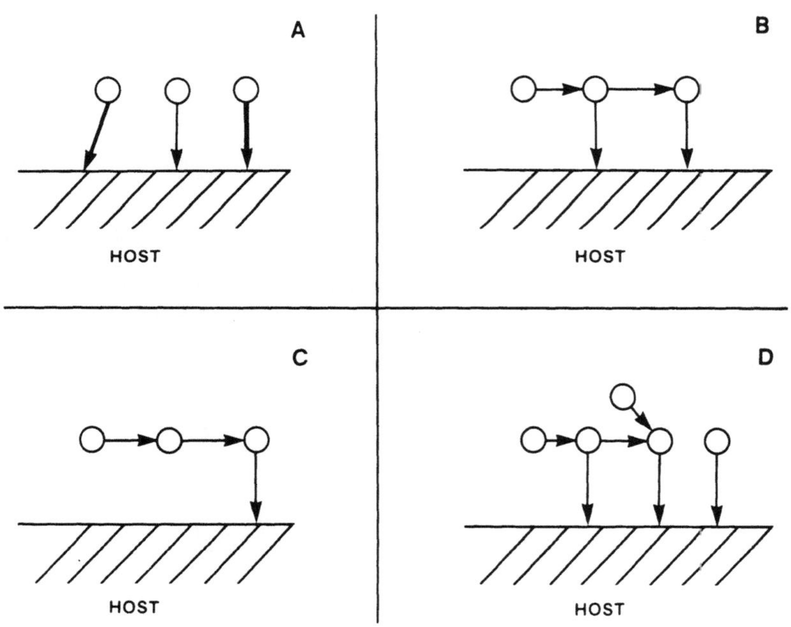

Fig. 2. Possible mechanisms of virulence promotion in mixed bacterial infections

The "addition" model (Fig. 2a) may reflect an acute situation where the infection is the net result of additive effects of bacteria which all possess the necessary abilities to penetrate host tissues, to survive, and to cause tissue damage. The sheer number of these bacteria or the increased proportion of all these specific bacteria enables them to resist the host defense system. The "cascade" model (Fig. 2b) might reflect a two-stage or multiple-stage reaction which can either be acute or manifest itself within days or a few weeks from initation. The intra-abdominal abscess model in rats [21] could serve as an example of this situation. On the other hand, the "sequential" model (Fig. 2c) can reflect a more chronic situation. The clinical symptoms may take months or years to manifest themselves.

Some periodontal disease entities can fall within this category and results from ligature-induced periodontitis in monkeys [14, 15], along with studies of combinations of oral bacteria on periapical tissues of monkeys [8], indicate that this model may be common for mixed bacterial infections in the oral cavity. Finally, several possible combinations of these basic models can be imagined. Figure 2d illustrates one such model which, in its turn, can be represented by the natural infection, sheep foot rot, studied by Roberts [22].

In summary, we can say that there is ample evidence to indicate that virulence can be enhanced within mixed bacterial populations. What remains to be determined is the pathway, or pathways, effecting the promotion of virulence. I think that any worker studying mixed infections in which each single bacterial component does not show overt pathogenicity is faced with a dilemma. On the one hand, dominant species within established lesions, endowed with a large set of pathogenic attributes, nevertheless require factors from other bacteria or the host to express their pathogenicity fully. On the other hand, one is forced to admit that, within the mixed bacterial population, species devoid of overt pathogenicity participate in the infectious process to establish the clinical lesion.

Acknowledgments. I wish to acknowledge the helpful comments and suggestions of G. Bourgeau, C. Mouton, and R.J. Bojanowsky. Work done by the author was supported by Canadian Medical Research Council grant MT-6799.

References

1. Attström R, Lindhe J (1983) Pathogenesis of plaque associated periodontal disease. In: Lindhe J (ed) Textbook of clinical periodontology, 1st edn. Munksgaard, Copenhagen
2. Bartlett JG (1982) Virulence factors of anaerobic bacteria. John Hopkins Med J 151:1-9
3. Brook I, Coolbaugh JC, Walker RI (1983a) Antibiotic and clavulanic acid treatment of subcutaneous abscesses caused by *Bacteroides fragilis* alone or in combination with aerobic bacteria. J Infect Dis 148:156-159
4. Brook I, Gillmore JD, Coolbaugh JC, Walker RI (1983b) Pathogenicity of encapsulated *Bacteroides melaninogenicus* group, *B. oralis* and *B. ruminicola* subsp. *brevis* in abscesses in mice. J Infect 7:218-226

5. Carlsson J, Herrmann BF, Höfling JF, Sundqvist GK (1984) Degradation of the human proteinase inhibitors alpha-1-antitrypsin and alpha-2-macroglobulin by *Bacteroides gingivalis*. Infect Immun 43:644-648
6. Dalhoff A (1982a) Therapy of infections caused by mixed cultures of *Escherichia coli* and *Streptococcus faecalis*. Curr Microbiol 7:275-280
7. Dalhoff A (1982b) Influence of beta-lactam antibiotics in vitro on mixed cultures of *Escherichia coli* and *Streptococcus faecalis*. Curr Microbiol 7:269-274
8. Fabricius L, Dahlen G, Holm SE, Moller AJR (1982) Influence of combinations of oral bacteria on periapical tissues of monkeys. Scand J Dent Res 90:200-206
9. Gorbach SL (1982) The pre-eminent role of anaerobes in mixed infections. J Antimicrob Chemother 10:1-6
10. Grenier D, Mayrand D (1983) Etudes d'infections mixtes anaêrobies comportant *Bacteroides gingivalis*. Can J Microbiol 29:612-618
11. Hill GB, Osterhout S, Pratt PC (1974) Liver abscess production by non-spore-forming anaerobic bacteria in a mouse model. Infect Immun 9:599-603
12. Holt SC (1982) Bacterial surface structures and their role in periodontal disease. In: Mergenhagen SE, Genco RJ (eds) Host-parasite interactions in periodontal diseases. ASM, Washington, pp 139-150
13. Kastelein P, van Steenbergen TJM, Bras JM, de Graaff J (1981) An experimentally induced phlegmonous abscess by a strain of *Bacteroides gingivalis* in guinea pigs and mice. Antonie van Leeuwenhoek 47:1-9
14. Kiel RA, Kornman KS, Robertson PB (1983) Clinical and microbiological effects of localized ligature-induced periodontitis on non-ligated sites in the cynomolgus monkey. J Periodontal Res 18:200-211
15. Kornman KS, Holt SC, Robertson PB (1981) The microbiology of ligature-induced periodontitis in the cynomolgus monkey. J Periodontal Res 16:363-371
16. Macdonald JB, Sutton RM, Madlener EM, Grainger RM (1956) The pathogenic components of an experimental fusospirochetal infection. J Infect Dis 98:15-20
17. Mayrand D, McBride BC (1980) Ecological relationships of bacteria involved in a simple mixed anaerobic infection. Infect Immun 17:44-50
18. Mayrand D, McBride BC, Edwards T, Jensen S (1980) Characterization of *Bacteroides asaccharolyticus* and *B. melaninogenicus* oral isolates. Can J Microbiol 26:1178-1183
19. McCallum RE, Rohrer MD, Urbaschek R, Urbaschek B (1982) Histopathology of mixed anaerobic intraabdominal infection in mice. Klin Wochenschr 60:702-704
20. Mergenhagen SE, Thonard JC, Scherp HW (1958) Studies on synergistic infections. J Infect Dis 103:33-44
21. Onderdonk AB, Bartlett JG, Louie T, Sullivan-Seigler N, Gorbach SL (1976) Microbial synergy in experimental intra-abdominal abscess. Infect Immun 13:22-26
22. Roberts DS (1969) Synergic mechanisms in certain mixed infections. J Infect Dis 120:720-724
23. Rosebury T, Clark AR, Engel SG, Tergis F (1950) Studies of fusospirochetal infection. J Infect Dis 87:217-225
24. Slots J (1979) Subgingival microflora and periodontal disease. J Clin Periodontol 6:351-382
25. Slots J (1982) Importance of black-pigmented *Bacteroides* in human periodontal disease. In: Genco RJ, Mergenhagen SE (eds) Host-parasite interactions in periodontal diseases. ASM, Washington, pp 27-45

26. Slots J, Genco RJ (1984) Black-pigmented *Bacteroides* species, *Capnocytophaga* species, and *Actinobacillus actinomycetemcomitans* in human periodontal disease: virulence factors in colonization, survival, and tissue destruction. J Dent Res 63:412-421
27. Slots J, Hausmann E (1979) Longitudinal study of experimentally induced periodontal disease in *Macaca arctoides*: relationship between microflora and alveolar bone loss. Infect Immun 23:260-269
28. Socransky SS (1979) Criteria for the infectious agents in dental caries and periodontal disease. J Clin Periodontol 7:16-21
29. Socransky SS, Gibbons RJ (1965) Required role of *Bacteroides melaninogenicus* in mixed anaerobic infections. J Infect Dis 115:247-253
30. Socransky SS, Haffajee AD, Goodson JM, Lindhe J (1984) New concepts of destructive periodontal disease. J Clin Periodont 11:21-32
31. Socransky SS, Tanner ACA, Haffajee AD, Hillman JD, Goodson JM (1982) Present status of studies on the microbial etiology of periodontal diseases. In: Genco RJ, Mergenhagen SE (eds) Host-parasite interactions in periodontal diseases. ASM, Washington
32. Spiegel CA, Hayduk SE, Minah GE, Krywolap GN (1979) Black-pigmented *Bacteroides* from clinically characterized periodontal sites. J Periodontal Res 14:376-382
33. Sundqvist GK, Eckerbom MI, Larsson AP, Sjogren UT (1979) Capacity of anaerobic bacteria from necrotic dental pulps to induce purulent infections. Infect Immun 25:685-693
34. Sundqvist GK, Carlsson J, Herrmann BF, Höfling JF, Väätäinen A (1984) Degradation in vivo of the C3 protein of guinea-pig complement by a pathogenic strain of *Bacteroides gingivalis*. Scand J Dent Res 92:14-24
35. Takazoe I, Tanaka M, Homma T (1971) A pathogenic strain of *Bacteroides melaninogenicus*. Arch Oral Biol 16:817-822
36. Takazoe I, Nakamura T (1971) Experimental mixed infection by human gingival crevice material. Bull Tokyo Dent Coll 12:85-93
37. Tanner ACR, Haffer C, Bratthall GT, Visconti RA, Socransky SS (1979) A study of the bacteria associated with advancing periodontitis in man. J Clin Periodontol 6:278-307
38. White D, Mayrand D (1981) Association of oral *Bacteroides* with gingivitis and adult periodontitis. J Periodontal Res 16:259-265
39. Wilkins TD (1982) Chemotherapy of experimental anaerobic infections. J Antimicrob Chemother 9:249-251
40. Zambon JJ, Reynolds HS, Slots J (1981) Black-pigmented *Bacteroides* spp. in the human oral cavity. Infect Immun 32:198-203

Discussion

(pp. 281-291)

In the establishment of mixed infections, the aerobic component may be important for lowering the oxidation reduction potential so that the anaerobic component can proliferate. However, inter-bacterial nutritional relationships are at least as important. For example, one anaerobe supplied succinate to *B. gingivalis* in a mixed infection. In the dental plaque and the ginvival pockets, there is very little or no oxygen. Of the 50-100 species in the mouth, the important ones have not all been defined nor have any real toxins been identified.

Session 4

Tissue Invasion, Inflammation, and Immunopathologic Disease

Chairman: Ph. Y. Paterson

Bayer-Symposium VIII
The Pathogenesis of Bacterial Infections, 294-307 (1985)

Vascular Endothelium: The Interface Between the Site of Antigen and Cellular Immunity

D. R. Burger, C. R. Wagner, and R. M. Vetto

Summary

Endothelial cells line the vessels and lymphatics, forming a barrier between circulating T cells and the extravascular tissue site of antigen. We have suggested that circulating T cells recognize antigen on the surface of endothelial cells, resulting in the activation of the endothelium such that the endothelial cells then release the key mediators of a cell-mediated immune response. To test this hypothesis we have evaluated the extent to which endothelial cells can signal antigen-specific T cell activation. We have shown that cultured endothelial cells are as effective as macrophages in lymphocyte activation and that this activation is HLA-DR restricted. In additional experiments, we have established that endothelial cells synthesize both Ia and IL-1 early in the signaling process. To eliminate any possible contribution of other cell types participating in the T cell-endothelial cell interaction, we have shown that cloned endothelial cells present antigen to cloned T cells. These experiments document that endothelial cells are independently competent antigen-presenting cells.

Introduction

Endothelial cells (EC) line the vessels and lymphatics, forming a barrier between circulating T cells and the extravascular tissue site of antigen. The fact that this barrier must be transgressed in a cell-mediated immune (CMI) response has stimulated our interest in the role of the endothelium in CMI. We have recently published a hypothesis suggesting that the vascular endothelium may be a major participant in T lymphocyte immunity [1]. We suggested that circulating T cells recognize antigen on the surface of EC, resulting in the activation of endothelium such that the EC then release the key mediators of a CMI response. These mediators would then promote lymphocyte activation and egress into the extravascular tissue. This theory would account for the brief cell-cell exposure which occurs during ordinary hemodynamics and for the rapid dilution of factors by blood flow. That is, the EC would become activated after brief contact with antigen-specific T cells and then the activated EC could focally release mediators. Thus, while antigen-specific T cells would still provide the specificity of the CMI response, the EC would be the central participant in the maturation of this response.

A crucial feature for the validity of this model is the extent to which endothelial cells can signal T cells. Recently we [2,3] and others [4,5] have provided preliminary evidence that endothelial cells fulfill the requirements that lead to the expression of T cell activation. We have have previously shown that cultured endothelial cells from umbilical veins are as effective as macrophages in signaling lymphocyte activation and that this activation is genetically restricted at the HLA-DR locus [2,3]. The experiments presented here are designed to evaluate the mechanism by which endothelial cells fulfill the antigen presentation requirements and activate antigen-specific T cells.

Endothelial cells are obtained by collagenase treatment of umbilical veins and are cultured in fibronectin-treated flasks in media containing EC growth factor (ECGF) [6]. As a result of these culture conditions, we have been able to maintain EC in culture for at least 20 subcultures and recover EC from liquid nitrogen storage. The capability to maintain EC in culture for extended periods has facilitated the experiments described subsequently. In this report we document that: (a) endothelial cells synthesize and express Ia upon contact with T cells or T cell factors; (b) endothelial cells produce IL-1 upon external stimulation; and (c) cloned endothelial cells present antigen to cloned T cells, thus eliminating concern that additional cell types participate in these activation events.

Materials and Methods

Isolation of Blood Mononuclear Cells

Mononuclear cells (MNC) were separated from heparinized (10 U/ml) peripheral blood from normal donors by Ficoll-Hypaque (Pharmacia Fine Chemicals, Piscataway, New Jersey) density gradient centrifugation [2]. Interface cells were subsequently washed twice with RPMI 1640 (Gibco, Grand Island, New York) and counted.

Macrophage Isolation

Cells of the mononuclear phagocytic series (MO) were isolated from MNC by adherence to plastic. Tissue culture flasks (No. 3013, Falcon, Oxnard, California) were pretreated for 30-60 min at 4°C with RPMI + 50% AB serum and rinsed. MNC (40-60 $\times$ 10^6 cells) were added to the pretreated flasks in RPMI with 5% AB serum. After a 1- to 2-h incubation at 37°C and 5% CO_2, the flasks were rinsed with medium to remove nonadherent cells. Subsequently, RPMI with 5% AB serum and 0.2% EDTA was added and the flasks were held for 10-20 min at room temperature. The macrophages were removed by shaking and vigorous pipetting, washed twice, and counted.

Macrophage Depletion

Macrophage depletion was accomplished by two sequential steps: adherence to plastic and passage over Sephadex G-10 (Pharmacia

Fine Chemicals, Piscataway, New Jersey). The MNC, routinely containing 5%-15% monocytes, were first subjected to adherence on serum-pretreated plastic flasks as described. After 1-2 h, the nonadherent cells were washed from the flasks and resuspended in 2 ml RPMI with 5% AB serum. Sephadex G-10 was resuspended to 2-3 times its bed volume in RPMI and autoclaved for 20 min. A column consisting of a plastic 20-ml syringe barrel was prepared and used as previously described [7]. Briefly, the column was packed by gravity flow with 15 ml swollen Sephadex G-10 and washed with 2 volumes RPMI with 5% AB serum. Cells (2 ml) were added to the top of the column and followed by 1 ml RPMI (5% AB serum). The column was then incubated for 30 min at 37°C and 5% CO_2. The cells were eluted with RPMI (5% AB serum) in 5-10 ml and washed (10 min at 250 *g*). The isolated cells characteristically contained less than 0.2% monocytes by esterase staining and would not support antigen-induced lymphocyte proliferation without macrophage addition.

Endothelial Cells

Endothelial cells were isolated from the vein of umbilical cords by a modification of the technique described by Jaffe et al. [8]. The fresh cords were cannulated, flushed with saline, and then filled with 0.2% collagenase (Sigma Chemical Company, No. C-0131, St. Louis, Missouri). After a 20-min incubation at 37°C, the endothelial cells were expressed with 20 ml RPMI and washed (10 min at 250 *g*). The cells were dispersed into culture plates (approximately 10^4 cells per well) and cultured in RPMI with 20% heat-inactivated fetal calf serum and 4 µg/ml ECGF [6] at 37°C and 5% CO_2. Approximately 10% of the cultures grew vigorously, becoming monolayers within 4-6 days. The cells were released from the plastic by a brief treatment (3 min) with trypsin-EDTA at room temperature, centrifuged (10 min at 500 *g*), and replated into human fibronectin-coated (4 µg/ml, Collaborative Research Products) 25-cm^2 culture flasks. The endothelial cell cultures were expanded by repetitive subculturing (splitting the cells 1:4 within a week of reaching a monolayer). To confirm that the cultured cells were endothelial cells, cytocentrifuged cells were stained with monoclonal antibody to factor VIII related antigen (Cappel Laboratories, West Chester, Pennsylvania) followed by FITC-conjugated goat anti-mouse IgG (Cappel Laboratories) and then examined by fluorescent microscopy.

Standard Lymphocyte Proliferation Assay

MO-depleted MNC were diluted to 10^6 cells/ml in RPMI supplemented with antibiotics and 30% AB serum and 100 µl (10^5 cells) distributed in flat-botted, 96-well microplates. Additional 100-µl preparations containing antigen dilutions, other cells, or media alone were added in quadruplicate to appropriate wells, depending upon the experimental design. The antigens used were measles (30-850J), mumps - viral and soluble (30-848J), and varicella (30-149J), (complement fixation antigens from M.A. Bioproducts, Walkersville, Massachusetts) and tuberculin PPD (Connaught Laboratories Limited, Willowdale, Ontario, Canada). The microplates were incubated in a 5% CO_2, humidified atmosphere for 4 days, the last 24 h with 0.1 µCi thymidine ^3H (specific activity 6.7 Ci/mmol, New England Nuclear, Boston, Massachusetts). The cultures were harvested and counted by commonly used automated techniques [9].

HLA-DR Typing of MNC

Cell donors were healthy volunteers whose HLA-DR phenotypes were established by standard serologic techniques [10] in a commercial laboratory (Epitope Incorporated, Portland, Oregon).

Antisera/Monoclonal Antibodies

Monoclonal antibodies to monomorphic HLA-DR determinants: NEI-011 (clone 7.2), was obtained from New England Nuclear, Boston, Massachusetts; and BRL DR.1, was obtained from Bethesda Research Laboratories, Rockville, Maryland. Monoclonal antibodies to HLA-DS framework determinants, Genox 3.53, was the gift of Frank Bodner, Imperial Cancer Research Fund, London; and Anti-Leu-10, was obtained from Becton Dickinson, Mountain View, California. Monoclonal antibody specific for human monocytes, Mac-120, was a gift of Howard Raff, Department of Microbiology, University of Washington, Seattle. All antibodies used in culture were extensively dialysed against RPMI prior to use.

T Cell Cloning

T cells were expanded in continuous culture by alternate exposure to IL-2 and antigen-pulsed MO for 7- to 10-day periods. After three rounds, the cells were cloned by limiting dilution on irradiated monocyte monolayers as previously described [11]. Antigen-responsive clones were recloned in IL-2-containing media without monocytes at least once prior to use in these experiments.

Thymidine Suicide Technique

The thymidine suicide technique for elimination of dividing cells was a modification of that described by Hirschberg et al. [12]. The MNC were cultured in tissue culture tubes (10^6 cells/ml, 2-5 ml) in RPMI supplemented with 15% heat-inactivated (56°C for 30 min) fetal calf serum with and without antigen added in the optimal dose-response range. Monocytes isolated from the MNC (described previously) were distributed into microplates (10^4 cells/100-µl/well) and the plates held at 37°C until needed. After 2-5 days of incubation (37°C and 5% CO_2), the tube cultures received 10 µCi thymidine ^3H (specific activity 44 Ci/mmol, The Radiochemical Centre, Amersham, England) for an additional 24 h. The tube-cultured cells were washed (two or three times), diluted with RPMI so that 50 µl dispensed 10^5 cells into each well of the microplate which had been set aside with monocytes previously added. An additional 50 µl containing antigen dilutions was then distributed to quadruplicate wells and the microplate was incubated for 2-4 days, pulsed with 0.1 µCi thymidine ^3H (specific activity 6.7 Ci/mmol), and harvested 24 h later.

EC Cloning

Endothelial cells from the 14th subculture were cloned twice by limiting dilution in the presence of ECGF. Less than 2% of the cloning attempts survived to yield the cell numbers required for a single experiment. None produced more than 2 × 10^6 cells before exhibiting failure to thrive.

IL-1 Assessment

IL-1 assessment was accomplished by the use of IL-1-dependent LBRM-33-1A5 production of IL-2 [13] performed by Steven Hefeneider (Immunex Corporation, Seattle, Washington). A volume of 100 µl LBRM-33-1A5 cells (5 × 10^5 cells/ml) inactivated by mitomycin C (50 µg/ml, 1 h, 37°C), was cultured in 96-well, flat-bottomed plates in the presence of equal volumes of tissue culture medium alone, PHA (phytohemmagglutinin M; 0.1% final concentration by volume, Gibco), IL-1 (at several dilutions) or both PHA and IL-1. After 24 h of incubation, IL-2 activity was determined by the direct addition of 50 µl CTLL-2 cells (8 × 10^4 cells/ml). The microwell cultures were incubated for an additional 20 h, followed by a 4-h pulse with 0.5 µCi thymidine ^{3}H.

Results

Antigen Presentation by Subcultured Endothelial Cells

The capability to maintain endothelial cells in culture for extented periods of time (up to 20 subcultures) has facilitated many of the experiments described here. The basic experimental design (Fig. 1) involves addition of endothelial cells to lymphocyte cultures which have been previously depleted of antigen-presenting cells (APC). An analysis of MO depletion is detailed in Fig. 2 which shows that MO-depleted T cells could not respond to antigen without subsequent MO addition. When antigen-pulsed EC were used to reconstitute the MO-depleted cultures, lymphocyte activation was observed in all experiments evaluated (Fig. 3) MO-depleted T cells did not respond to antigen alone (Fig. 3, column one) whereas addition of either macrophages or EC fully reconstituted the response (Fig. 3, columns 2 and 3). In these experiments, the EC were from the subcultures 2-3. In control experiments, we showed that fibroblasts or smooth muscle cells cultured from the same umbilical veins could not reconstitute these responses (Fig. 4, column 2). Moreover, the reconstitution of the response with EC was not due to macrophage contamination of either cell preparation since it was not blocked by monoclonal antibodies [14] against macrophages (Fig. 4, column 3), but was blocked by endothelial-specific monoclonal reagents (Fig. 4, column 4). In previous experiments [2], we have shown that the anti-macrophage monoclonal antibody completely blocked macrophage presentation of antigen. The presentation of antigen by EC was HLA-DR restricted since polymorphic antisera against HLA-DR blocked presentation in a restricted fashion (Fig. 5).

When endothelial cell cultures were maintained by serial subculture, the cells continued to be endothelial by morphological criteria, general growth patterns, and specific marker analysis (e.g., factor VIII-related antigen). The results presented in Fig. 6 demonstrate that endothelial cells from subcultures 5-18 were effective at antigen presentation. Additional experiments

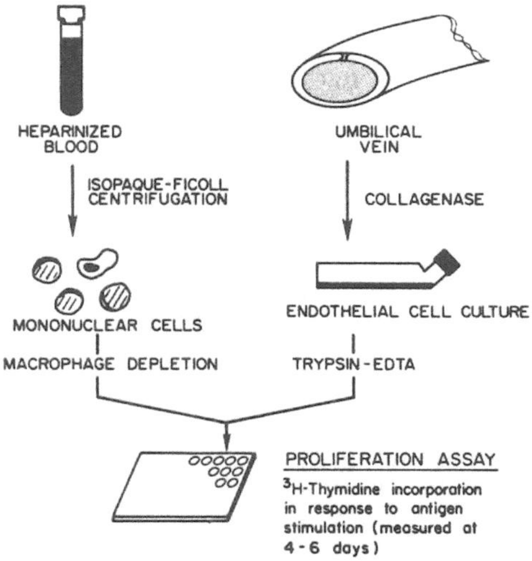

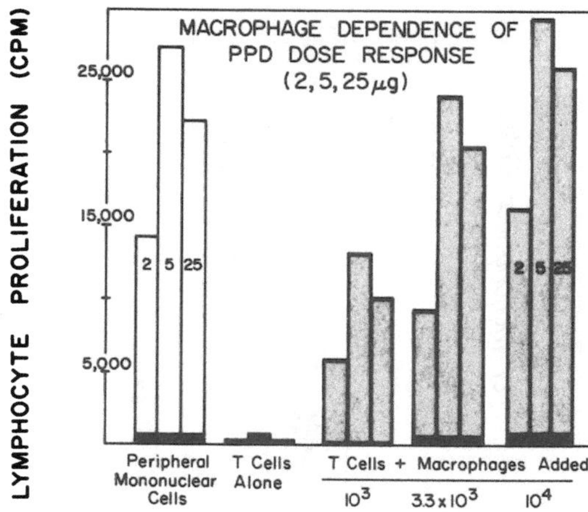

Fig. 1

Fig. 2

Fig. 1. Experimental design for evaluating the capability of endothelial cells to present antigen

Fig. 2. Demonstration that lymphocyte proliferation is dependent on macrophages for optimal responses. T cells are cultured at 10^5 cells per culture

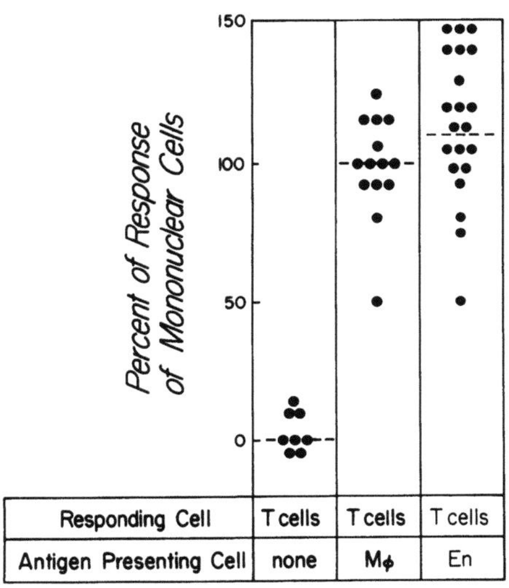

Fig. 3. Scatter diagram comparing presentation of antigen by endothelial cells with presentation of antigen by macrophages. The proliferation response is expressed as a percentage of the response obtained with autologous macrophages. *Broken line* represents the mean response

suggested that the variation in responses seen when subcultured EC were used is due to problems with the precise enumeration of the number of EC added to the cultures and not changes in presentation efficiency (Fig. 6, tuberculin response, subculture 5,6,7, 18). Overall, these results support the idea that EC can themselves fulfill all of the requirements of APC.

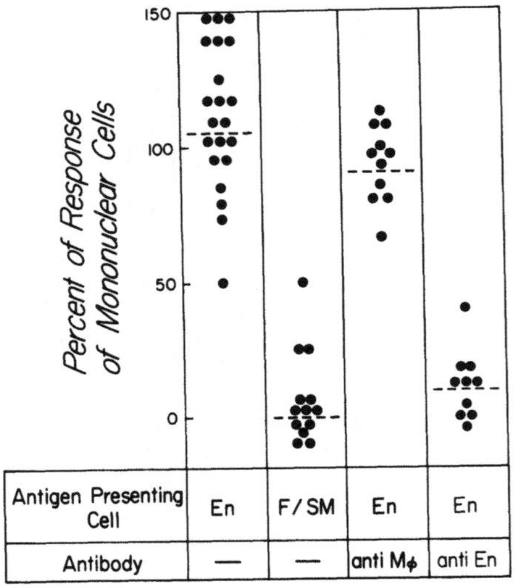

Fig. 4

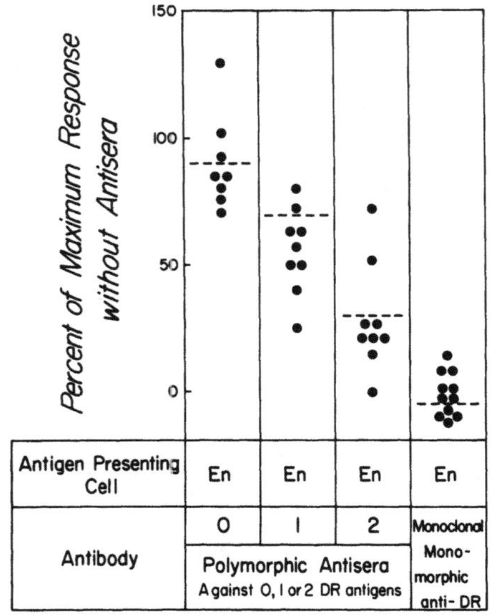

Fig. 5

Fig. 4. Scatter diagram depicting the effects of a monoclonal anti-macrophage antibody or monoclonal anti-endothelial cell antibody on lymphocyte proliferation induced by antigen-pulsed endothelial cells (EC). The effect of fibroblasts and smooth muscle cells (F/SM) as antigen-presenting cells is also shown. The 100% response was the proliferation obtained with antigen-pulsed macrophages and a control monoclonal antibody added to cultures. *Broken line* represents the mean response

Fig. 5. Scatter diagram depicting the effects of polymorphic HLA-DR antisera on lymphocyte proliferation in secondary cultures induced by antigen-pulsed endothelial cells. The maximum response was the proliferation obtained with antigen-pulsed endothelial cells and normal human sera added to cultures rather than the alloantisera. *Broken line* represents mean response

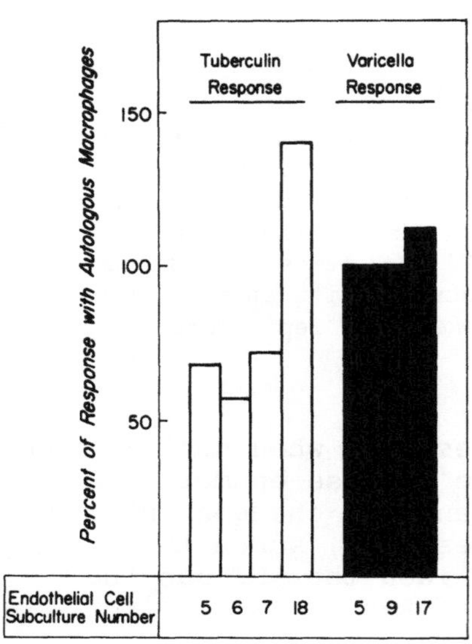

Fig. 6. Comparison of antigen presentation by various subcultures of EC with antigen presentation by fresh macrophages

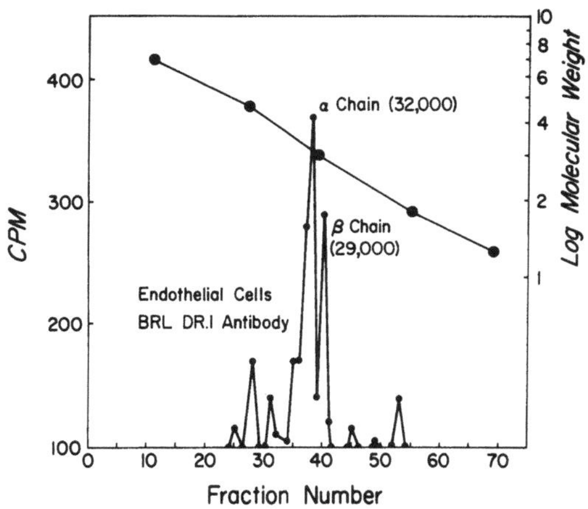

Fig. 7. Synthesis of HLA-DR antigen by human endothelial cells. Data points represent CPM of ^{14}C-labeled amino acids incorporated into immunoprecipitated proteins in SDS-polyacrylamide gel following electrophoresis

MHC Class II Determinants on Endothelial Cells

It is currently thought that T cells recognize antigen in the context of Ia (MHC class II) determinants on the surface of APC. Therefore, if subcultured EC are capable of presenting antigen without the aid of other "accessory" cells, EC should be able to synthesize Ia determinants (HLA-D region determinants in humans). After exposure of subcultured EC to either T cells (depleted of APC) and antigen or T cell factors, we have been able to immunoprecipitate radiolabeled EC membrane proteins with antibody to HLA-DR (BRL DR.1). By SDS-PAGE (reducing conditions), the immunoprecipitated proteins were found to have the characteristic molecular weights of traditional human class II MHC determinants with an α chain of 32 000 and a β chain of 29 000 (Fig. 7).

Recently, an additional human class II locus, HLA-DS has been recognized [15]. Using the same protocol, it was possible to immunoprecipitate EC membrane proteins (with molecular weights of 31 000 and 29 000) using Genox 3.53 antibody to HLA-DS (data not shown). Consequently, it appears that EC are capable of synthesizing both HLA-DR and HLA-DS determinants.

IL-1 and Signals for Activation

In addition to antigen and Ia determinants, macrophage-derived IL-1 is thought to be a requirement for T cell activation. MO IL-1 activity has been assayed by the LBRM cell line assay system described by Conlon [13]. In the presence of IL-1, LBRM cells secrete IL-1 which can then be assayed on IL-2-dependent cells. As can be seen in Table 1, our results show that when subcultured EC are stimulated with bacterial lipopolysaccharide (5 µg/ml, *Escherichia coli* 055:B5, Difco Laboratories) that they produce an activity that is positive in this IL-1 assay. These results are consistent with the conclusion that EC produce functional IL-1 although isolation and characterization of this activity will be required to conclude that it is the same structure. In preliminary experiments, macrophage IL-1 activity and endothelial cell IL-1 activity cochromatograph on reverse phase HPLC.

Table 1. Assay of cell culture supernatants for IL-1 using LBRM-33-1A5 cells[a,b]

Cell supernatant dilution	Culture media with 5 μg LPS	MO-conditioned media (5 μg LPS)	EC-conditioned media (5 μg LPS) 24 h	48 h
1:3	3456	10 330	24 594	34 762
1:6	4390	12 960	23 612	30 470
1:50	3214	23 578	17 718	26 304
1:400	2854	30 722	4 064	12 602
1:3000	4242	30 650	2 430	5 970

[a] Assay controls: media alone = 521 (LBRM + CTLL-2); IL-1 alone = 562; PHA alone = 2062; IL-1 + PHA = 36 100; IL-2 = 85 846.

[b] The length of MO or EC exposure to 5 μg/ml LPS (*E. coli* 055:B5, Difco Laboratories) prior to collection of the conditioned media was 48 h

Antigen Presentation Using Cloned Cells

One of the subcultured endothelial cell lines (EC-38) was cloned by limiting dilution and the clones were tested for their capacity to present antigen. Five EC clones survived two rounds of limiting dilution cloning and were available for these experiments. All cells from each of the clones tested were positive for factor VIII-related antigen. Since these EC clones were derived from a line that was HLA-DR 4,7 positive, antigen presentation was evaluated on both histocompatible (HLA-DR 4) and histoincompatible (HLA-DR 6) T cells. EC line 38 and the derived clones presented antigen only to the histocompatible T cells (Table 2). These results eliminated any contribution from other cell types in the EC preparations. In order to exclude any contribution from non-T cells in the T cell preparation, we established several T cell clones from T cell lines maintained by alternate cycles of IL-2 and antigen-pulsed MO stimulation [11]. The T cell lines were cloned by limiting dilution and shown to be responsive in antigen presentation experiments (Table 3). The response of two of the T cell clones (M6 and M18) to presentation of antigen by EC was significant. However, each of these T cell clones responded better to antigen presented by MO than antigen presented by EC. When T cell clone M18 was used in additional experiments to test presentation of antigen by the EC clones, antigen-specific activation occurred with each of the five EC clones evaluated (Table 4). When T cell clone E13 was used, antigen-specific activation was more pronounced when EC rather than MO were the APC.

Discussion

T cells are responsible for a diverse group of immune reactions all of which fall under the heading of cell-mediated immunity (CMI). T cells are thought to provide the specificity of the

Table 2. Antigen presentation by endothelial cell clones

T cells	Antigen-presenting cells	Antigen -	Antigen +
PBL (MO-depleted) histocompatible	None	186[a]	176
	MO	211	2308
	EC-38	286	1811
	EC-38 clone 1A5	256	1921
	2A7	288	2640
	2F3	412	3111
	3C3	196	1796
	3F6	241	1899
PBL (MO-depleted) histoincompatible	None	202	189
	MO	313	675
	EC-38	322	667
	EC-38 clone 1A5	381	711
	2A7	295	582

[a]Mean cpm of thymidine ^{3}H uptake

Table 3. Response of T cell clones to antigen presented by endothelial cells

T cells	Antigen-presenting cells	Antigen -	Antigen +
PBL (MO-depleted)	None	156[a]	161
	MO	138	2183
	EC-38	206	1454
Clone M6	MO	421	6240
	EC-38	540	3850
Clone M18	MO	386	16950
	EC-38	310	6220
Clone M32	MO	510	7151
	EC-38	538	1062

[a]Mean cpm of thymidine ^{3}H uptake

Table 4. Responses of T cell clones to antigen presented by cloned endothelial cells

T cells	Antigen-presenting cells	Antigen	
		-	+
Clone M18	None	169[a]	211
	MO	561	14510
	EC-38	610	5850
	EC-38 clone 1A5	658	6150
	2A7	586	3650
	2F3	313	3280
	3C3	621	5400
	3F6	606	4280
Clone E13	None	136	141
	MO	388	14600
	EC-38	422	22650
	EC-38 clone 1A5	512	21860
	2A7	826	14582
	2F3	588	23466
	3C3	436	22831
	3F6	581	26510

[a] Mean cpm of thymidine ^3H uptake

CMI response while their mediators stimulate cellular exudates and the histologic findings at the site of antigen. T cells require the antigen to be displayed on Ia-bearing APC and require the involvement of IL-1 and IL-2 for maximal activity. Antigen-specific T cells in an immune individual circulate within the vasculature at an approximate frequency of 10^{-3}-10^{-4} [16]. Some of these cells must be triggered for activation and development of the CMI response. To account for the involvement of the low frequency, antigen-specific T cell, we have considered two basic alternatives. First, the nonspecific inflammatory response induced by antigen alone produces endothelial changes which allow thousands of cells to egress from blood to tissue. When enough antigen-specific cells are present at the extravascular site of antigen, the specific T cells become activated and, via mediators, induce and/or direct the development of classic CMI pathology. A second possibility is that antigen is taken up by the endothelium and presented on the luminal surface of capillaries. An intravascular display of antigen could provide the recognition site for triggering of antigen-specific T cells. Even though it may occur at low frequency, the specific T cell would eventually come in contact with the antigen at this intravascular site. These two alternatives are distinguished by where the T cell first encounters antigen. We favor the second hypothesis since it seems to account in an efficient manner for the earliest events in recognition.

After specific T cell activation, the accumulation of mononuclear cells in the tissue can be accounted for in at least two ways. The activated T cell could release mediators which would affect endothelium, inducing changes in vascular permeability, or the endothelium could be activated by the T cell contact to undergo structural changes and to elaborate EC mediators (endokines) which would lead to classic CMI histology. This latter theory [1] would account for the brief cell-cell exposure which occurs during ordinary hemodynamics, the low frequency of antigen-specific T cells in blood, and for the rapid dilution of factors by the blood flow. In this model, EC could become activated after brief contact with antigen-specific T cells and then the activated EC could focally release mediators (Fig. 8). Thus, while antigen-specific T cells would still provide the specificity to the CMI response, the EC would be the central participant in the CMI response.

Several findings support this theory. First, EC are known to express MHC determinants, including Ia [5,17]. Second, EC have been shown to (a) activate lymphocytes in allogeneic mixed-cell culture reactions [18,19]; (b) present conventional antigen to antigen-specific T cells in an HLA-DR-restricted manner [2,3]; and (c) function as accessory cells for mitogen-induced responses [20]. There is also the suggestion that EC and T cells interact in the development of delayed-type hypersensitivity (DTH) in that histologic examination of DTH sites showed lymphocytes attached to vascular endothelium within the lumen of the venule

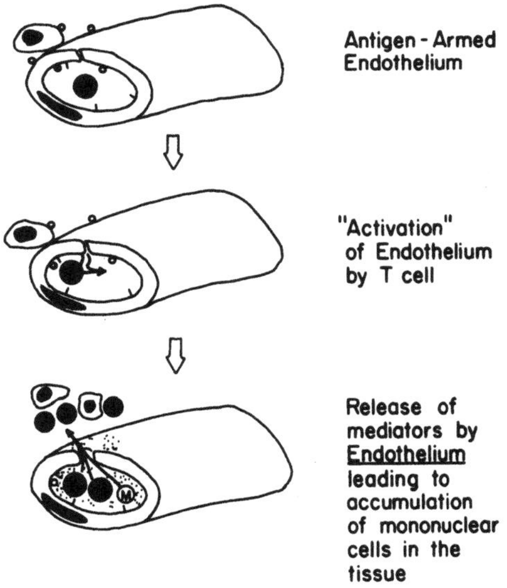

Fig. 8. General model for the T cell-endothelial cell interaction leading to mononuclear cell egress into the extravascular tissue

at the DTH site [21]. Also, lymphocytes have been shown to adhere to cultured endothelium and migrate through the EC if sensitized [21]. Finally, EC are known to produce metabolites of arachidonic acid such as prostacyclin, a mediator of vasodilation [22,23].

While these findings support a major role for EC in CMI responses, the experiments are not conclusive. For example, the requirement of other cell types for EC presentation of antigen has not been previously excluded. Also, while Ia determinants have been found on the surface of EC, there has only been preliminary evidence that EC themselves synthesize Ia determinants. Moreover, EC have not been previously shown to produce IL-1 activity. These questions have been the central theme of this work.

A significant factor in all of our experiments has been the long-term serial culture of endothelial cells. We have been able to demonstrate that extensively subcultured EC (up to 20 subcultures) present antigen as effectively as fresh EC (see Fig. 5) and do so in an HLA-DR-restricted manner (see Fig. 6). Additional experiments confirmed our earlier observations that other cell types (macrophages, fibroblasts, and smooth muscle cells) were not participating in these presentation experiments (see Figs. 3,4). Moreover, we have now provided formal evidence that EC express the two critical signals required by APC. We have shown that, when exposed to appropriate stimuli, they synthesize Ia determinants (see Fig. 7) and secrete IL-1 (see Table 1). To eliminate any final concern that either the T cell or EC populations still contained a small number of contributory cell components, we cloned both cell populations. The cloned EC presented antigen to the cloned T cells in a restricted fashion (see Tables 2,3,4). This further clarified the independent presentation capacity of EC.

References

1. Burger DR, Vetto RM (1982) Vascular endothelium as a major participant in T-lymphocyte immunity. Cell Immunol 70:357
2. Burger DR, Ford D, Vetto RM, Hamblin A, Goldstein A, Hubbard M, Dumonde DC (1981) Endothelial cell presentation of antigen to human T cells. Hum Immunol 3:209
3. Burger DR, Vetto RM, Hamblin A, Dumonde DC (1982) T-lymphocyte activation by antigen presented by HLA-DR compatible endothelial cells. In: Nossel, Vogel (eds) Pathobiology of the endothelial cell. Academic Press, London, pp 387-407
4. Hirschberg H, Bergh OH, Thorsby E (1980) Antigen-presenting properties of human vascular endothelial cells. J Exp Med 152:249
5. Hirschberg H, Moen T, Thorsby E (1979) Specific destruction of human endothelial cell monolayers by anti-DRw antisera. Transplantation 28(2):116
6. Maciag T, Cerundolo J, Ilsley S, Kelley PR, Forand R (1979) An endothelial cell growth factor from bovine hypothalamus: Identification and partial characterization. Proc Natl Acad Sci USA 76(11):5674
7. Jerrells TR, Dean JH, Richardson GL, Herberman RB (1980) Depletion of monocytes from human peripheral blood mononuclear leucocytes: Comparison of

the Sephadex G-10 column method with other commonly used techniques. J Immunol Methods 32:11
8. Jaffe EA, Nachman RL, Becher CG, Minick CR (1973) Culture of human endothelial cells derived from umbilical veins. Identification by morphologic and immunologic criteria. J Clin Invest 52:2745
9. Votila K, Marnela M, Hamblin A, Krohn K (1978) Human transfer factor in vitro: Identification of L-serine and glycine as components with augmenting effect in lymphocyte transformation assay. Scand J Immunol 7:495
10. Brand DL, Roy JR, Jr., Kayhoe DB, McClelland JD (1970) Preliminary trials towards standardization of leucocyte typing. In: Terasaki P (ed) Histocompatibility testing. Munksgaard, Copenhagen, pp 357-567
11. Kurnick JT, Altevogt P, Lindblom J, Sjoberg O, Danneus A, Wigzell H (1980) Long-term maintenance of HLA-D restricted T cells specific for soluble antigens. Scand J Immunol 11:131
12. Hirschberg H, Bergh OJ, Thorsby E (1979) Clonal distribution of HLA-restricted antigen-reactive T cells in man. J Exp Med 150:1271
13. Conlon PJ (1983) A rapid biologic assay for the detection of interleukin 1. J Immunol 131(3):1280
14. Raff HV, Picker LJ, Stobo JD (1980) Macrophage heterogeneity in man. A subpopulation of HLA-DR bearing macrophages required for antigen-induced T cell activation also contains stimulators for autologous-reactive T cells. J Exp Med 152:581
15. Tanigaki N, Tosi R, Duquesnoy RJ, Ferrara GB (1983) Three Ia species with different structures and alloantigenic determinants in an HLA-homozygous cell line. J Exp Med 157:231
16. Ford D, Burger D (1983) Precursor frequency of antigen-specific T cells: Effects of sensitization in vivo and in vitro. Cell Immunol 79:334
17. Pober JS, Gimbrone MA, Sr, Cotran DS, et al. (1983) Ia expression by vascular endothelium is inducible by activated T cells and by human interferon. J Exp Med 157:1339
18. Vetto RM, Burger DR (1972) Endothelial cell stimulation of allogeneic lymphocytes. Transplantation 14(5):652
19. Hirschberg H, Evensen SA, Henriksen T, Thorsby E (1975) The human mixed lymphocyte-endothelium culture interaction. Transplantation 19(6):495
20. Ashida ER, Johnson AR, Lipsky PE (1981) Human endothelial cell-lymphocyte interaction. J Clin Invest 67:1490
21. Dvorak HF (1974) Delayed hypersensitivity. In: Zweifach BW, Grant L, McClusky RT (eds) The inflammatory process. Academic Press, New York, pp 291-345
22. DeBono D (1976) Endothelial-lymphocyte interaction in vitro: I. Adherence of nonallergized lymphocytes. Cell Immunol 26:78
23. DeBono D (1979) Endothelial-lymphocyte interaction in vitro: II. Adherence of allergized lymphocytes. Cell Immunol 44:64
24. Gryglewski RJ, Bunting S, Moncada S, Flower RJ, Vane JR (1976) Prostaglandins 12:685
25. Williams TJ (1979) Br J Pharmacol 65:517

Bayer-Symposium VIII
The Pathogenesis of Bacterial Infections, 308-319 (1985)

Augmenting Interactions of the Clotting System and Immune Responses in Inflammatory Tissue Injury

Ph. Y. Paterson

Summary

Activation of the clotting cascade is intimately associated with immunologic and inflammatory host responses to bacterial infections and other antigenic stimuli. Although clotting and its inevitable fibrinolytic end result rarely may have detrimental effects, the diverse consequences of clotting-fibrinolysis usually are beneficial for the host. The biologic ramifications of the clotting cascade encompass a wide spectrum of events, ranging from cellular differentiation through induction of microbicidal lysins to modulation of host inflammatory-immune response. Specific examples of beneficial effects of the coagulation cascade include enhanced permeability of vascular barriers of the central nervous system and the capacity of microbes to induce platelet-derived microbial lysins. Examples of how the coagulation system also may augment immunologically mediated tissue injury include the role of the coagulation system in immune glomerulonephritis and autoimmune disease involving the epidermis. On balance, the coagulation cascade represents an evolutionarily conserved system pari passu with the immunologic-inflammatory systems, with important adaptive-selective influences on host antimicrobial immune and inflammatory defense responses.

Background and Orientation

The coagulation cascade, like the immunologic and inflammatory systems, represents an evolutionarily conserved interlocking enzymatic gridwork of immense adaptive-selective importance with respect to species adaptation, selection, and survival. While origins of the clotting process can be found in primitive arthropods, fibrinogen and other marker enzymes comprising the coagulation cascade of contemporary mammals are relatively young proteins within a phylogenetic context [1].[1]

[1] This paper is an abbreviated perspective, not an inclusive review, and for this reason a limited number of references have been selected somewhat arbitrarily for the purpose of highlighting main points of the innumerable excellent publications concerning this topic.

Interdependence of the Clotting and the Immunologic-Inflammatory Systems

There is increasing evidence that host immune responses to bacteria, other microbes, and a diverse array of nonmicrobial signals usually activate the coagulation system in a manner which facilitates inflammation and augments antimicrobial defenses [2,3]. It also should be stressed that activation of the coagulation cascade usually occurs in concert with activation of several other biologically pivotal enzyme systems, e.g., the complement and kallikrein-kinin systems [3,4]. Dictates of space and the preselected focus of the present perspective does not permit a discussion of these systems and of how they often serve to amplify many of the effects of clotting on host defense against injury.

As illustrated in Fig. 1, clotting, immune activity, and inflammation in fact enjoy a mutual interdependence, whether viewed in terms of host mobilization and deployment of antimicrobial defense or other contexts, including autoreactive tissue injury. Immune responses variably activate and modulate the coagulation pathways; coagulation and its resulting fibrinolytic products similarly modulate host immune and inflammatory responses. When "*Alles ist wunderbar,*" the net result is augmentation of host antimicrobial defenses.

Initiation of Clotting by Activated Lymphoid Cells

Specific, major pathways of initiation of clotting by activated lymphoid cells are depicted in Fig. 2. Each of the three major participants of the immune system, viz., monocyte-macrophages (Mϕ), thymus-derived and/or -influenced T lymphocytes, and/or bone marrow-derived B lymphocytes, when suitably activated, synthesize and secrete a membrane surface-associated procoagulant capable of activating the coagulation cascade [5-9]. Activation of the cascade via procoagulant (also variously known as tissue factor, tissue thromboplastin, and coagulation factor III) occurs via the extrinsic pathway involving factor VII [10]. Note that mere initiation of an immune response at the monocyte or antigen presentation phase is sufficient to result in procoagulant secretion in all three classes of lymphoid cells.

Coagulation-Fibrinolysis: A Two-Sided Coin

As illustrated in Fig. 3, the bad side of the coin, of course, is microbial infection leading to disseminated intravascular coagulation (DIC), uncontrollable bleeding, and irreversible shock [11]. Fortunately, this life-threatening syndrome is comparatively uncommon. The good side of the coin, and the side most commonly seen, has beneficial effects on host defenses, e.g., chemotaxis, physiologic degrees of increased vasopermeability and generation of powerful microbicidal lysins with the general properties of β lysins.

Biologic Ramifications of Coagulation-Fibrinolysis

Some of the diverse end results of clotting-fibrinolysis are listed in Table 1. Activation of a multiplicity of different

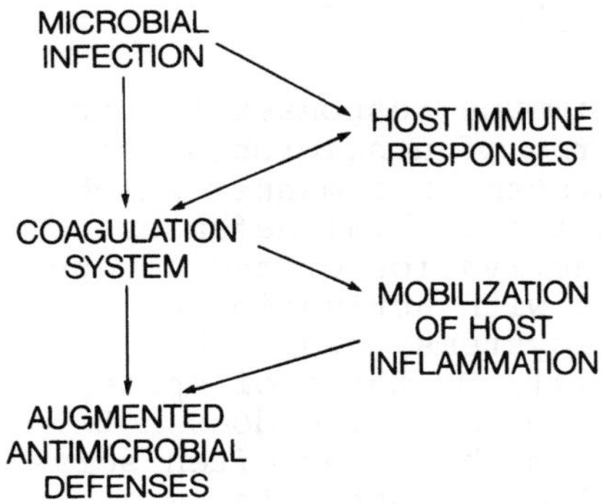

Fig. 1

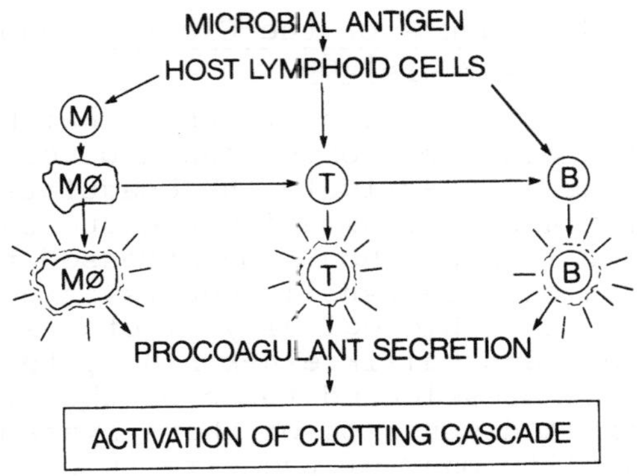

Fig. 2

Fig. 1. Mutual interdependence of the coagulation, immunologic, and inflammatory systems in terms of antimicrobial host defenses

Fig. 2. Specific pathways whereby host antimicrobial immune responses involving monocytes-macrophages ($M\phi$), T lymphocytes, and B lymphocytes activate the clotting cascade

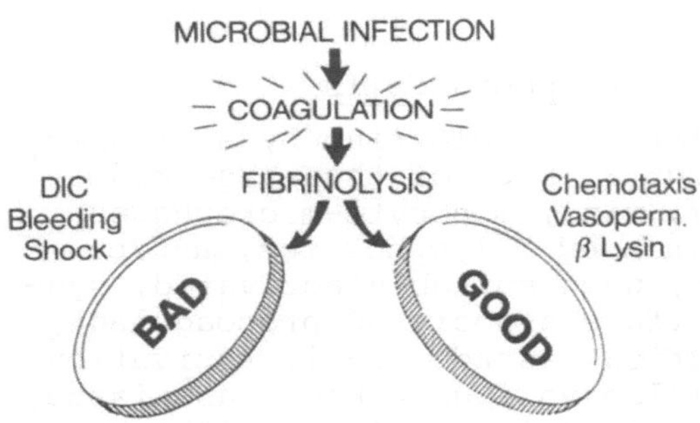

Fig. 3. The coagulation system as a "two-sided coin," with effects which are occasionally detrimental to host survival and other effects, happily much more frequent, which benefit the infected host

types of host cells leads to plasminogen activator and generation of plasmin, a mild serine protease, which may provide an important signal for embryogenesis, cellular differentiation, loss of cell-cell contact or adhesiveness, and activation of endothelial cells with augmented antigen-presenting capacity [12]. Peptides resulting from fibrinolysis exhibit potent chemotactic and permeability-increasing properties [13], which help mobilize and deploy host inflammatory cells to extravascular sites of bacterial colonization and tissue invasion. Certain microbes themselves can produce platelet-derived microbicidal products or lysins [14]. In various ways, clotting may result in mitogenic signals which augment proliferation of infiltrating lymphocytes and other inflammatory cells [15], thereby bolstering antimicrobial defenses. Finally, certain products of fibrinolysis have been shown to exert appreciable immunosuppressive effects [16], allowing the coagulation cascade to participate in the all-important job of "fine tuning" or regulating the immunologic system.

Table 1. Ramifications of coagulation-fibrinolysis

Modulation of embryogenesis, differentiation, and cell adhesion
Enhanced endothelial cell activation
Increased interendothelial cell permeability
Augmented mobilization of inflammatory response
Platelet-derived antimicrobial β lysins
Mitogenic stimulation of infiltrating lymphoid cells
Regulatory feedback immunosuppressive activity

Specific Perspectives to be Discussed

Many different examples (beyond the restricted listing set out in Table 1) could be presented and discussed, illustrating how the clotting system directly or indirectly augments host inflammatory-immune responses in either a beneficial or detrimental manner. Again, because of page limitations and time constraints, I will focus on only four situations, viz., two examples of how the clotting system amplifies such responses so as to reinforce host defenses against bacterial infection and two examples of how the coagulation cascade may potentiate immunologically mediated tissue injury, seemingly to the host's disadvantage.

How Clotting Factors May Augment Inflammatory Antimicrobial Host Defenses

Clotting and Vascular Permeability

One obvious prerequisite for effective deployment of host antimicrobial defenses is rapid ingress of immune effector cells and nonimmune inflammatory cells to specific anatomic sites where unrestrained, replicating bacteria are forming microcolonies and causing tissue injury. This prerequisite almost invariably requires circulating lymphoid cells to traverse endothelial cell barriers in the process of arriving at the site (or sites) of extravascular microbial infection. As illustrated in Fig. 4, nowhere in the body is this crucial early phase of host defense more important and more difficult than in acute bacterial infections of the central nervous system (CNS). Comparatively ineffective delivery of cellular and humoral defense mediators to intra-CNS microbial targets is largely due to the strikingly restrictive vascular barriers demarcating the cerebrospinal fluid (CSF) and CNS parenchymal tissue compartments, viz., the well-known blood-CSF and blood-brain barriers [17]. Soluble immune effector components, such as the third complement component (C3) as well as other complement components, immunoglobulin G (IgG), and β lysin, are incapable of traversing the exceptionally tight interendothelial cell junctions which account, at least in large part, for the unrivaled restrictive permeability of the cerebrovasculature [17]. Host phagocytes represented by segmented neutrophils as well as Mϕ, and T or B lymphocytes, although endowed with the locomotive advantage assured by inherent active motility, gain ingress to the CNS with considerable difficulty. Whether T lymphocytes truly "pass

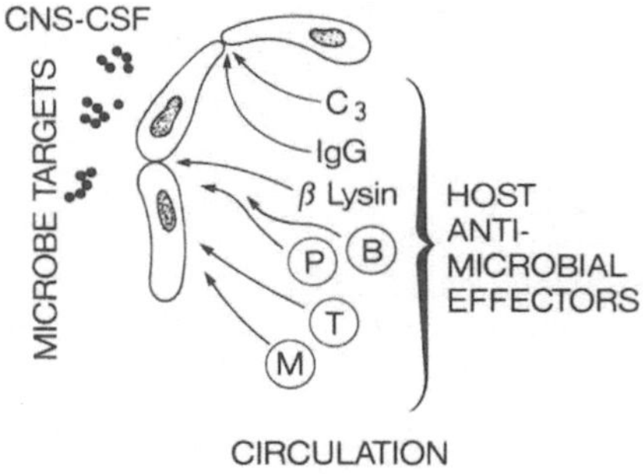

Fig. 4

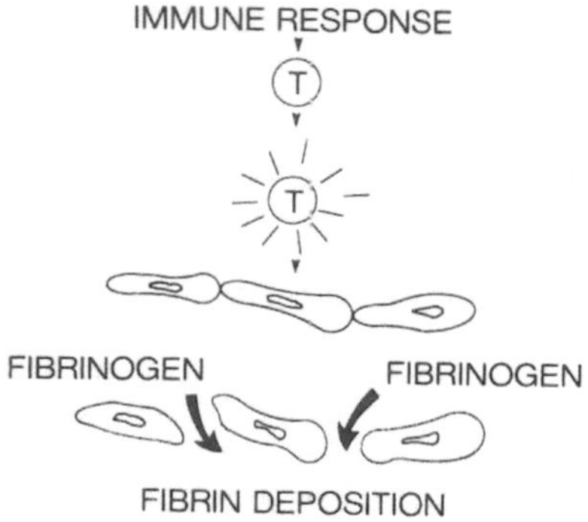

Fig. 5

Fig. 4. Blood-cerebrospinal fluid (*CSF*) and blood-central nervous system (*CNS*) vascular barriers, in part due to inordinately tight interendothelial junctions, restrict delivery of host immune effector proteins and phagocytic lymphocyte immune effectors to intra-CNS microbial targets

Fig. 5. Prevailing view of events leading to accumulation of fibrin in areas of enhanced vascular permeability resulting from release of activated T cells and/or activated endothelial cells. In this context, accumulation of fibrin is strictly a passive, secondary event, reflecting increased vasopermeability

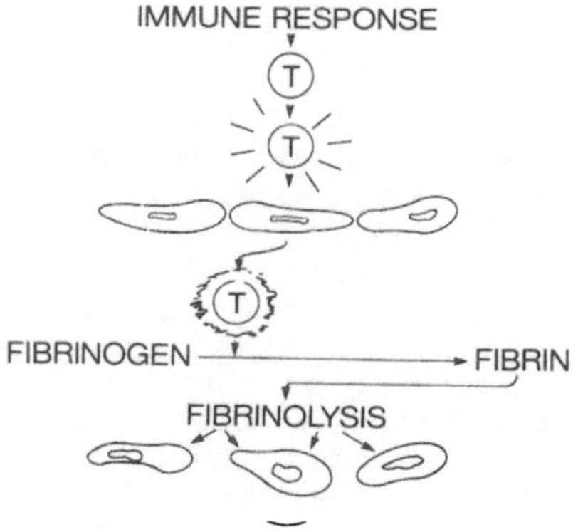

Fig. 6

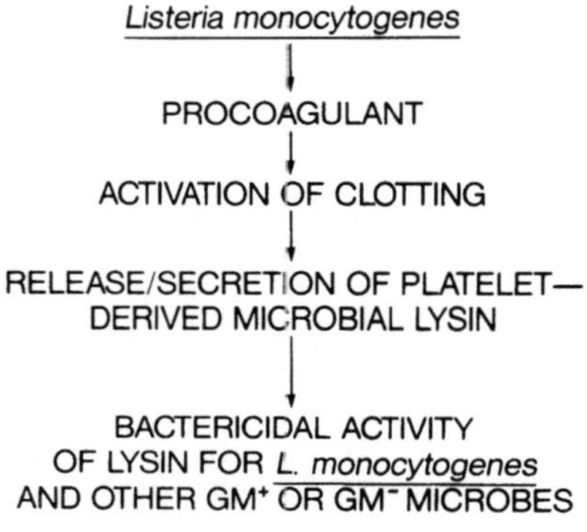

Fig. 7

Fig. 6. Alternative view of accumulation of fibrin at sites of ongoing immune and inflammatory responses. In this context, activation of the coagulation pathway by procoagulant-secreting lymphoid cells and generation of vasoactive fibrin cleavage peptides has a primary role in increasing vasopermeability

Fig. 7. Schematic depiction of events underlying production of a platelet-derived microbial lysin by procoagulant-secreting *Listeria monocytogenes*

through" endothelial cell membranes and cytosol or, like all other classes of motile cells, must traverse the endothelial barriers by inserting themselves through the tight intercellular junctions remains a polemical issue.

For some time, my laboratory has been studying determinants of cerebrovascular permeability in rats with presumed T lymphocyte immunologically mediated CNS disease [18,19]. In this work, occurrence of perivascular deposits of fibrin, detected by direct immunofluorescence in crystat sections of brain and spinal cord, has been found to be directly correlated with development of clinical neurologic signs. In the early phases of this work, carried out with Dr. Hau Kwaan, Department of Medicine, Northwestern University, we demonstrated that deposition of fibrin in the immediate vicinity of CNS vessels resulted in vigorous secretion of plasminogen activator [18]. More recently I, my graduate student, Mr. John Gausas, and my postdoctoral research assistant, Dr. Chang-Sung Koh, have uncovered additional evidence for the coagulation system being intimately linked to development of clinical signs and increased permeability of the blood-brain barrier. In this work, cerebrovascular permeability has been quantitatively assessed using ^{125}I and ^{131}I iodinated proteins, as described by other investigators [20]. Using the day of initial appearance of hindleg paralysis or other neurologic abnormalities as a convenient reference point (day 0) and focusing on that region of the neuraxis most susceptible to ongoing autoreactive immunologic injury, viz., the lumbosacrococcygeal segment of the spinal cord, we have made the following observations: (a) increased permeability of spinal cord vasculature begins 1 day before appearance of clinical signs, peaks on day 0 and then returns to normal; (b) fibrin deposition also begins on day -1, but doesn't peak until day +1, and then rapidly disappears (presumably due to increased in situ plasminogen activator and fibrinolysis); and (c) focal, perivascular infiltration of host inflammatory cells is evident at the time increased vascular permeability and accumulation of fibrin are noted, but continues to increase long after permeability has returned to normal and the fibrin deposition process had ended.

The conventional view of this sequence of events is illustrated in Fig. 5. According to this view, autoreactive, activated T cells interact with the vascular bed of the CNS target and release lymphokines, including permeability factor which causes a transient loss of tight endothelial cell-cell abutment which in turn allows fibrinogen and other plasma proteins to pass through the widened intercellular junctions; fibrinogen, unlike the other traversing plasma proteins, is converted into an insoluble product owing to unusual amounts and availability of CNS thromboplastin. In the context of this perspective, accumulation of perivascular deposits of fibrin has no biologic relevance beyond its presence signaling increased permeability of the blood-CNS barrier. An alternative interpretation of the events described is illustrated in Fig. 6. This latter perspective also underlines the autoreactive and activated T lymphocyte as a primary immune effector, but puts special emphasis on the secretion of procoagulant by the T lymphocyte as it gains access to the CNS compartment, where, in the presence of low levels of fibrinogen and other essential clotting factors, it induces formation of fibrin. As already indicated, the presence of fibrin would trigger release of plasminogen activator and initiate fibrinolysis with resulting vasoactive peptides directly causing increased permeability of the cerebrovasculature. Support for this alternative hypothesis has been obtained through experiments utilizing either ancrod-treated hypofibrinogenemic rats [18,19] or, more recently, rats treated with trans-4-aminomethylcyclohexane carboxylic acid (AMCA), a potent inhibitor of plasminogen activator. Should our thesis (see Fig. 6) involving the clotting system as a primary determinant of increased cerebrovascular permeability ultimately be verified, drug-mediated manipulation of clotting-fibrinolysis could be envisioned as a means for augmenting and accelerating delivery of antimicrobial drugs and host antibacterial defense factors to infected CNS tissues.

Production of Platelet-Derived Microbial Lysin

Listeria monocytogenes, when actively growing in vitro or in vivo, produces a procoagulant-like product which activates the clotting system [14]. This is one of several different mechanisms whereby microbes in general, and not just gram-negative bacteria, can cause DIC in patients with infectious diseases. But to stay with our present theme and as illustrated in Fig. 7, the *L. monocytogenes*-derived procoagulant which activates clotting results in release of a platelet product with striking bactericidal activity for this bacterium as well as other gram-positive or gram-negative bacteria [14]. Properties of the platelet-derived microbial lysin indicate that it is a β lysin, a long-known class of proteins in normal mammalian sera with remarkable lytic activity against a wide array of bacteria.

Data indicating the in vivo significance of clotting system-induced microbial lysin are shown in Table 2. Normal rats injected with 1.3×10^9 colony-forming units of *L. monocytogenes* had no evidence of bacteremia 48 h later and none died. In contrast, rats treated with heparin to prevent clotting and which received the same infecting dose of *L. monocytogenes* developed bacteremia 48 h later, with relatively large numbers of this bacterium in the circulation. In addition, the majority of animals, i.e., 75%, went on to die of *Listeria* bacteremic infection. Activation of the clotting system and production of platelet-derived β lysin appears to be one reason for the extraordinary resistance of rats to infection by this and many other types of bacteria. Data strictly analogous to those set out in Table 2 are not available for human beings, to the best of my knowledge. But since low levels of β lysins are present in plasma samples of clinically well human subjects, there is every reason to believe that the clotting-platelet-microbial lysin pathway system undoubtedly plays some role in the resistance of human beings to bacterial infection.

Table 2. *Listeria monocytogenes* infection in rats[a]

Treatment	Bacteremia[b]	Mortality
None	0	0%
Heparin	9.7-36.8 × 10^3	75%

[a]From reference [14].

[b]Colony-forming units of *L. monocytogenes* 48 h after injection of 1 × 10^9 colony-forming units.

How the Clotting System May Augment Immunologic-Inflammatory Respones Causing Host Injury

Clotting and Nephrotoxic Nephritis

There is a relatively large literature implicating the clotting system as an important pathogenic determinant of immunologically mediated glomerulonephritis in experimental animals and human beings [21,22]. Naish and his colleagues in England have been important contributors to this body of information over the years. In fact, periodic enthusiasm has existed at one time or another for utilizing anticoagulants in the therapeutic approach to managing nephritis in human beings [23].

Data from a paper [24] bearing on this subject and involving nephrotoxic glomerulonephritis (NTN) in rabbits are set out in Table 3. As expected, untreated rabbits injected with sheep anti-rabbit glomerular membrane antiserum developed nephritis, with rising creatinine as evidence of renal function impairment, accumulation of fibrin, periglomerular cellular crescents, and innumerable Mϕ within Bowman's space. In contrast, rabbits rendered hypofibrinogenemic as a result of treatment with ancrod, a polypeptide constituent of the venom of the Malayan pit viper *Agkistrodon rhodostoma*, and incapable of generating normal amounts of fibrin irrespective of how intensely their clotting cascades may have been activated, had creatinine values in the normal range, little or no demonstrable fibrin, and few or no cellular crescents among isolated glomeruli studied in culture by light and electron microscopy.

It must be stressed that, in the study described, the glomeruli contained the expected array of immunologic and inflammatory components associated with NTN, viz., sheep anti-rabbit glomerular antibody, rabbit anti-sheep immunoglobulin antibody, complement, and an admixture of infiltrating segmented neutrophils and mononuclear cells. Of considerable importance, few or no Mϕ were demonstrable within Bowman's space, prompting the authors to postulate that the cellular crescents depicting immune glomerular injury arise from intraglomerular monocyte-Mϕ-infiltrating inflammatory cells which migrate through Bowman's space and accumulate around Bowman's capsule as transformed epithelioid cells. This postulate conflicts with the traditional view that crescent formation results from in situ proliferation of glome-

Table 3. Role of clotting system in nephrotoxic glomerulonephritis in rabbits[a]

Treatment	Serum creatinine (mmol/l)	Glomerular changes Fibrin score	Crescent score	Mϕ in Bowman's space
Nil	1.3 ± 0.3	2.21 ± 0.32	2.81 ± 0.12	Numerous
Ancrod	0.8 ± 0.07	0.08 ± 0.005	0.61 ± 0.35	Rare

[a]From reference [24] . Data recorded 14 days after treatment with sheep anti-rabbit glomerular membrane antiserum, and 10 days after initiating ancrod treatment, when all animals were killed.

rular epithelial cells in response to injury and associated inflammation. Such a divergent perspective would never have been considered without knowledge that the clotting system plays a significant note in the immunopathogenesis of NTN and other forms of immun glomerulitis

Clotting and Autoimmune Disease

As depticted schematically in Fig. 8, microbes of all classes share antigenic determinants with cell- or tissue-specific antigens of mammalian tissues [25]. Infection by such microbes not infrequently results in loss of immunologic tolerance to the corresponding "self-antigen" by the infected host, with clonal proliferation of autoreactive cells to a degree which may result in clinically manifest autoimmune disease. As might be expected from what already has been stated in this exposition, development of autoreactive immune responses and autoimmune disease usually is accompanied by activation of the clotting system.

Evidence from certain quarters has suggested that the clotting process per se may be responsible for at least some of the manifestations of developing autoimmune disease. At least some data, for example, indicate that it is the perivascular accumulations of fibrin and excessive fluid in the CNS of animals with experimental allergic encephalomyelitis (EAE) which had been induced by a single injection of neural antigen combined with some type of immunologic adjuvant, that causes the paralytic and other clinical neurologic abnormalities of this neuroautoimmune disorder [18,19].

Studies over a period of many years have indicated that the human dermatologic disease known as pemphigus has, in all probability, an autoimmune pathogenesis [26]. As depicted in Fig. 9, host autoreactive immune responses directed against epidermal cells are demonstrable in patients with pemphigus, e.g., circulating anti-epidermal antibody and intracutaneous deposits of specifically reactive IgG in the skin [26,27]. Deposits of IgG and complement can be shown to occur with greatest regularity within the cutaneous lesions characterizing this disease, with the presence of these immune reactants being most intense at

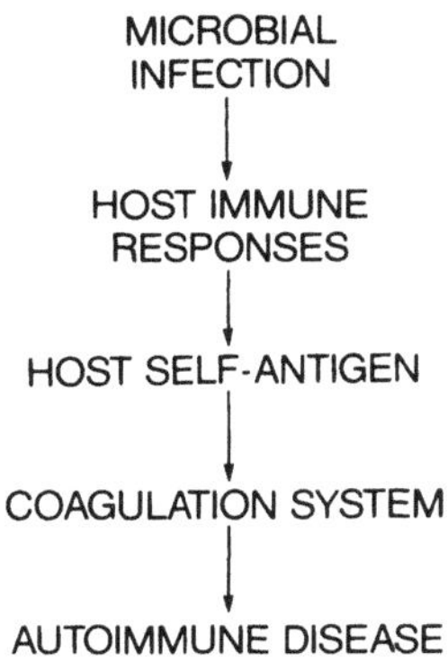

Fig. 8

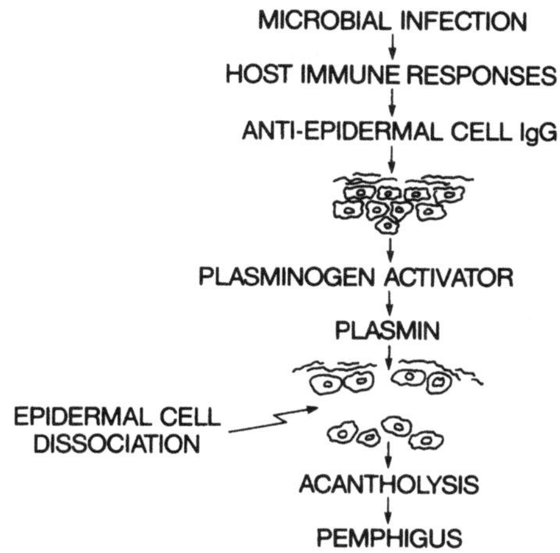

Fig. 9

Fig. 8. Postulated sequence of events whereby cross-reacting microbes induce autoreactive host immune responses which result in coagulation system augmentation of autoimmune disease

Fig. 9. Role of activation of the clotting system with resulting plasmin causing epidermal cell dissociation (acantholysis, the fundamental lesion of pemphigus - an autoimmune disease of humans)

precisely those sites of epidermal cell dissociation which give rise to the pemphigus lesions [26]. The event (or events) which initially trigger and perpetuate such autoimmune host responses directed against one's own "ectodermal envelope" remain undefined, but persistent infection with a microbe cross-reacting with epidermal cell antigen would seem to be a reasonable possibility. Binding of IgG to epidermal cells, probably in concert with complement, stimulates the epidermal cells to produce plasminogen activator which results in formation of plasmin which in turn causes loss of cell adhesiveness with cell-cell dissociation, a process termed acantholysis [28]. What is especially germane to this discussion is the primary role of the terminal portion of the coagulation cascade, not the autoreactive immune response per se, in causing the basic lesion of this human autoimmune disease.

Conclusions

In this necessarily abbreviated overview, the diverse biologic ramifications of the coagulation pathways and the mutual interdependence of the clotting and immune-inflammatory response systems have been highlighted. Specific examples of how concomitant activation of the coagulation cascade may augment host immune-inflammatory responses so as to potentiate antibacterial defenses are presented. Additional examples of how the clotting system also may augment immunologically mediated tissue injury and enhance host inflammatory responses leading to autoimmune disease also are discussed. There are good reasons for believing that greater understanding of how the coagulation system acts in concert with host immune and inflammatory responses ultimately will translate to greater insights concerning the molecular basis of antibacterial host defense and tissue injury of an immunologic nature and lead to novel therapeutic approaches to the management of disease.

Acknowledgment. Research referred to in this paper which was carried out by the author and his associates was supported in part by USPHS Research Grants NS06262 and NS 19028, and in part by Grant RG1501 from the National Multiple Sclerosis Society.

References

1. Zimmermann E (1983) Zur Evolution des Gerinnungssystems aus primitiven Abwehrmechanismen. Behring Inst Mitt 73:1-12
2. Barnhart MI, Sulisz L, Bluhm GB (1971) Role for fibrinogen and its derivates in acute inflammation. In: Forscher BK, Houck JC (eds) Immunopathology of Inflammation, Excerpta Medica, Amsterdam, pp 59-65
3. Pesce AJ, Dosekun AK (1983) Interrelationships between the immune systems, complement, coagulation and inflammation. Clin Physiol Biochem 1:92-116
4. Prydz H, Allison AC, Schorlemmer HU (1977) Further link between complement activation and blood coagulation. Nature 270:173-174
5. Chapman HA Jr, Vavrin J, Hibbs JB Jr (1983) Coordinate expression of macrophage procoagulant and fibrinolytic activity in vitro and in vivo. J Immunol 130:261-266
6. Helin HJ, Fox RI, Edgington TS (1983) The instructor cell for the human procoagulant monocyte response to bacterial lipopolysaccharide is a Leu-$3a^+$ T cell by fluorescence-activated cell sorting. J Immunol 131:749-752
7. Schwartz BS, Edgington TS (1981) Lymphocyte collaboration is required for induction of murine monocyte procoagulant acitivity by immune complexes. J Immunol 127:438-443
8. Toullet F, Maillard JL, Favreau C (1983) Release of a lymphokine-like plasminogen activator by stimulated B lymphocytes. J Immunol 130:254-260
9. Edgington TS et al. (1981) A unidirectional pathway of lymphocyte-instructed macrophage and monocyte function characterized by the generation of procoagulant monokines. In: Weigle WO (ed) Advances in immunopathology, Elsevier North Holland, Amsterdam, pp 173-196
10. Carson SD (1984) Tissue factor-initiated blood coagulation. In: Shefanini M, Gorstein I, Fink IM (eds) Progress in clinical pathology, vol 9, Grune and Stratton, New York, pp 1-14
11. Young LS (1979) Gram-negative sepsis. In: Mandell GL, Douglas AG Jr, Bennett JE (eds) Principles and practice of infectious diseases. Wiley, New York, pp 571-608
12. Kalderon N (1982) Role of the plasmin-generating system in the developing nervous tissue: I. Proteolysis as a mitogenic signal for the glial cells. J Neurosci Res 8:509-518
13. Richardson DL, Pepper DS, Kay AB (1976) Chemotaxis for human monocytes by fibrinogen-derived peptides. Br J Haematol 52:507-513
14. Davies WA, Ackerman VP, Nelson DS (1981) Mechanism for nonspecific immunity to *Listeria monocytogenes* in rats mediated by platelets and the clotting system. Infect Immun 33:477-481
15. Cohen SD, Israel E, Spiess-Meier B, Wainberg MA (1981) Plasminogen activator is an apparent lymphocyte mitogen. J Immunol 126:1415-1420

16. Girmann G, Pees H, Schwarze G, Scheurlen PG (1976) Immunosuppression by micromolecular fibrinogen degradation products in cancer. Nature 259: 399-401
17. Bradbury M (1979) The concept of a blood-brain barrier. Wiley, New York
18. Paterson PY (1976) Experimental allergic encephalomyelitis: Role of fibrin deposition in immunopathogenesis of inflammation in rats. Fed. Proc 35:2428-2434
19. Paterson PY (1982) Molecular and cellular determinants of neuroimmunologic inflammatory disease. Fed Proc 41:2569-2576
20. Leibowitz S, Kennedy L (1972) Cerebral vascular permeability and cellular infiltration in experimental allergic encephalomyelitis. Immunology 22:859-869
21. Naish P, Penn GB, Evans DJ, Peters DK (1972) The effect of defibrination on nephrotoxic serum nephritis in rabbits. Clin Sci 42:643-646
22. Vassalli P, McCluskey RT (1971) The pathogenetic role of the coagulation process in glomerular diseases of immunologic origin. Adv Nephrol 1: 47-63
23. Kincaid-Smith P, Laver MC, Fairley KF (1970) Dipyridamole and anti-coagulants in renal disease due to glomerular and vascular lesions. A new approach to therapy. Med J Aust 1:145-151
24. Holdsworth SR, Thomson NM, Glasgow EF, Atkins RC (1979) The effect of defibrination on macrophage participation in rabbit nephrotoxic nephritis: Studies using glomerular culture and electronmicroscopy. Clin Exp Immunol 37:38-43
25. Paterson PY (1981) Microbial parasitism cross-reactive with host antigens: Implications concerning loss of "self" tolerance and development of autoimmune disease. Recomb DNA Tech Bull 4:98-107
26. Patel HP, Anhalt GJ, Provost TT, Diaz LA (1983-84) Immunopathology of pemphigus vulgaris, bullous pemphigoid and related bullous dermatoses. Clin Immunol Rev 2:157-186
27. Beutner EH, Jordon RE (1964) Demonstration of skin antibodies in sera of pemphigus vulgaris patients by indirect immunofluosescent staining. Proc Soc Exp Biol Med 117:505-510
28. Singer KH, Hashimoto K, Lazarus GS (1984) Autoantibody-mediated alteration of cellular adhesion: the role of plasminogen activator. Clin Immunol Newsletter 5:20-23

Discussion

(pp. 294-319)

In response to queries from *Blake* and *Morrison* concerning activation of endothelial cells, *Burger* indicated that one can see that these cells express both Ia and IL-1 in response to activated T cell products, followed by detectable outpouring of arachidonic acid metabolites and other factors influencing permeability which are morphologically expressed in vitro by the viable cells curling up and lifting off plastic surfaces. Whether endothelial cells bear small amounts of Ia which current technology does not allow us to detect, are triggered to produce more of this product which we can clearly discern or, alternatively, whether the cells receive a signal to express Ia products de novo is not known. As *Paterson* indicated, the same situation exists for another class of antigen-presenting cell, the astrocyte in central nervous system tissues.

Prompted by *Devey*, *Burger* explained that by using the F1 to parent rat chimera cell transfer system, antigens of residual parental cells other than endothelial cells would be histocompatible with adoptively transferred F1 cells and, therefore, unable to participate actively in the response observed.

Burger allayed *Hahn's* concern over whether antigen-specific T cells interacting with endothelial cells leave the circulation as one might expect, based on what is known about their circulatory kinetics, by stating that there really is no problem with that concept. In the *Burger* model, the specific T cells are provided with a means for egress to extravascular tissues, viz., through increased permeability of endothelial cell barriers, distinct and apart from migrating to such sites in the context of a general inflammatory response where most of the infiltrating cells have no antigen specificity. *Burger* reminded everyone that one of the "endokine" products of activated endothelial cells has chemotactic activity and that it might facilitate both T cells and monocytes entering extravascular tissues. This would be particularly so if, just by chance, a greater concentration of chemotactic signals arose on the abluminal than on the luminal surfaces of activated endothelial cells, thereby establishing a chemotactic gradient favoring movement of host inflammatory cells from vascular to extravascular compartments.

In responce to questioning *McGee*, *Burger* indicated that it is assumed that antigenic determinants enter abluminal surfaces of endothelial cells by pinocytosis and, in the process of being presented, appear on the luminal surfaces where they are in favorable position to bind circulating T cells. A Symposium participant, on the basis of work he knew to have been done at the University of Virginia, suggested that appropriate signaling of endothelial cell membranes causes microvillus-like structures to appear on the cell surfaces, which may facilitate intracellular uptake.

Moxon suggested that the *Listeria* experiments in rats presented by *Paterson* employed such large numbers of microorganisms as to have little relevance for human beings. *Paterson* countered by reemphasizing that rats are more resistant to infection by *L. monocytogenes* that humans, perhaps in part because of the powerful platelet-derived microbicidal factors these microbes are able to induce in this mammalian species, and that the significant point of the experiments was the profound, relative decrease in ID_{50} when the clotting system was blocked and β lysins were not produced.

Burger responded to *McGee's* queries concerning interleukin-1 (Il-1) by indicating that it was detected using human umbilical vein endothelial cells and that it is produced by these cells following stimulation with bacterial endotoxin, viz., about 5 μg per milliliter culture fluid. Much less IL-1 is produced by endothelial cells compared with macrophages. Whether endothelial cells are susceptible to ultraviolet light, as is the case with some of the other types of antigen-presenting cells, is not known.

Devey and *Karnovsky* asked for a clarification of "antigen processing" by any cells, including endothelial cells. Several important points emerged in *Burger's* response: (a) endothelial cells possess little or no phagocytic activity, but yet can present antigenic determinants associated with simple or complex, soluble or insoluble antigens such as erythrocytes; (b) endothelial cells may resemble dendritic cells by "processing" antigen via extracellular membrane enzymes; and (c) *Paterson's* suggestion that extracellular processing and presentation conceivably occur as a result of specific surface cell receptors was ruled out, this strong denial prompting *Paterson* to comment that its vehemence might be the clue to the suggestion having validity.

Bayer-Symposium VIII
The Pathogenesis of Bacterial Infections, 322-333 (1985)

Fever, Interleukin-1, and the Defense Against Bacterial Pathogens

P. A. Murphy

Summary

Monocytes and macrophages exposed to bacteria or bacterial products secrete proteins which mediate a large number of different biologic actions. They were first described as mediators of fever (endogenous pyrogens, or EP) and subsequently as powerful T cell mitogens (interleukin-1, or IL-1). Other actions of IL-1 include specific granule release by polymorphonuclear neutrophils (PMN), collagenase secretion by synovial cells, increased proteolysis by muscle cells, and increased mitotic rate by fibroblasts. Finally, IL-1 appears to mediate systemic acute phase responses such as neutrophil leukocytosis, lowered serum iron, and increased synthesis of plasma fibrinogen and other proteins.

We found that IL-1 action on T cells was remarkably temperature sensitive, with Q_{10} between 100 and 200, whereas IL-1 secretion, and IL-2 action were much less sensitive to temperature ($Q_{10}<10$). This finding suggests that fever could well serve as a powerful regulatory mechanism of the immune response to infections.

Fever has been recognized as a sign of infectious illness since antiquity. Ever since Wunderlich's monograph [1], an accurate chart of the patients temperature, pulse, and respiratory rate has been an indispensable guide to the diagnosis and prognosis of infectious illnesses. However, an understanding of how fever occurs during bacterial infections has developed only during the last 40 years. And while we can now give a reasonable account of the pathophysiology of fever, there is still much uncertainty about whether the febrile response is beneficial to the host, and if so, why?

Clinicians have always been divided into these who, like Sydenham, regarded fever as a "mighty engine" which was vital to host defense; and those like Bennett and Nicastri [2], who regarded fever as either neutral or harmful. There is no question that hyperpyrexia may be lethal, and that there are people for whom even modest degrees of fever are harmful, such as children subject to febrile convulsions. The question is whether fever is more useful than deleterious in most people who develop it. My prejudice will be stated at the outset: I do not believe that such an intricate and well-controlled response to infection could possibly have evolved and persisted in all vertebrates investigated unless it was, on the whole, useful to the host.

If fever is admitted to be useful, the next question is whether it is so because fever has an unfavorable effect on the invading bacteria, or because fever somehow enhances the host defenses. Mackowiak [3], has thoroughly reviewed several instances where fever either prevents bacterial replication, or induces changes which render bacteria less virulent. The alternative viewpoint is that a generalized response to all infections, such as fever, could not have evolved in response to a few selected infections. Most bacteria are little affected by temperature variation over the range 37°-$41^{o}C$ in which most clinical fevers occur. It is probable, therefore, that fever somehow enhances the host defense.

In the nineteenth century, Billroth showed that animals developed fever when they were injected with pus from patients. Hort and Penfold [4] and Siebert [5] showed that gram-negative aerobic rods contained a powerful pyrogen, which was later identified as the lipopolysaccharide, endotoxin. Since endotoxin was shown to contaminate almost all solutions, it became widely accepted that fever was a response to bacterial endotoxin. Still, fever occurred during infections with gram-positive organisms which contained no endotoxin. It also accompanied diseases such as rheumatoid arthritis, drug allergies, and Hodgkin's disease, where infection seemed improbable. The idea grew that there might be a host factor, presumably a protein, whose secretion was stimulated by infection and which served as the common mediator of all fevers, however caused.

The first person to describe an EP which could be shown to be independent of bacterial products was Beeson [6]. He injected specially purified sodium chloride solution into the peritoneal cavity of rabbits, and removed the fluid 16 h later. The cells in the fluid were shown to contain a substance which caused fever when injected intravenously into rabbits, and which could be distinguished from endotoxin by several biologic tests. Subsequently, Wood and his co-workers [7] showed that EP could be obtained from leukocytes exposed to gram-positive organisms and viruses. Atkins and co-workers [8] showed that antigen-antibody complexes and antigens of cell mediated immunity were also effective stimuli, and Bodel et al. [9] demonstrated spontaneous EP secretion by a variety of tumors. Wood [7] and his co-workers demonstrated circulatory EP in the blood of rabbits suffering from a variety of experimental infections. Numerous workers demonstrated that EP could be obtained from the leukocytes of all mammalian species investigated, and it was found that EP from one species would frequently cause fever when injected into another. Jackson [10] in the cat, and Cooper et al. [11] in the rabbit, showed that minute amounts of EP caused fever when injected into the anterior hypothalamic nuclei which were known to be concerned with temperature regulation.

As a result of all this evidence, it seemed reasonable [12] to suppose that EP was a hormone released by phagocytic cells when they encountered bacteria or bacterial products, certain other infectious agents such as viruses and fungi, and antigens of cellular and humoral immunity. EP was released in the infected tissues, traveled in the bloodstream to the hypothalamus, and altered the behavior of anterior hypothalamic neurons in a way which led to regulation of the body temperature at a higher level than normal. Two problems remained unresolved: there was no detailed knowledge of the cellular source of EP, and virtually nothing was known about its nature, except that it was heat labile and trypsin sensitive, and was therefore presumably a protein.

Beeson [6] had supposed that because more than 95% of the cells in his preparations were polymorphonuclear leukocytes, that these cells made EP. The first step toward correcting this natural mistake was taken by Atkins et al. [13], who showed that various mononuclear cell populations were good sources of EP. It was assumed for many years that neutrophils also made EP, but attempts to obtain EP from purified neutrophil preparations always failed. Finally, Hanson et al. [14] purified rabbit neutrophils and showed that they retained all the traditional neutrophil properties such as chemotaxis and bacterial killing. However, they did not make EP. This observation has been confirmed, and it is now widely agreed that monocytes and macrophages are the source of EP from inflammatory exudates. EP can also be obtained from certain other cells such as keratinocytes, giant cells, mesangial cells, and macrophage cell lines.

Meanwhile, Murphy et al [15] had succeeded in purifying the principal EP from rabbit acute peritoneal exudates to apparent homogeneity. The purified protein caused a fever of 1°C when 20-30 ng was injected into a rabbit. They also found that macrophages secreted several molecular forms of EP [16] and that these forms were chemically and immunologically distinct [17]. The two main forms of EP had isoelectric points (pI) of 7.3 and 4.8. Both had molecular weights of approximately 15 000 daltons. The PI 7.3 form had a free sulfhydryl group which was essential to its activity, whereas the pI 4.8 form did not. Both forms of EP were synthesized de novo from amino acids when macrophages were suitably stimulated [16,18].

These molecular properties were very similar to those described for lymphocyte activating factor (LAF). This was a protein originally discovered by Gery and co-workers [19] which was a powerful T cell mitogen. It was found to be able to replace the macrophage requirement in several immunologic reactions [20], and was shown to be secreted by macrophages in response to the same stimuli as those which caused the secretion of EP. Exchange of materials between laboratories working on LAF and those working on EP showed that these very different biologic activities seemed to be properties of the same molecules [21,22]. Recently, IL-1 activity has been demonstrated in EP purified to apparent homogeneity [23,24].

LAF has since been renamed interleukin-1 (IL-1) [25]. This step was taken because it was discovered that a large number of different immunologic reactions depended upon this molecule. Each biologic activity had originally been described as a separate entity, and the realization that they were all mediated by the same molecule was a great step forward. It was hoped that IL-1 would be the prototype of a series of messenger molecules which collectively mediated immune responses. So far, interleukins-2 and 3 have also been described. Interleukin-2 is a mature T cell product which promotes the clonal expansion of immature T cells into effector cells of several types: helper cells, suppressor cells, and cytotoxic cells. IL-1 acts on mature T cells to promote IL-2 secretion [26]. Thus, the sequence of events during bacterial infection is now thought to be as follows: bacteria stimulate macrophages to secrete IL-1; IL-1 acts on a mature T cell population to cause the secretion of IL-2; IL-2 drives the clonal expansion of immature T cells which is fundamental to any immune response. If a great deal of IL-1 is formed in the infected site, some of it will escape into the bloodstream, travel to the hypothalamus, and cause fever.

EP/IL-1 has turned out to have several other totally unexpected actions. At the cellular level, it has been shown to stimulate the release of proteolytic enzymes from synovial cells; this proteolytic activity is thought to mediate the destruction of articular cartilage characteristic of rheumatoid arthritis [27]. Also, IL-1 causes neutrophils to release their specific granules into the medium [28]. These granules contain lactoferrin, which is a very strong chelator of iron. It is thought that iron chelation is a powerful antibacterial defense mechanism [29] and that the specific degranulation of PMN mediates the hypoferremia characteristic of infections [30]. Bacteria counter the action of host iron chelators (lactoferrin and transferrin) by synthesizing chelators of their own (siderophores). Siderophores are essential to bacterial virulence, and it is of some interest that siderophore synthesis has been shown to be strongly repressed by quite modest elevations of temperature [31,32].

Other cells which are directly acted on by IL-1 include fibroblasts, which are stimulated to divide at an increased rate [33], and skeletal muscle cells, which break down large quantities of their intracellular proteins into amino acid monomers which are excreted into the medium [34]. It is thought that IL-1 may be responsible for pathologic fibrosis such as occurs in the acute respiratory distress syndrome, or around schistosome eggs. Breakdown of protein in muscle and in bone matrix is characteristic of all severe infections, and leads to severe muscle wasting and spontaneous fractures if the febrile state is prolonged.

It is thought that the action of IL-1 on these various cells is probably mediated by a stimulation of arachidonic acid release from cell membranes, followed by the generation of active products by either the cyclooxygenase or the lipoxygenase pathway. In the case of the action on lymphocytes and the degranulation of PMN, the mediator is probably a leukotriene, since inhibitors of prostaglandin synthesis do not abolish the actions of IL-1 on those cells. This field is rapidly expanding, and has been recently reviewed [35].

Finally, EP/IL-1 has been shown to cause a variety of systemic effects when injected into whole animals. Most of this work has been done by Kampschmidt [36] and his associates. They showed that a substance originally described as leukocyte endogenous mediator (LEM) was secreted by phagocytic cells when they were exposed to bacteria or to bacterial products. LEM was subsequently shown to copurify with EP and IL-1, and is currently regarded as being the same molecule or molecules [37]. The effects of intravenous injections of EP/IL-1/LEM are many and various. They include fever, neutrophil leukocytosis, striking falls in the serum iron and serum zinc, virtual cessation of albumin synthesis by the liver, and increased synthesis of several plasma proteins, most of which are made by the liver. The plasma proteins include fibrinogen, ceruloplasmin, and the haptoglobins, which are found in normal plasma, but whose concentration is greatly increased when an animal is given injections of LEM. Other proteins such as C-reactive protein and the serum amyloid associated protein are present in low or zero concentrations in normal serum, but accumulate very rapidly after injections of LEM. Under the usual experimental conditions, when only single injections of LEM were given, these changes in serum protein concentration are transitory, being maximal at 24 h after injection, and completely resolved by 48-72 h. However, sustained changes in serum proteins, entirely comparable to those seen in infected patients, could be produced by sustained infusions of EP/IL-1/LEM [38]. Naturally, when a substance produces an effect when infused into a whole animal, one does not know whether the effect is directly mediated, or is a secondary consequence of some primary change. In the case of the hypoferremia, it seems reasonable to suppose that it is a consequence of the action of IL-1 on polymorphonuclear neutrophils. In the case of most of the other actions, the mechanism is unknown.

The evidence reviewed to this point makes it appear that IL-1 is a key molecule which mediates the response to bacterial infections, as well as to viral and fungal infections, immunologic reactions, and even certain tumors. It has both local and systemic actions: locally it acts on various cells to cause enhancement of the immune response, degranulation of PMN, muscle proteolysis, proteolytic enzyme release, and fibrosis. Systemically, it causes fever and all the other acute phase responses which are characteristic of infection. Some of the consequences of IL-1 production during bacterial infection are clearly of adaptive value. It is obviously useful to lower the serum iron during infection, because that interferes with microbial growth. It is also clearly useful to induce a PMN leukocytosis, because that makes more phagocytes available for mobilization into infected tissues. It is not so clear why it is useful to lower the serum zinc, or to increase the concentration of serum C-reactive protein. However, it was well said that teleology is a mistress that no biologist can live without, even though he may not wish to be seen with her in public. I feel confident that future research will show that each of the changes which accompany acute infection is of some adaptive value to the host.

We have recently become interested in the interactions between LAF and the fever-inducing actions of IL-1 [39]. It seemed a remarkable fact that two such very different activities should have been conserved in the same molecules, and we therefore wondered if the central action of IL-1 (fever) enhanced the peripheral action (stimulation of the immune response). We had purified the pI 4.8 form of rabbit EP/IL-1 to apparent homogeneity [24] and therefore studied the effects of small temperature changes on the action of this form of IL-1 on T cells. We found that the activity of IL-1 on unfractionated thymocytes in the presence of phytohemagglutinin (PHA) was greatly enhanced by small changes in temperature over the range 32°-38°C. Thymocytes selected as being peanut agglutinin negative were greatly enriched in IL-1 target cells. These cells responded to IL-1 without the necessity for a concomitant lectin stimulus. Again, the response was powerfully enhanced by slight increases in temperature over the range 32°-38°C. We also studied the effects of temperature on the release of IL-1 from macrophages, and on the action of the next interleukin in the sequence, IL-2. Both of these activities were much less temperature sensitive.

Any biologic process will increase in speed as the temperature is raised. Obviously, there will be a limit to that process, which occurs when the temperature is high enough to denature the enzyme or kill the cell which is being studied. In order to compare the effect of temperature on different biologic processes, one can derive numerical coefficients from the data which measure how much the rates increase for a standard temperature rise. The most commonly used coefficient is the Q_{10}, the rate increase which occurs when the temperature is changed by 10°C. If, as is usual, the process cannot be studied over a 10°C range, one studies it over a smaller range and then calculates what the Q_{10} would have been, assuming that the observed rate change had been maintained over 10°C [40].

Chemical reactions and simple enzymatic reactions generally have Q_{10} values in the range 2-5. In other words, the rate doubles to quintuples when the temperature is raised by 10°C. Biologic processes depend on very large numbers of concatenated reactions, most of which are unknown and cannot be measured. However, it is a remarkable fact that many biologic processes, ranging from heart rate to nerve conduction velocity, also have Q_{10} values in the 2-5 range. The simplest explanation of this behavior would be that a single reaction is rate limiting, and that the overall behavior of the whole process is dependent on it.

Because of the obvious connection of fever with infectious illnesses, many aspects of the immune response have been studied at different temperatures, in an attempt to find a mechanism which is strikingly enhanced by temperature. Neutrophils have been most often investigated; chemotaxis, phagocytosis, and bacterial killing by these cells have been reported to have Q_{10} values between 1.0 and 5.3, with most lying between 2 and 3. Opsonization, as measured by complement fixation, also has Q_{10} values in that range. Lymphocyte effector functions such as cytotoxicity were also not greatly enhanced by temperature (Q_{10} =2.5).

On the other hand, immunologic processes which were macrophage mediated and involved the clonal expansion of lymphocytes had sometimes been reported to have huge temperature coefficients. The data were inconsistent, but Q_{10} values ranging up to 7000 could be derived from published figures (references in [39]). Our own data showed that the average Q_{10} value for the action of IL-1 on thymocytes in the presence of PHA was 190, and the mean value for the action of IL-1 on partially purified IL-1 target cells was 72. By contrast, Q_{10} values for IL-2 action on thymocytes averaged 9.0, and the value for IL-1 release from macrophages averaged 2.5. It thus seemed that IL-1 action was far more temperature sensitive than were other components of the immune response.

On reflection, this arrangement seemed to make a great deal of teleological sense. Much of the body is normally below 37°C, and it is peripheral areas which are most likely to sustain minor injuries through which bacteria are introduced into the tissues. These infections are mostly mopped up locally by phagocytes either resident in the tissue or mobilized from the blood. One could not afford to design these cells so that they worked sluggishly at the temperature of hand skin (30°C), and indeed, they are not particularly temperature sensitive. Similarly, the binding of antibodies, and complement fixation by both pathways, are not greatly affected by temperature.

On the other hand, the immune response occurs when an infection has got out of hand, when a considerable local population of organisms has developed. It might be very useful to arrange that increased temperature stimulated the immune response in a major way. Trivial infections, which caused little or no inflammation, would not stimulate an immune response. Serious infections would first raise the local temperature, because of increased blood flow. In the case of frankly invasive infections, fever would develop, and the immune response would be enhanced all over the body, especially in the local lymph nodes. Temperature would then be a regulatory mechanism which ensured that the full resources of the immune system were only mobilized when it was necessary.

At the time we were doing our work, similar observations were being made at Yale University by Duff, Durum and Atkins. They studied slightly different aspects of the immune response, but the final message was the same. Temperature greatly enhanced proliferative immune reactions such as antibody synthesis, and the effect was mediated by the T cell rather than the B cell [41].

We have now investigated the temperature sensitivity of the form of IL-1 which has a pI of 7.3. It seems to be entirely comparable to that of the pI 4.8 form. Increased temperature strongly enhances its activity both on thymocytes in the presence of PHA (Fig. 1) and on partially purified IL-1 target cells (Fig. 2).

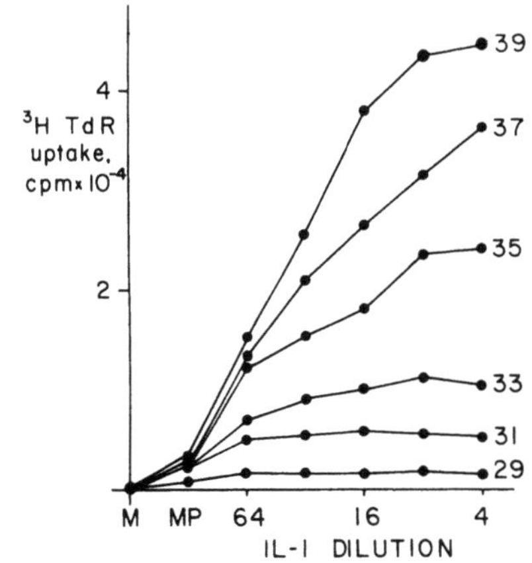

Fig. 1

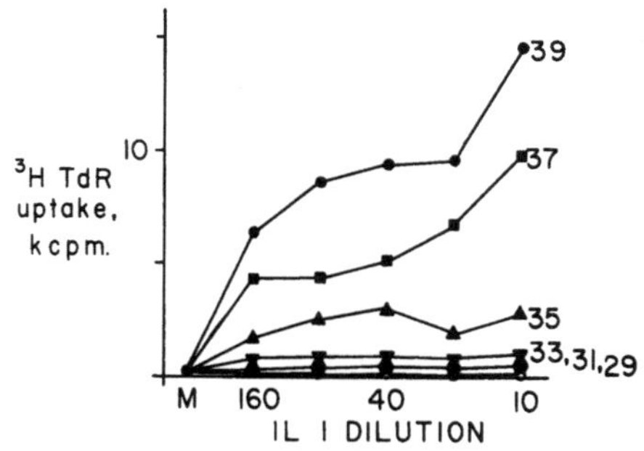

Fig. 2

Fig. 1. ^{3}HTdR uptake by thymocytes exposed to 5 µg/ml PHA plus various concentrations of the pI 7.3 form of IL-1, at different temperatures. The temperatures, in ^{O}C, are given on the right-hand side of the figure. *M* medium alone, *MP* medium plus 5 µg/ml PHA. All the IL-1 dilutions also contained 5 µg/ml PHA

Fig. 2. ^{3}HTdR uptake by IL-1 target cells (peanut aggulutinin-negative thymocytes) stimulated with various concentrations of pI 7.3 IL-1, in the absence of PHA, at different temperatures

Also, we have been able to clear up one problem with our initial paper [39]. We observed an optimum temperature of 38°C; responses at 40°C were considerably diminished. Obviously, we would have preferred to see a high optimum, because it would have been more "relevant" to events in living animals where febrile temperatures may range up to 41°C. However, the system we used was totally artificial because it involved cultivating the cells in vitro for 4 days before the observations were made. By that time, strongly stimulated cells at 40°C had exhausted the medium and the pH had dropped to levels which inhibited them. We showed that the action of both forms of IL-1 was exquisitely sensitive to pH (Fig. 3). If we controlled the pH by adding HEPES or other similar buffers, the observed temperature optimum was 39° or 40°C.

It is possible that the sensitivity of IL-1 action to pH provides another mechanism for regulating the immune response, this time at the local level. The pH of infected effusions such as empyemas frequently drops below 7.2, and sometimes below 7.0. This kind of pH drop occurs when the local battle has already been lost, a large microbial population has developed, and abscess formation has occurred. Under these circumstances it might be useful to downregulate local actions of IL-1, such as the degranulation of PMN and the stimulation of fibroblasts. It might perhaps minimize local tissue damage, while allowing the immune response to proceed at increased rates in less involved areas.

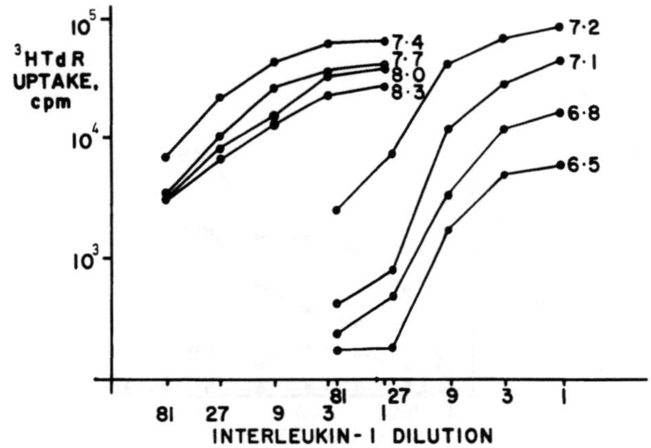

Fig. 3. The effect of pH on IL-1 activity. Cells were incubated in various concentrations of pI 7.3 IL-1 plus 5 μg/ml PHA at the pH indicated to the right of each curve

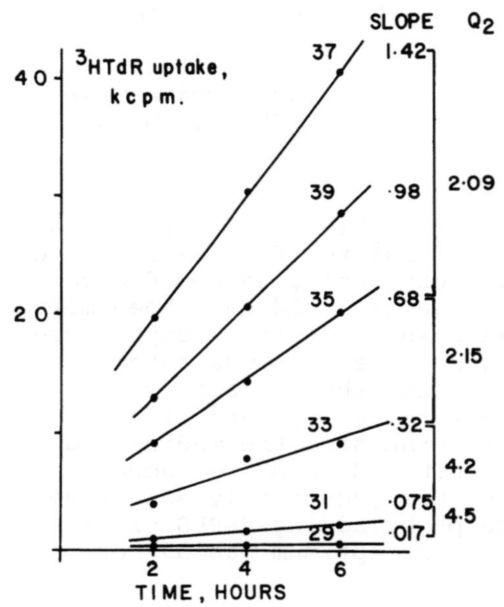

Fig. 4

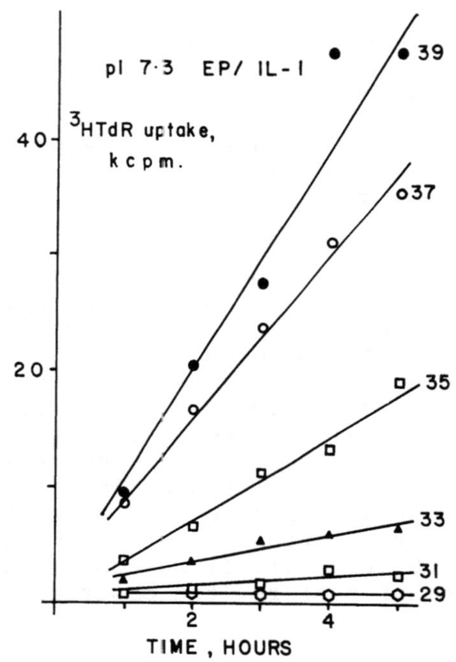

Fig. 5

Fig. 4. Rate study of ^{3}HTdR uptake by thymocytes incubated in 100 U/ml pI 7.3 EP plus 5 μg/ml PHA at the temperatures indicated. The slopes of the lines are given at the right. For each 2°C interval, a Q_2 value can be derived by dividing the slope of the *upper line* by that of the *lower line*. These values are given at the extreme right. The incubation medium was minimal essential medium

Fig. 5. Rate study of ^{3}HTdR uptake by thymocytes incubated in 100 U/ml pI 7.3 EP and 5 μg/ml PHA at the temperatures indicated. The medium was minimal essential medium buffered with 20 m*M* HEPES

Finally, we have devised a more elegant way of demonstrating temperature sensitivity. All our data to this point were derived from single observations of ^{3}HTdR uptake. The uptake rate was assumed to be linear, but that had not been demonstrated. We accordingly performed some timed ^{3}HTdR uptake studies at various temperatures. The uptake rates were indeed linear, and were strongly influenced by temperature. The slopes of the lines could be compared to get Q_{10} data. Using this technique, we were able to show that the same batch of thymocytes showed an apparent optimum temperature of IL-1 action of 37°C in bicarbonate-buffered medium (Fig. 4), and 39°C in the presence of HEPES (Fig. 5).

In summary, we think that the febrile reaction to bacterial infection is a purposive response whose function is to promote the activation and replication of T cells. We were led to that view by the apparent identity of endogenous pyrogen and interleukin-1. Our investigations have clearly shown that T cells are unusually temperature sensitive. So far, we have studied the effects of temperature on the mechanism for clonal expansion of T lymphocytes. It may well be that other temperature-sensitive aspects of T cell function are important, and remain to be discovered.

References

1. Wunderlich CA (1871) Medical thermometry. New Sydenham Society, London
2. Bennett IL Jr, Nicastri A (1960) Fever as a mechanism of resistance. Bacterial Rev 24:16-34
3. Mackowiak PA (1981) Direct effects of hyperthermia on pathogenic microorganisms. Rev Infect Dis 3:508-520
4. Hort EC, Penfold WJ (1911) The dangers of saline injections. Br Med J 2: 1589-1591
5. Siebert F (1923) Fever producing substance found in some distilled waters. Protein fevers. Am J Physiol 67:90-123
6. Beeson PB (1948) Temperature elevating effect of a substance obtained from polymorphonuclear leukocytes. J Clin Invest 27:524
7. Wood WB Jr (1958) Studies on the cause of fever. N Engl J Med 258:1023-1031
8. Chao P, Francis L, Atkins E (1978) The release of an endogenous pyrogen from guinea pig leukocytes *in vitro*. J Exp Med 145:1288-98
9. Bodel P, Ralph P, Wene K, Long JC (1980) Endogenous pyrogen production by Hodgkins disease and human histiocytic lymphoma cell lines *in vitro*. J Clin Invest 65:514-8
10. Jackson DC (1967) A hypothalamic region responsive to localized injection of pyrogens. J Neurophysiol 30:586-602
11. Cooper KE, Cranston WI, Honour AJ (1967) Observations on the site and mode of action of pyrogens in the rabbit brain. J Physiol 191:325-337
12. Bernheim HA, Block LH, Atkins E (1979) Fever: pathogenesis, physiology and purpose. Ann Int Med 91:262-270
13. Atkins E, Bodel P, Francis L (1967) Release of an endogenous pyrogen *in vitro* from rabbit mononuclear cells. J Exp Med 126:357-384
14. Hanson DF, Murphy PA, Windle BE (1980) Failure of rabbit neutrophils to secrete endogenous pyrogen when stimulated with staphylococci. J Exp Med 151:1360-1371

15. Murphy PA, Chesney PJ, Wood WB Jr (1974) Further purification of rabbit leukocyte pyrogen. J Lab Clin Med 83:310-322
16. Cebula TA, Hanson DF, Moore DM, Murphy PA (1979) Synthesis of four endogenous pyrogens made by rabbit macrophages. J Lab Clin Med 94:95-105
17. Murphy PA, Cebula TA, Levin J, Windle BE (1981) Rabbit macrophages secrete two biochemically and immunologically distinct endogenous pyrogens. Infect Immun 34:177-183
18. Moore DM, Murphy PA, Chesney PJ, Wood WB Jr (1973) Synthesis of endogenous pyrogen by rabbit leukocytes. J Exp Med 137:1263-1274
19. Gery I, Gershon RK, Waksman BH (1972) Potentiation of the T lymphocyte response to mitogens: I. The responding cell. J Exp Med 136:128-142
20. Koopman, WJ, Farrar JJ, Fuller-Bonar J (1978) Evidence for the identification of lymphocyte activating factor as the adherent cell derived mediator responsible for enhanced antibody synthesis by nude mouse spleen cells. Cell Immunol 35:92-98
21. Rosenwasser LJ, Dinarello CA, Rosenthal AS (1979) Adherent cell function in murine T-lymphocyte antigen recognition: IV. Enhancement of murine T-cell antigen recognition by human leukocytic pyrogen. J Exp Med 150: 709-714
22. Murphy PA, Simon PL, Willoughby WF (1980) Endogenous pyrogens made by rabbit peritoneal exudate cells are identical with lymphocyte activating factors made by rabbit alveolar macrophages. J Immunol 124:2498-2501
23. Pacak F, Siegert R (1982) Chemical characterization of a rabbit leukocyte pyrogen. Eur J Biochem 127:375-380
24. Hanson DF, Murphy PA (1984) Demonstration of Interleukin I activity in apparently homogenous specimens of the PI form of rabbit endogenous pyrogen. Infect Immun 45:483-490
25. Aarden LA et al. (1979) Revised nomenclature for antigen nonspecific T cell proliferation and helper factors. J Immunol 123:2928-9
26. Smith KA, Lachman LB, Oppenheim JJ, Favata M (1980) The functional relationship of the Interleukins. J Exp Med 151:1551-1556
27. Mizel SB, Dayer JM, Krane SM, Mergenhagen SE (1981) Stimulation of rheumatoid synovial cell collagenase by lymphocyte activating factor (Interleukin-1). Proc Natl Acad Sci USA 78:2474-2477
28. Klempner MS, Dinarello CA, Gallin JI (1978) Human leukocytic pyrogen induces release of specific granule contents from human neutrophils. J Clin Invest 61:1330-6
29. Bullen JJ (1981) The significance of iron in infection. Rev Infect Dis 3:1127-1135
30. Van Snick JL, Masson PL, Heremans JF (1974) The involvement of lactoferrin in the hyposideremia of acute inflammation. J Exp Med 140:1068-84
31. Garibaldi JA (1972) Influence of temperature on the biosynthesis of iron transport compounds by *Salmonella typhimurium*. J Bacteriol 110:262-265
32. Kluger MJ, Rothenburg BA (1979) Fever and reduced iron: their interactions as a host defense response to bacterial infection. Science 203: 374-376
33. Schmidt JA, Mizel SB, Cohen D, Green I (1982) Interleukin-1, a potential regulator of fibroblast proliferation. J Immunol 128:2177-2182
34. Baracos V, Rodemann HP, Dinarello CA, Goldberg AL (1983) Stimulation of muscle protein degradation and prostaglandin E_2 release by Interleukin 1. N Engl J Med 308:552-558
35. Dinarello CA (1984) Interleukin 1. Rev Infect Dis 6:51-95
36. Kampschmidt RF (1981) Leukocytic endogenous mediator/endogenous pyrogen. In: Powanda MC, Canonico PG (eds) The physiologic and metabolic responses of the host. Elsevier/North Holland, Amsterdam, pp 55-74

37. Merriam CR, Pulliam LA, Kampschmidt RF (1977) Comparison of leukocytic endogenous mediator and leukocytic pyrogen. Proc Soc Exp Biol Med 154: 224-227
38. Sobrado J, Moldawer LL, Dinarello CA, Blackburn GL, Biotrain BR (1983) Continuous infusion of human leukocytic pyrogen in the guinea pig. Fed Proc 42:699
39. Hanson DF, Murphy PA, Silicano R, Shin HS (1983) The effect of temperature on the activation of thymocytes by Interleukins I and II. J Immunol 130:216-221
40. Giese AC (1968) Cell physiology, 3rd edn, Saunders, Philadelphia, chap 10
41. Jampel HD, Duff GW, Gershon RK, Atkins E, Durum SK (1983) Hyperthermia augments the primary *in vitro* humoral immune response. J Exp Med 157: 1229-38

Discussion

(pp. 322-333)

Murphy was asked to speculate on whether the observations made with human cells can be carried over to mice in light of the fact that the murine response to bacterial products such as endotoxin often is hypothermia, not hyperpyrexia. With an undercurrent of humor, *Murphy* replied that mice were never intended to live in animal rooms and laboratories with temperatures in the range of 20°C, which makes them cold and huddle close together. We should remember that mice are designed to live in the much warmer milieu of mouse holes. In fact, *Bodel* (Yale University) showed that if mice are kept at 33°C, which approximates the temperature of mouse holes, they exhibit responses to endotoxin closely simulating those of human beings.

In response to comments by *Karnovsky* concerning the striking Q_{10} differential of Il-1, cross-reactivity of anti-muramyl dipeptide (MDP) monoclonal antibodies with Il-1 and somnogenicity of Il-1, *Murphy* indicated he also had thought about membrane physicochemical changes at increased temperatures that preferentially favor Il-1 binding, but has no data on the subject. Indeed, it is not yet certain whether the Q_{10} reflects an effect on the mediator, Il-1, or the target cell it interacts with. No comment was made about the MDP-Il-1 cross-reactivity. As to the somnogenicity of Il-1, *Murphy* said he wasn't surprised since from time immemorial, when we are febrile we tend to cuddle up and go to bed, rest being perhaps another indirect beneficial effect of fever on host defense.

Murphy pointed out, in response to *Paterson's* comment about certain rickettsiae growing optimally at temperatures of 32°-33°C, that this makes sense in terms of where the rickettsiae spend most of their lives: (a) the rickettsiae causing Rocky Mountain spotted fever live virtually all their lives in ticks living in nature at lower temperatures, only occasionally feeding on humans to get a needed blood meal. It is not surprising, therefore, that when these rickettsiae infect human beings they tend to infect those parts of the body that are at lower temperature, i.e., a rash that begins peripherally; and (b) in the case of epidemic typhus rickettsiae whose natural habitat is the human body louse, the cutaneous eruption of this rickettsial disease begins centrally.

Several questions were raised by *Hahn* and *McGee* concerning the source and reason for two types of Il-1. *Murphy* indicated he had looked for production of Il-1 by restricted subsets of monocytes-macrophages or by Ia-positive versus Ia-negative cells, but that all the evidence was against the idea. Since there is evidence for dissociability of fever production and other effects of the higher molecular weight species of Il-1, there is reason to think that the most pyrogenic Il-1 molecules are the lower molecular weight species and that they may represent cleavage products derived from the higher molecular weight Il-1. Alternatively, it may be that we have two populations of Il-1 which differ in the degree of fever they elicit and, furthermore, they are preferentially released in different types of infection.

Inevitably, the question arose as to whether suppression of fever by pharmacologic drugs is a good thing to do in terms of tryping to help host immune defenses. *Murphy* responded by saying that for certain febrile infectious disorders where effective antimicrobial drugs are not available, existence of fever or even raising body temperature is more advantageous than detrimental. For example, in cases of sporotrichosis of the fingers or hand, wrapping the fingers or putting the hand in a glove accelerates recovery.

Bayer-Symposium VIII
The Pathogenesis of Bacterial Infections, 336-348 (1985)

The Immunological Significance of Antibody Affinity

M. E. Devey and M. W. Steward

Summary

Mice selectively bred to produce low affinity antibodies are more susceptible to immune complex glomerulonephritis induced by daily injections of a foreign protein antigen than are mice selected to produce high affinity antibody. Development of disease is associated with an inability to produce the normal maturational switch from low to high affinity antibody. Low affinity NM mice, selected by their failure to show affinity maturation after injection of adjuvantised antigen showed an even greater susceptibility to disease. Sucrose density gradient ultracentrifugation studies showed that immune complexes formed in high affinity mice were large (19 *S*) and cleared rapidly from the circulation. Immune complexes in low affinity mice were significantly smaller. We propose that immune complex diseases may result from an inherited or acquired form of immunodeficiency favouring a predominantly low affinity antibody response. Immune complexes formed from low affinity antibody have a tendency to dissociate and form small (12-17 *S*) complexes in antigen excess which may deposit in filtering membranes such as the renal glomerulus.

Introduction

Antibody Affinity

A fundamental characteristic of the immune response is the ability to eliminate foreign antigens and infectious agents from the body. Antibodies are clearly important in this process and, under normal circumstances, they combine with antigen to form immune complexes. The interaction of an antibody combining site Ab with an antigenic determinant Ag is reversible and the association Ka and dissociation rate constants Kd can be measured.

$$\text{Ab} + \text{Ag} \underset{K_d}{\overset{K_a}{\rightleftharpoons}} \text{AbAg}$$

The equilibrium constant or affinity K can be determined from the formula

$$K = \frac{K_a}{K_d} = \frac{[\text{AgAb}]}{[\text{Ag}]\ [\text{Ab}]}$$

Ideally, measurement of affinity should be carried out using homogeneous reagents in terms of both antigenic determinants and antibody binding sites, for example a monoclonal antibody to a monovalent hapten. When both the antigen and antibody are monovalent the terms "affinity" or "intrinsic affinity" may be used to describe the interaction of a single antibody combining site with its antigenic determinant. In the case of multivalent antigen and antibodies, the equilibrium constant depends not only on the intrinsic affinity of the binding site, but also on the valence of the antigen and antibody and also on other contributory factors not necessarily associated with the primary antigen-antibody reaction. Under these circumstances, the terms "avidity" or "functional affinity" have been used to describe the equilibrium constant.

The measurement of antibody affinity in serum is complicated by the extreme heterogeneity of the antibody response in terms of amount, isotype, and affinity. Under such circumstances perhaps the technically simplest method of affinity determination is that of Steward and Petty [1,2] which employs saturated ammonium sulphate to separate bound from free antigen over a defined range of antigen concentrations in antigen excess. This method has recently been validated experimentally by comparison with several other methods, including equilibrium dialysis, using a panel of monoclonal anti-DNP antibodies [3].

Genetic Control of Antibody Affinity

Antibody affinity is under the control of genes independent of those governing antibody levels and it has been shown that the affinity of antibodies produced to human serum albumin (HSA) injected in saline differs in different inbred strains of mice [4]. These differences were also observed in responses to other antigens and were independent of antibody levels, but could be overcome by injecting the antigen with adjuvant [5]. Back-cross studies with inbred strains and with selectively bred mice suggest that the control of antibody affinity is polygenic, but the cellular level at which it operates is far from clear at the present time, and is likely to be complex. Major histocompatibility complex typing suggests that the genes controlling antibody affinity are not linked to the H-2 loci K and D [6].

Antibody Affinity and Biological Activity

Many studies indicate that antibody affinity increases with time after immunisation and this phenomenon is known as "affinity maturation". As high affinity antibody forms more stable bonds with antigen, it would seem to be highly advantageous for an animal to produce a high affinity antibody response to an immunological challenge. Indeed it has been shown that high affinity antibody is superior to low affinity antibody in many biological reactions, including several which are of importance in providing effective immunity in the host such as neutralisation of toxins and viruses, complement fixation and immune elimination (references in [7]). Of particular interest in the context of the pathogenesis of bacterial infection is the finding that low affinity antibodies are less protective than high affinity antibodies in *Escherichia coli* infection in mice [8].

Inability to produce a predominantly high affinity antibody response has thus been considered an expression of immunodeficiency. Chronic infections are frequently associated with immune complex glomerulonephritis (GN) and it has been proposed that such diseases may result from an inability to eliminate antigen from the circulation with the subsequent formation of immune complexes which localise in tissue [9]. The first evidence in support of this hypothesis came from the finding that the inbred strains of mice (SWR and B10D2) that were susceptible to GN after neonatal LCM virus infection were strains producing low affinity antibodies whereas strains producing high affinity antibodies (A/Jax and C3H) were not susceptible to GN [9]. An association has also been shown between low affinity antibody-producing strains and GN after *Trypansoma brucei* infection [10].

Selection of Mice for High and Low Affinity Antibody Production and the Nonmaturing Affinity Response

Mice from an initially random-bred population were selectively bred on the basis of the affinity of the antibody produced after four injections of a protein antigen in saline. At each generation mice producing high affinity antibody ($K > 10^6$ L/M) were mated and similarly those producing low affinity antibody ($K < 0.7 \times 10^6$ L/M) were mated to produce the high and low affinity lines, respectively [11]. At present selective breeding has been carried out for 22 successive generations and has resulted in a gradual and progressive divergence of the two lines with regard to their antibody affinity. In contrast, antibody levels did not show a corresponding separation and there was no relationship between levels and affinity.

Daily injections of a small dose of HSA (3 mg kg/day) in these mice for up to 17 weeks results in a chronic immune complex GN in 35%-55% of the low affinity mice, but only rarely (< 13%) in high affinity mice [12-14]. The disease was characterised by high levels of proteinuria (up to 60 mg/ml mouse serum albumin in urine), a decreased glomerular filtration rate in the later stages of the disease, massive deposition of immune complexes (antigen, C3 and mouse immunoglobulin) in the kidneys and eventual death from renal failure. Immunofluorescent studies showed that immune complex deposition in the renal glomeruli was diffuse and predominantly capillary (Fig. 1) and electron microscopy showed deposits in the subepithelial region of the glomerular basement membrane [15]. In contrast, high affinity mice showed a low incidence of proteinuria and, when present, renal deposits were focal and predominantly mesangial. Both high and low affinty mice receiving daily antigen injections had circulating immune complexes by two solid phase binding assays (C1q and conglutinin), but levels of these showed no correlation with development of GN and instead reflected the amount of antibody produced, which was significantly higher in low affinity female mice compared with the other groups [14].

The affinity of free antibody in the serum increased in high affinity mice with time and the increasing number of antigen

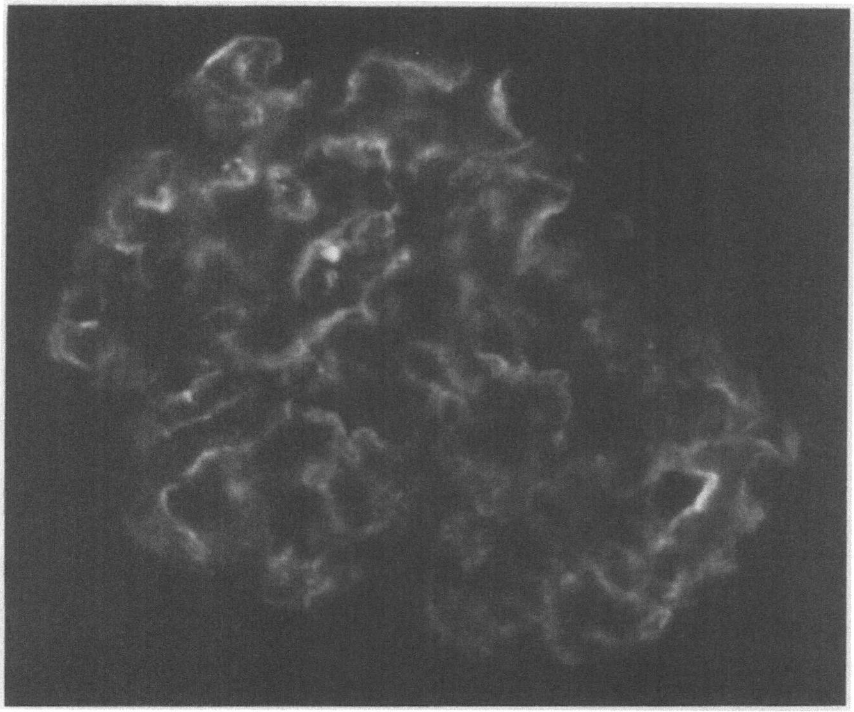

Fig. 1. Predominantly capillary localisation of immunoglobulin in the renal glomerulus of a low affinity mouse after 51 daily injections of HSA

injections and a similar increase was also seen in low affinity mice (Fig. 2a), although individual animals showed a wide range of affinity values. However, most of the low affinity mice that developed GN had died by the 11th week of the experiment and did not show affinity maturation and it was therefore the surviving low affinity mice that did not develop GN that were responsible for the increase in affinity seen after week 11. This suggested that the low affinity line contained a subpopulation that lacked the ability to produce the normal maturational transition from low to high affinity antibody and that it was this population that was particularly susceptible to chronic GN. Injection of low affinity mice with antigen in Freund's adjuvant showed that they fell into two groups, one (60%) producing antibody of increasing affinity and the other producing only low affinity antibody - a nonmaturing antibody response (Fig. 2b). Both of these groups produced identical amounts of antibody. Mice producing the nonmaturing affinity response were interbred and their progeny termed low affinity nonmaturing mice (NM mice). A similar regimen of daily antigen injections in these mice produced a more rapid and severe GN that was observed in the low affinity line, particularly in male NM mice (Fig. 3). Mice that developed GN did not show affinity maturation and in addition had significantly lower antibody levels than those that did not develop GN. The antibody index (obtained by the product of the

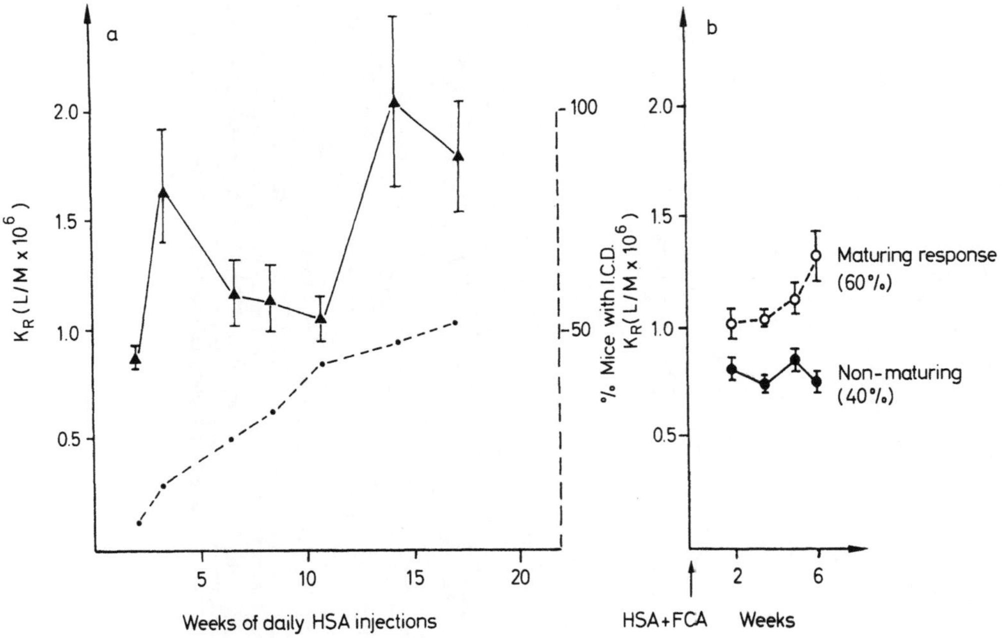

Fig. 2. (a) Affinity maturation (mean ± standard errcr) and incidence of immune complex disease in low affinity mice. (b) Affinity maturation (mean ± standard error) in low affinity mice after a single injection of HSA in Freund's complete adjuvant

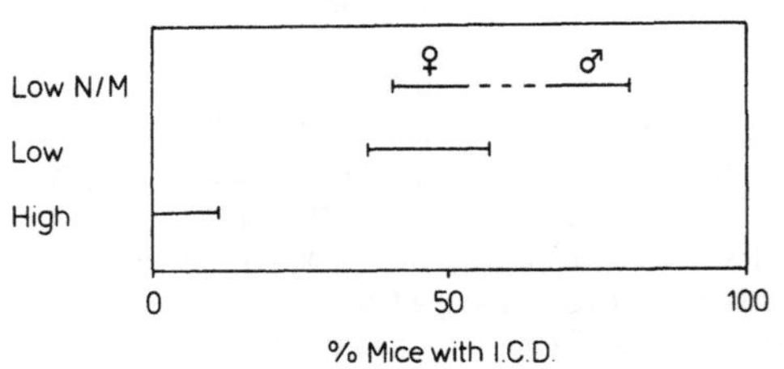

Fig. 3. The incidence of immune complex glomerulcnephritis in high affinity, low affinity and low affinity in NM mice

Ab_t and *K* values) was significantly lower in both male and female NM mice with GN than in those without (Fig. 4) suggesting that a functionally poor antibody response in terms of both the amount and affinity of the antibody produced is likely to result in the formation of pathogenic immune complexes. However, an alternative explanation for the low antibody levels in these proteinuric mice is loss of antibody in the urine, although it is unlikely that this should affect antibody affinity. Female NM mice did not have a significantly increased incidence of GN and this may have been due to their capacity to produce very high amounts of antibody which may have overcome the disadvantage of low affinity (Fig. 5).

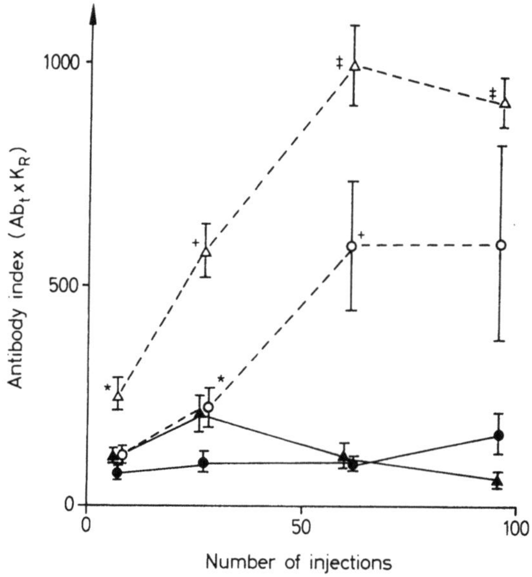

Fig. 4. Mean antibody index $K_R \times Ab_t \pm$ standard error in low affinity NM male mice with ICD *(full circles)* and without ICD *(open circles)* and in low affinity NM female mice with ICD *(full triangles)* and without ICD *(open triangles)*; * P < 0.05, + P < 0.01, ‡ < 0.001. (From reference [16] with permission)

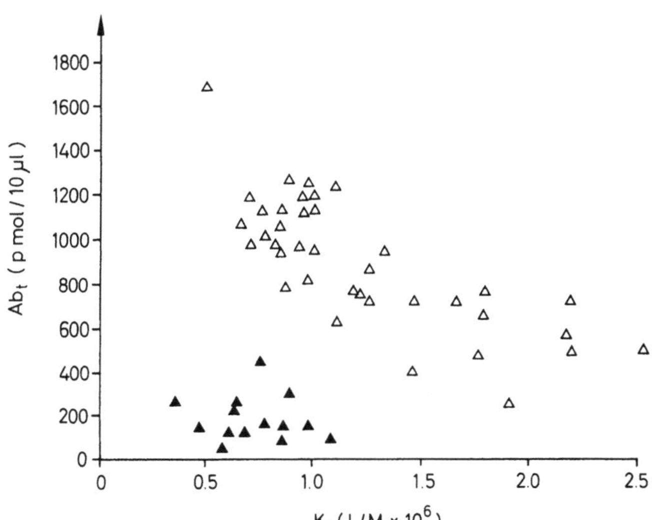

Fig. 5. Antibody affinity K_R and amount Ab_t in low affinity NM female mice with ICD *(full triangles)* and without ICD *(open triangles)*. (From reference [16] with permission)

Experimental Results

High affinity male mice and low affinity NM male mice were given daily intraperitoneal injections of 10 mg/kg HSA in saline. After 40 injections, 44% of the low affinity NM mice, but none of the high affinity mice had proteinuria. In order to determine the handling of the daily antigen dose by the two groups of animals, mice were injected intraperitoneally with ^{125}I-labelled HSA in saline and bled from the retro-orbital venous plexus after 1, 2, 5 and 24 h. The clearance of bound and free antigen from the circulation was calculated after precipitation of bound

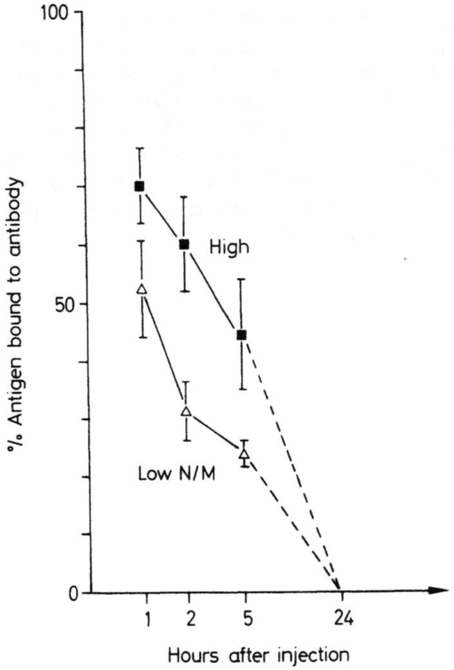

Fig. 6. The percentage of antigen bound to antibody in the sera of high affinity and low affinity NM mice after 40 daily antigen injections taken 1, 2, 5 and 24 h after an intraperitoneal injection of ^{125}I-labelled HSA. Results expressed as mean ± standard error. Differences at 2 and 5 h are significant ($P < 0.01$)

and free antigen from the circulation was calculated after precipitation of bound antigen (immune complexes) with saturated ammonium sulphate. In both groups of mice, blood levels of bound and free antigen were maximum between 1 and 2 h and >98% of the injected dose of ^{125}I-labelled HSA had been cleared from the circulation by 24 h. There were no significant differences in immune complex clearance between the two groups, although similar experiments reported previously [15] showed some differences in antigen handling in high and low affinity mice. In the present experiment, however, at 2 and 5 h after antigen injection there were significant differences in the proportions of antibody-bound antigen and free antigen in low affinity NM compared with high affinity mice, suggesting that there was greater dissociation of the immune complexes in low affinity NM mice (Fig. 6).

Sucrose Density Gradient Ultracentrifugation

Pooled serum samples from high affinity mice, low affinity NM mice or ^{125}I-labelled molecular weight markers were applied to sucrose density gradients (10%-40% w/v in phosphate-buffered saline) and centrifuged in a vertical rotor at 50 000 rpm for 5 h at 4°C. Sequential samples were removed from the top of the gradients and counted in a gamma counter. At 1 h (Fig. 7a), 2 h (Fig. 7b) and 5 h (Fig. 7c) there were significant differences in the size distribution of the circulating immune complexes in the two groups of mice, low affinity NM mice having predominantly small to medium sized complexes (< 19 *S*) and high affinity mice having predominantly larger complexes (> 19 *S*). The high molecular weight complexes in high affinity mice were rapidly cleared between 2 and 5 h (Fig. 8). In low affinity NM mice there was also rapid clearance of the low molecular weight peak seen at 2 h, but at 5 h there were higher levels of low molecular weight material remaining in the sera compared with high affinity mice (Fig. 9).

Antibody Levels and Isotype

Measurement of antibody levels showed that low affinity NM male mice had similar antibody levels to those previously reported, but these were significantly higher than those in high affinity mice although the affinity was significantly lower (Table 1). The isotype of the specific antibodies to HSA was measured by an enzyme-linked immunosorbent assay using rabbit antisera specific for mouse IgG1, IgG2a, IgG2b, IgM and IgA and a peroxidase-labelled goat antiserum to rabbit IgG. There were no differences between the isotype of antibodies produced by the two groups which was predominantly IgG1 (Table 1).

Table 1. Levels, affinity and isotype of antibodies to HSA in high affinity and low affinity NM male mice after 41 daily injections (value are mean ± standard deviation)

	Mean antibody titre		Mean affinity	Predominant isotype
	HA ($\log_{10}$)	Ab_t (pM/10 µl)	K_R (L/M x 10^6)	
High affinity	2.83 ± 0.52	56 ± 13	1.12 ± .28	IgG1
Low affinity NM	3.81 ± 0.56	345 ± 216	0.78 ± .33	IgG1
Significance (P)	< 0.005	< 0.005	< 0.05	

Discussion and Conclusions

Circulating immune complexes have been demonstrated in many chronic diseases and complex deposition in tissues such as the kidneys, arteries and joints have been implicated in the disease pathology. However, it is clear that not all circulating complexes deposit in tissue causing inflammatory reactions and injury and that, in general, immune complex formation is a normal event leading to the rapid removal of foreign antigens by the mononuclear phagocyte system (MPS). The mechanisms of immune complex deposition are not well understood, but appear to include intrinsic properties of the immune complexes themselves as well as host and environmental factors. The demonstration that mice selectively bred to produce low affinity antibodies are highly susceptible to chronic immune complex glomerulonephritis induced by daily injections of a protein antigen and that this susceptibility is associated with an inability to produce the normal maturational switch from low to high affinity antibody supports the hypothesis that the genetically controlled production of antibody of low affinity is an important host factor in the development of immune complex disease.

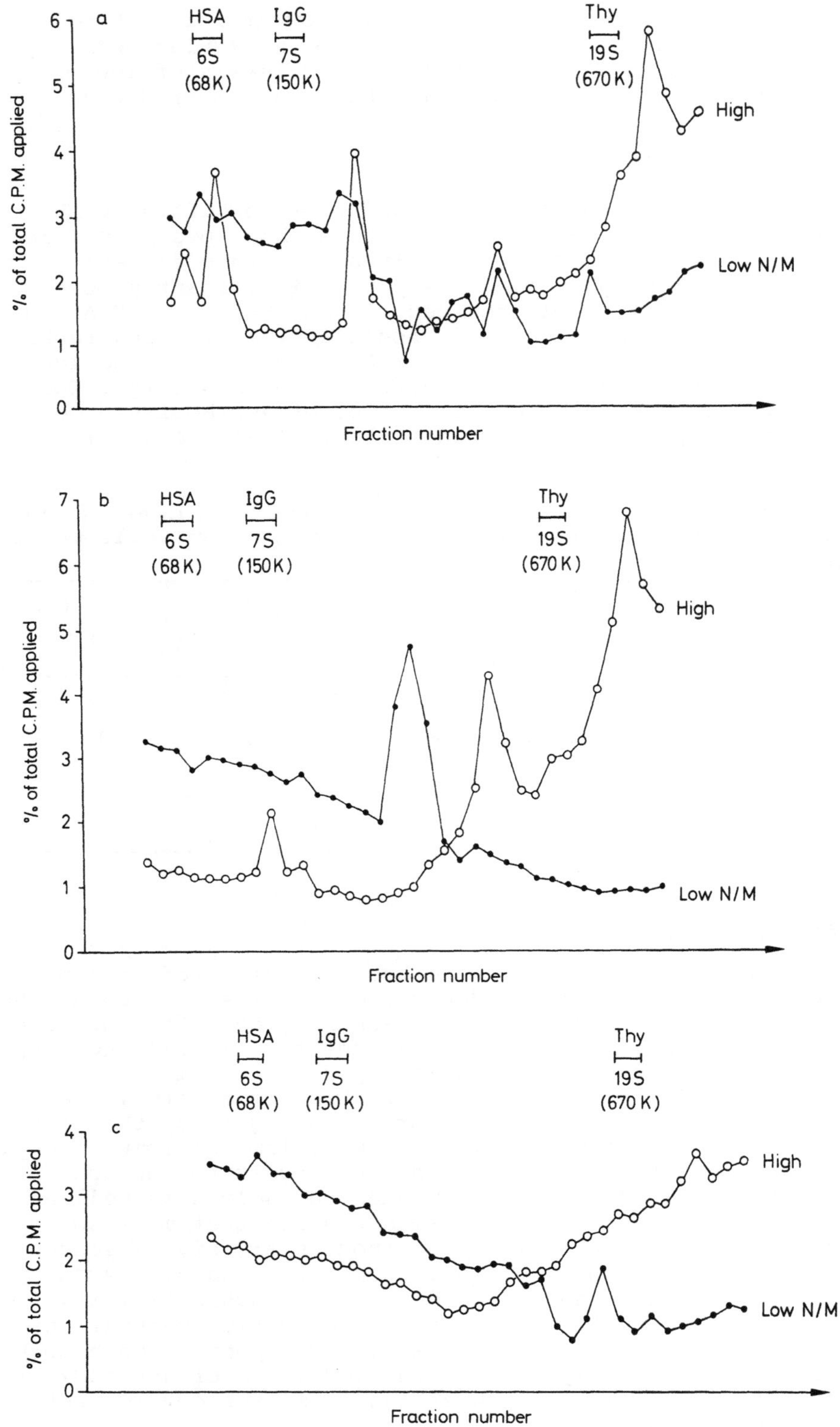
a
HSA
6S
(68K)
IgG
7S
(150K)
Thy
19S
(670K)
High
Low N/M
% of total C.P.M. applied
Fraction number
b
HSA
6S
(68K)
IgG
7S
(150K)
Thy
19S
(670K)
High
Low N/M
% of total C.P.M. applied
Fraction number
c
HSA
6S
(68K)
IgG
7S
(150K)
Thy
19S
(670K)
High
Low N/M
% of total C.P.M. applied
Fraction number

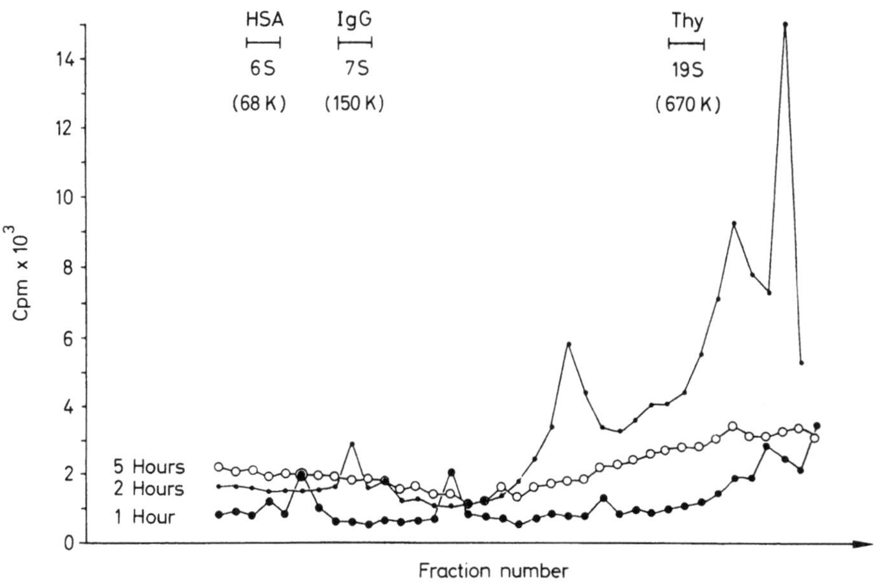

Fig. 8. Sucrose gradient ultracentrifugation of sera from high affinity mice after 40 daily antigen injections taken 1, 2 and 5 h after an intraperitoneal injection of ^{125}I-labelled HSA. The positions of the molecular weight markers are shown

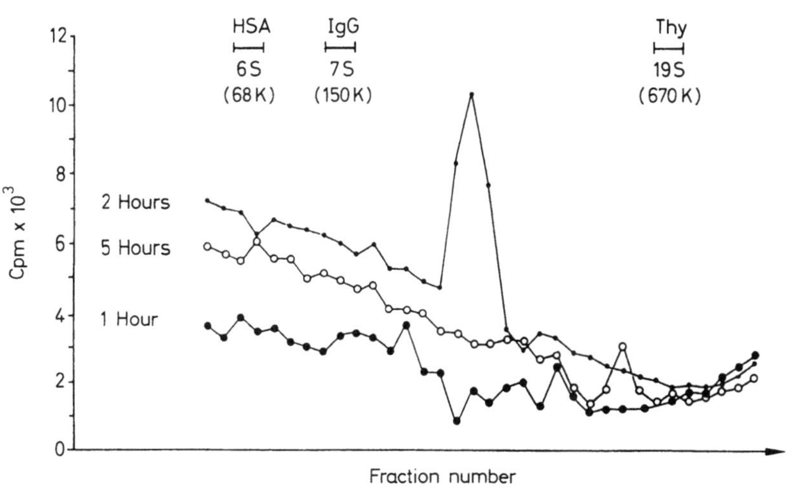

Fig. 9. Sucrose gradient ultracentrifugation of sera from low affinity NM mice after 40 daily antigen injections taken 1, 2 and 5 h after an intraperitoneal injection of ^{125}I-labelled HSA. The positions of the molecular weight markers are shown

Fig. 7a-c. Sucrose gradient ultracentrifugation of pooled sera from high affinity and low affinity NM mice after 40 daily antigen injections (a) 1 h, (b) 2 h and (c) 5 h after an intraperitoneal injection of ^{125}I-labelled HSA. Results are expressed as a percentage of the total cpm applied to the gradient. The positions of the molecular weight markers are shown

The studies reported here, and others employing preformed immune complexes formed from monoclonal antibodies of defined affinity [17,18] suggest that immune complexes containing low affinity antibodies are cleared more slowly from the circulation than those formed with high affinty antibodies. However in all these studies the differences in complex clearance were most apparent between 1 and 5 h after injection and complexes were usually completely cleared from the circulation by 24 h. This suggests that early events in immune complex formation are important in determining their eventual fate and perhaps explains why conventional immune complex tests have been shown to be of limited clinical usefulness. Sucrose gradient ultracentrifugation studies showed that the circulating immune complexes 1, 2 and 5 h after an intraperitoneal injection of ^{125}I-labelled antigen were predominantly large (> 19 *S*) in high affinity mice, but predominantly small (< 19 *S*) in low affinity NM mice and it is likely that the large immune complexes are rapidly cleared from the circulation by the MPS and do not localise in the renal glomeruli. Low affinity NM male mice, despite producing higher levels of antibody, were not able to form these large complexes, but instead formed complexes of 12-17 *S* which are thought to be capable of localising in the glomerular basement membrane [19,20] Alternatively, it is possible that failure of immune elimination of antigen as a consequence of the dissociation of the complexes formed with low affinity antibodies may have led to a primary deposition of free antigen followed by subsequent in situ immune complex formation [21]. Our findings do not argue for or against either of these mechanisms, but it may be relevant that small (550K) covalent immune complexes (which cannot dissociate) have been shown to be capable of penetrating the glomerular basement membrane and localising subepithelially [22]. The differences between the high and low affinity mice were not due to differences in their MPS function as no inherent differences have been shown in the ability of the two lines to clear polyvinylpyrrolidone (PVP), aggregated IgG or preformed immune complexes in unimmunised mice [23]. However, after 40 daily injections of antigen, low affinity mice were less able to clear PVP from their circulation than were high affinity mice [15], perhaps due to "fatigue" of the MPS.

In conclusion, we suggest that, in chronic infections and other situations where there is prolonged exposure to foreign antigens, a predominantly low affinity antibody response may result in the formation of potentially tissue-damaging immune complexes. Production of low affinity antibody may be an inherited form of immunodeficiency or, in view of the fact that factors such as protein deprivation [23], parasitic infections [24,25] and ageing [7] cause a significant reduction in antibody affinity, it may be acquired. The superiority of high affinity to low affinity antibody in a number of biological activities has been well documented, but very little is known about the importance of affinity in protection against infection and this surprising omission must surely be corrected soon.

Acknowledgments. We should like to thank Miss K. Bleasdale, Miss C. Stanley and Mr. P. Stephenson for technical assistance and the Wellcome Trust for financial support. M.E.D. is a Wellcome Trust Senior Lecturer.

References

1. Steward MW, Petty RE (1972) The use of ammonium sulphate globulin precipitation for determination of affinity of anti-protein antibodies in mouse serum. Immunology 22:474
2. Steward MW, Petty RE (1972) The antigen-binding characteristics of antibody pools of different relative affinity. Immunology 23:881
3. Stanley C, Lew AM, Steward MW (1983) The measurement of antibody affinity: a comparison of five techniques using a panel of monoclonal anti-DNP antibodies and the effect of high affinity antibody on the measurement of low affinity antibody. J Immunol Methods 64:119
4. Petty RE, Steward MW, Soothill JF (1972) The heterogeneity of antibody affinity in inbred mice and its possible immunopathologic significance. Clin Exp Immunol 12:231
5. Petty RE, Steward MW (1977) The effect of immunological adjuvants on the relative affinity of antiprotein antibodies. Immunology 32:49
6. Steward MW, Reinhardt MC, Staines NA (1979) The genetic control of antibody affinity: Evidence from breeding studies with mice selectively bred for either high or low affinity antibody production. Immunology 37:697
7. Steward MW, Steensgaard (1983) Antibody affinity: Thermodynamic aspects and biological significance. CRC Press, Boca Raton
8. Ahlstedt S, Holmgren J, Hanson LA (1974) Protective capacity of antibodies against *E. coli* O antigen with special reference to the avidity. Int Arch allergy 46:470
9. Soothill JF, Steward MW (1971) The immunopathological significance of the heterogeneity of antibody affinity. Clin Exp Immunol 9:193
10. Soothill JF, Smith MD, Morgan AG (1975) Immunodeficiency and the allergic effects of parasitic infection. In: Taylor AER, Miller R (eds) Pathogenic processes in parasitic infections, vol 13. Blackwell, Oxford, p 59
11. Katz FE, Steward MW (1976) The genetic control of antibody affinity in mice. Immunology 29:543
12. Steward MW (1979) Chronic immune complex disease in mice. The role of antibody affinity. Clin Exp Immunol 38:414
13. Devey ME, Steward MW (1980) The induction of chronic antigen-antibody complex disease in selectively bred mice producing either high or low affinity antibody to protein antigens. Immunology 41:303
14. Devey ME, Bleasdale K, Collins M, Steward MW (1982) Experimental antigen-antibody complex disease in mice: the role of antibody levels, antibody affinity and circulating antigen-antibody complexes. Int Arch Allergy Appl Immunol 68:47
15. Steward MW, Collins MJ, Stanley C, Devey ME (1981) Chronic antigen-antibody complex glomerulonephritis in mice. Br J Exp Pathol 62:614
16. Devey ME, Bleasdale K, Stanley C, Steward MW (1984) Failure of affinity maturation leads to increased susceptibility to immune complex glomerulonephritis. Immunology 52:377
17. Lew AM, Staines NA, Steward MW (1984) Glomerulonephritis induced by preformed immune complexs containing monoclonal antibodies of defined antibody and isotype. Clin Exp Immunol 47:413
18. Lew AM, Steward MW (1984) Glomerulonephritis: the use of grafted hybridomas to investigate the role of epitope density, antibody affinity and antibody isotype in active serum sickness. Immunology 52:367

19. Haakenstad AO, Striker GE, Mannik M (1976) The glomerular deposition of soluble immune complexex prepared with reduced and alkylated antibodies and with intact antibodies in mice. Lab Invest 35:293
20. Germuth FG, Rodriguez CA, Wise OL (1982) Passive immune complex glomerulonephritis in mice III. Clearance kinetics and properties of circulating complexes. Lab Invest 46:515
21. Couser WG, Salant DJ (1980) In situ immune complex formation and glomerular injury. Kidney Int 17:1
22. Lew AM, Tovey DG, Steward MW (1984) Localisation of covalent immune complexes on the epithelial side of the glomerular basement membrane in mice. Int Arch Allerg Appl Immunol 75:242
23. Reinhardt MC, Steward MW (1979) Antibody affinity and clearance function studies in high and low antibody affinity mice. The effect of protein defificiency. Immunology 38:735
24. Steward MW, Voller A (1973) The effect of malaria on the relative affinity of mouse anti protein antibody. Br J Exp Pathol 54:198
25. Pattison JR, Steward MW, Target GAT (1983) Trypanosome infection depresses antibody affinity and delays affinity maturation. Clin Exp Immunol 53:175

Discussion

(pp. 336-348)

Several questions bearing on the definition of affinity, technical aspects of capturing immune complexes of varying size containing antibody of different affinity binding, and potential problems of injection of such large amounts of antigen were raised by *Bhakdi*. *Devey* redefined affinity binding, emphasizing that it is a variable, qualitative characteristic of different populations of antibodies directed against the same antigenic determinant. She stressed that the method used for measuring immune complexes is the classical Farr type, using 50% saturated ammonium sulfate, which precipitates only antibody, not antigen; the size of the complex would not introduce artifacts. *Devey* also made it clear that the amount of foreign protein injected per day into the average sized mouse is not unreasonable and in no way accounts directly for their death; immune complexes are present in renal glomeruli of low affinity mice by 12 days and they start to die because of immune complex-induced nephritis, not antigen per se, as early as 20 days.

In answering other queries concerning the basis for preferential production of low affinity antibodies soon after immunization and high affinity antibodies later on, *Devey* explained that it can best be understood in terms of antigen presentation and how well the B lymphocytes are tolerized to the antigen at the point immunization commences. One would expect high affinity receptors on B cells to be extensively tolerized or blocked by large amounts of antigen whereas low affinity receptors would be more responsive. Thus, by necessity, the first antibodies produced will possess lower affinity binding. Only later on, when antigen becomes limiting (owing to catabolism and immune clearance), will antibodies of this degree of affinity binding begin to be found to an increasing extent in proportion to low affinity antibodies.

In answering questions by *Bhakdi*, *Anderson*, *Jackson* and *Schoolnik*, respectively, *Devey* responded, as follows: (a) evidence does exist from the work of one of *Steward's* graduate students, *Andrew*, that preformed covalent immune complexes which are unable to dissociate, are capable, when injected, of passing through the glomerular basement membrane of mice and can be localized on the epithelial side of the membrane by electron microscopy; (b) because immune complexes may dissociate, especially when the antibody is of low affinity, an alternative mechanism of immune complex deposition may be by in situ formation in the host organs; (c) really striking differences in affinity binding properties of antibodies to an antigen are observed when the antigen is injected *without* adjuvant; as soon as one resorts to the use of immunologic adjuvants for immunization, distinctions in affinity binding characteristics of different antibody populations become increasingly difficult to demonstrate; and (d) the situation, indeed, may become more complicated by production of anti-idiotypic antibodies, and their affinity binding features; so far attempts to identify and measure such antibodies have not been made and, hence, no information concerning the subject is available at this time.

Bayer-Symposium VIII
The Pathogenesis of Bacterial Infections, 351-363 (1985)

Trigger Mechanisms for the Release of Tissue Active Products of Phagocytic Cells

M. L. Karnovsky

Summary

Oxygen radicals, important in the cidal function of phagocytic leukocytes, are reviewed in terms of the specific types of cell that produce them, and the biologic history of those cells. The different types of stimuli necessary for their release are outlined. *Cis*-Polyene fatty acids are specially interesting stimuli, because their action may be reversed by withdrawing them from the cells with albumin, and because their activity can be correlated precisely with the kinetics of their cellular uptake and with their melting points. Protein kinase and calmodulin are probably involved in the phenomenon. The role of another class of small molecules, the muramyl peptides, in protecting the organism against infection is examined, but in a different context. These substances, exemplified by muramyl dipeptide, are of bacterial origin and exhibit several interesting activities, viz., adjuvanticity, pyrogenicity, and somnogenicity. Expression of these activities is a consequence of specific binding of the peptides to host macrophages.

Introduction

This paper is concerned mainly with the release of active oxygen radicals and of muramyl peptides by phagocytic leukocytes, and the roles of those substances in the host-parasite relationship. Although phagocytic leukocytes are overwhelmingly the main source of oxygen radicals in the body, muramyl peptide monomers are probably derived from other sources as well (e.g., gut wall). Both classes of substance are involved in antibacterial (and antitumor) action. The former class operates directly on the target, and the latter substances operate via further action of macrophages and lymphocytes. An overall aspect of the way animals may handle infectious diseases, involving both the nervous system and the immune system, is suggested in the last part of this paper.

Oxygen Radicals

In the past several years, there has been enormous interest in the nature and function of active oxygen radicals [2,4,15,16].

Table 1. Consumption of oxygen and release of active oxygen species by leukocytes

Reaction[a]	Active product
(1) $O + 2e + 2H^+ \rightarrow \underline{H_2O}$	
(2) $O_2 + e \rightarrow \underline{O_2^-}$	Superoxide
(3) $O_2 + 2e + 2H^+ \rightarrow \underline{H_2O_2}$	Hydrogen peroxide
(4)[b] $O_2^- + O_2^- + 2H^+ \rightarrow \underline{H_2O_2} + O_2$	Hydrogen peroxide
(5)[b] $O_2^- + H_2O_2 \xrightarrow{metal} \underline{OH^{\cdot}} + OH^- + O_2$	Hydroxyl radical
(6) $2H_2O_2 \xrightarrow{catalase} 2H_2O + O_2$	
(7) $O^-_2 + X_{ox} \rightarrow X_{red} + O_2$	

[a] Reactions 1-3 lead entirely to oxygen consumption; reactions 4-7 each return some molecular oxygen to the system.

[b] May be via singlet oxygen (see Fig. 1).

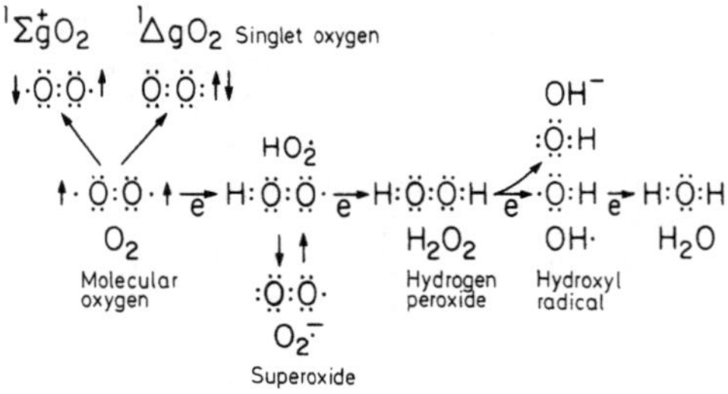

Fig. 1. Reduction and excitation of oxygen. The *vertical arrows* next to singlet oxygen and molecular oxygen indicate the directions of spin of the outer electrons. Adapted from [22]

These substances may be depicted as shown in Table 1 and Fig. 1, where specific reactions are listed. It may be noted that molecular oxygen can be raised to a higher energy level to give two forms of singlet oxygen - the Δ and the Σ forms. Decay to the ground state is accompanied by chemiluminescence, and this has formed the basis of many attempts to follow the responses of phagocytic leukocytes that produce these substances upon stimulation [4,20]. The oxygen atom may be reduced to water, in a conventional way, by a two-electron reduction (Table 1, reaction 1). Upon accepting a single electron, molecular oxygen gives rise to superoxide, which may be in the undissociated form, with a proton, as $HO_2^{\cdot}$, or it may be dissociated as superoxide anion O_2^- (Table 1, reaction 2). Superoxide may be dismutated by the enzyme (or enzymes) superoxide dismutase - among the most interesting and most discussed enzymes of the past decades - to form hydrogen peroxide [15,16] (Table 1, reaction 4). Hydrogen peroxide may originate directly as well (reaction 3). It is split to oxygen and water by a well-known reaction catalyzed by catalase (reaction 6). Peroxide and superoxide together may give rise to a hydroxyl radical, especially under the influence of iron and certain other metals (reviewed in [4] (reaction 5). This substance is considered to be the most potent agent in the cidal functions discussed later [4,16]. Finally, superoxide may reduce other substances (reaction 7) in cells or tissues, or in artificial reaction mixtures, or it may itself be reduced further (example not given, but in reaction 4, one O_2^- oxidizes another; the one may be considered as reducing the other). These reactions are dealt with in more detail in various reviews [2,4,16]. A matter that deserves further comment is the net versus total oxygen consumption of cells producing oxygen radicals. In Table 1, it is shown that oxygen is either consumed by a given (primary) reaction, or partially returned to the system by subsequent (secondary) reactions.

Oxygen radicals are produced by granulocytes when they are stimulated, but only by certain macrophages. In these phagocytic leukocytes, the active oxygen species is released at the outer plasmalemmal surface of the cell, or the inner surface of internalized vesicles (phagosomes) [4,5,9]. Resident peritoneal macrophages do not produce significant superoxide or hydrogen peroxide when they phagocytize or are stimulated in other ways (Table 2). On the other hand, inflammatory macrophages (e.g., from a sterile abscess), or those washed from the peritoneum after infection of the animal with organisms such as BCG or *Listeria monocytogenes*, are able to produce superoxide and other activated oxygen species when stimulated. Furthermore, macrophages "activated" in vitro with a lymphokine also manifest this activity [21,36].

Table 2. Release of superoxide by murine peritoneal phagocytes upon stimulation with PMA[a]

Cells	Treatment	O_2^- release (nmol/min per 10^7 cells)
<u>Granulocytes</u>	Sodium caseinate (6 h)	82.9 ± 10.0 (4)
<u>Macrophages</u>		
Resident	-	1.1 ± 2.0 (3)
Activated	*L. monocytogenes* (5-7 days)	17.7 ± 3.5 (7)
	BCG-PPD	14.1 ± 6.6 (4)
Elicited	Sodium caseinate	33.4 ± 3.6 (5)
	Proteose-peptone	35.0 ± 8.7 (3)
	Thioglycollate	4.1 ± 2.4 (5)

[a] The data are expressed as the mean ± standard deviation. The numbers of cell preparations employed (experiments) are given in parentheses. Each experiment was performed in triplicate. In no case was release of O_2^- detected in unstimulated cells. BCG-PPD refers to cells from animals first infected with Calmette-Guérin bacillus, and then injected intraperitoneally with purified protein derivative (tuberculin) [7]. Courtesy of Allan Liss Incorporated, New York.

Whereas it is well accepted that a key microbicidal process in granulocytes hinges on the availability of peroxide and of myeloperoxidase, an enzyme that constitutes about 5% of the protein of such cells [2,23], the situation is less clear in macrophages, since the availability and role of peroxidase are less evident [8,13,35]. However, it is clear that the history of particular macrophages is an important determinant of their respiratory behavior when they are stimulated. This is also reflected in the behavior of macrophages other than peritoneal, such as alveolar macrophages. There, smoking (exposure to particles and/or irritants) may cause greatly enhanced oxygen consumption upon later stimulation of the cells, accompanied by superoxide production and production of hydrogen peroxide, as seen in Fig. 2 [14]. This "modulation" of macrophage respiratory behavior is of extreme practical (as well as academic) importance as it underlies some aspects of the importance of macrophage function.

Stimuli and Trigger Mechanisms

It is commonly believed now that the system in phagocytic leukocytes that produces superoxide and other oxygen radicals consists of a trigger mechanism as well as the "oxidase" per se (i.e., the actual enzyme proteins responsible for conveying electrons from cytoplasmic reduced pyridine nucleotides to molecular oxygen). Both trigger and oxidase are at the cell membrane, although some contribution from granular membranes has been postulated (reviewed in [4,20]).

Some instigators of the production of superoxide are listed in Table 3. These range from free fatty acids, or detergents (surfactants), which have a general effect on the membrane of the cell, to more specific substances that bind to special receptors, such as phorbol myristate acetate, the activator of protein kinase C, and finally to phagocytizable particles, whose effects may involve immunologic factors. Contact of phagocytic leukocytes with some other cells (e.g., tumor cells) may also elicit a respiratory response [2].

Roles of Polyene Fatty Acids in the Functions of Phagocytic Leukocytes

Certain polyene fatty acids are precursors of prostaglandins (containing a five-carbon ring structure), thromboxanes, and prostacyclins (cyclooxygenase products), and of hydroxypolyenoic fatty acids and leukotrienes (lipoxygenase products). The latter group of compounds includes thioethers of the tripeptide glutathione, relevant derived dipeptides, or even cysteine [17]. All these substances are of interest in the context of this paper; the leukotrienes have multiple effects on polymorphonuclear leukocytes, particularly [17,37]. They and other products of the polyenoic fatty acid, arachidonate, have been reported to be secreted by macrophages (reviewed in [37]). These matters are receiving enormous current attention, but it is a more direct function of polyenoic fatty acids that will be discussed

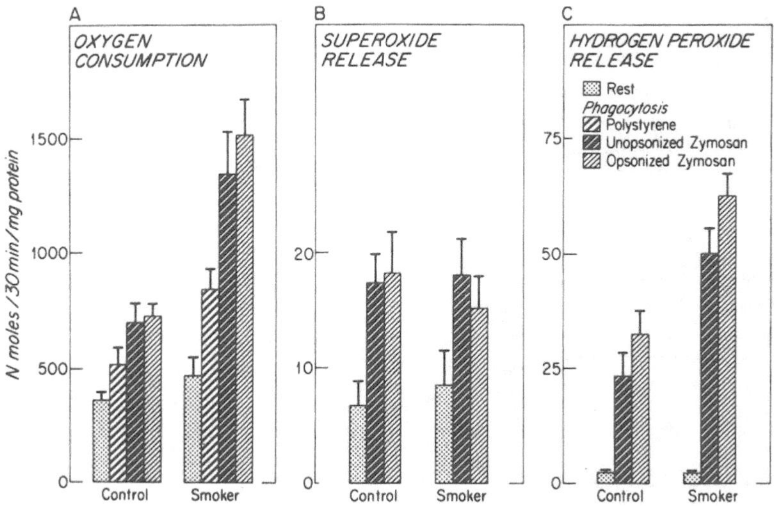

Fig. 2A-C. The effects of tobacco smoke on the respiratory burst of rat alveolar macrophages. The rats were subjected to 30 consecutive days of smoke inhalation. Values for consumption of oxygen and release of superoxide and hydrogen peroxide by cells at rest are shown by *stippled bars;* those for phagocytizing cells are *cross-hatched,* as indicated in panel C. All data are mean ± standard error for a minimum of three experiments, each comprised of multiple replicates [14]

Table 3. Instigators of release of oxygen radicals from phagocytic leukocytes

(1)	*cis*-Polyenoic fatty acids (direct increase of plasmalemma liquid crystalline fraction)
(2)	Detergents and surfactants (disruption of lipid bilayer)
(3)	Phorbol myristate actetate (through receptors and protein kinase C)
(4)	Lectins, antibodies, components of complement system and chemotactic factors (e.g., F-Met-Leu-Phe; some leukotrienes; receptors on cell surface)
(5)	Phagocytosis (aspects of all of the above)

here, that bears on the cidal activities of phagocytic leukocytes and may have physiologic importance.

It has recently been found that *cis*-polyene fatty acids trigger superoxide production by phagocytic leukocytes, whether these be granulocytes or the appropriate macrophages [7,10]. This is illustrated in Fig. 3. There are two schools of thought about the role of fatty acids in this regard. Some believe that the effect is purely physical, brought on by dissolution of the fatty acids in the plasmalemma lipid phase. This may lead to a modification of the properties of the lipid bilayer such that crucial membrane proteins (a cytochrome reductase; an autooxidizable cytochrome *b* [4,20]) might interact more easily. The idea is backed up by a demonstration that the phenomenon can be turned off by removing the fatty acid with delipidated albumin [7]. Further, the

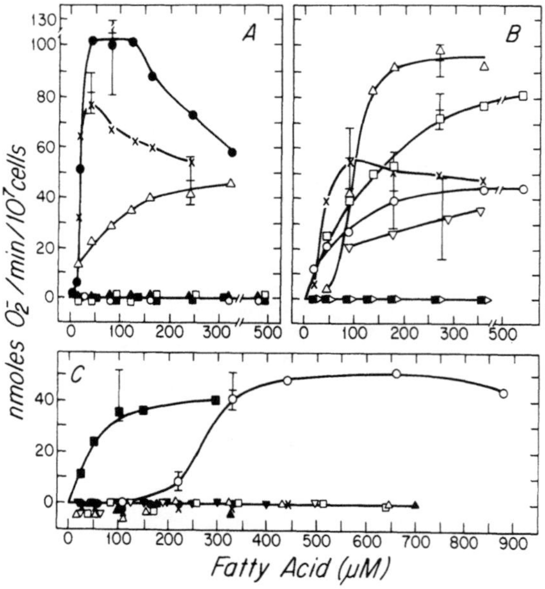

Fig. 3A-C. Ability of different concentrations of various fatty acids to stimulate superoxide release by human neutrophils. Superoxide release from human neutrophils was monitored after stimulation of the cells (1.5×10^6/ ml) with different concentrations of fatty acids. (A) 20-carbon fatty acids: arachidonate (*full circles*); 8,11,14-all-*cis*-eicosatrienoate (*crosses*); 11-*cis*-14-*cis*-eicosadienoate (*open triangles*); *trans*-11-*trans*-14-eicosadienoate (*full triangles*); 8-*cis*-eicosaenoate (*open circles*); 11-*cis*-eicosaenoate (*open squares*); and 13-*cis*-eicosaenoate (*full squares*), (B) 18-carbon fatty acids: 6,9,12-all-*cis*-octadecatrienoate (*upward triangles*); 9,12,15-all-*cis*-octadecatrienoate (*crosses*); *trans*-9-*trans*-12-octadecadienoate (*downward triangles*); 6-*cis*-octadecenoate (*open squares*); *trans*-6-octadecenoate (*full squares*); *cis*-11-octadecenoate (*circles*); and *cis*-9-octadecenoate (*sideways triangles*), (C) fatty acids of < 16 carbon atoms: *cis*-9-hexadecenoate (*full squares*); *cis*-9-tetradecenoate (*open circles*); *trans*-9-tetradecenoate (*full circles*); 11-dodecenoate (*open squares*); hexadecenoate (*full downward triangles*); tetradecenoate (*crosses*); dodecanoate (*open downward triangles*); *n*-hexanoate (*full upward triangles*); and *n*-octanoate (*open upward triangles*). The mean response ± standard deviation at an optimum concentration for each fatty acid is indicated by *error bars* [4]

use of a fluorescent probe has allowed determination of an increase of the fraction of the lipid bilayer that is liquid crystalline rather than gel-like, and this correlates with the increased production of oxygen radicals. There is excellent correlation of O_2^- release with the melting point of the fatty acid used - the lower this is, the greater the maximal stimulation of cellular O_2^- release [7]. It has been shown, by the use of *cis*-polyenoic fatty acids that do *not* give rise to prostaglandins, thromboxanes, lipoxygenase products, etc., that the effect does not depend upon production of such substances, as well as by the fact that preformed oxidation products of arachidonate are not active [7]. That the phenomenon can be directly related to the binding characteristics of the fatty acid is shown in Fig. 4.

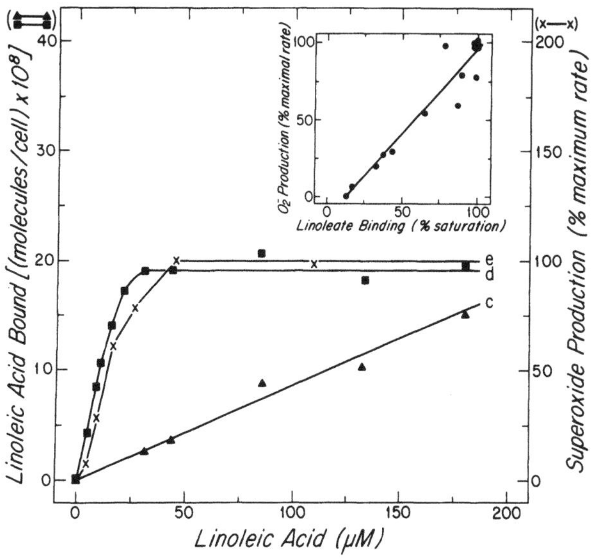

Fig. 4. Binding of linoleate to human neutrophils and stimulation of superoxide release. The binding curves for saturated fatty acids were linear and similar to the line labeled (*c*). Binding curves of *cis*-polyene fatty acids exhibited two components: the linear component mentioned, and a rapid saturable component labeled (*d*). These curves relate to the ordinate on the left, and were obtained by subtracting the linear component (*c*) from an overall binding curve (*c* + *d*). Curve (*e*) reflects the release of superoxide as a function of fatty acid concentration, and clearly is virtually superimposable on the rapid saturable component for the binding of polyene fatty acids, i.e., curve (*d*). The *inset* illustrates the correlation between the rate of O_2^- released (expressed as percentage of maximal rate) and the percentage of maximal binding to the saturable component [4]

Other workers have averred that the *cis*-polyenoic fatty acids are potentially a "second" messenger" [10,28] in the activation of a calcium dependent protein kinase of human neutrophils, which, in turn, is responsible for stimulation of the respiratory phenomenon. It would, in this author's opinion, not be difficult to reconcile the two views. That protein kinase C is involved in the phenomenon under scrutiny here is suggested by several lines of evidence, including the observation that those fatty acids that stimulate O_2^- production also directly stimulate the kinase [28]. Even more cogent, the same list of phorbol derivatives that stimulate that enzyme, stimulate O_2^- release from leukocytes [30].

Calmodulin also plays a significant role in "turning on" oxygen radical production by granulocytes and, presumably, macrophages as well [18,19]. This has been demonstrated with such calmodulin inhibitors as phenothiazine, and, in particular with trifluoperazine. Active inhibitors could be controlled by checking inactive analogs closely resembling them in structure, as illustrated in Table 4.

Table 4. Effects of calmodulin inhibitors, and inactive analogs on O_2^- release by neutrophils[a]

Additions (m*M*)	Activity (%)
None (control)	100
Trifluoperazine[b]	6.8 ± 7.6
Trifluoperazine sulfoxide	99.7 ± 0.6
Chlorpromazine	53.9 ± 7.3
Promethazine	107.8 ± 11.5
W_7 (5-chloro-W_5) (0.05)	3.6 ± 3.0
W_5 (0.05)[c]	102.2 ± 3.8

[a] Neutrophils were incubated in the standard assay mixture for 3 min with the compounds listed prior to stimulation with arachidonate (82 μ*M*). Data are expressed as the mean ± standard deviation for 3-12 different preparations of cells; 100% activity is that observed in the absence of drugs. None of the drugs utilized affected cell viability under the conditions employed, or inhibited O^-_2 production in an O_2^- generating system (i.e., xanthine oxidase plus purine).

[b] All at 0.01 m*M*, except W_5 and W_7 at 0.05 m*M*.

[c] W_5 = *N*-(6-aminohexyl)-1-naphthalenesulfonamide.

Relevance of Ability to Produce Oxygen Radicals to the Activation Process in Macrophages, and Their Cidal Power

The role of activation of macrophages in combating microbial and tumor cells as well as parasites has been viewed as hinging significantly on the ability of these cells to produce oxygen radicals [4,29,36,39]. As stated earlier, the key radical, in terms of lethality toward targets, is rather generally considered to be the hydroxyl radical, OH· [4]. Definition of an "activated" macrophage in terms of its biochemical capabilities has been attempted on several occasions (e.g., [21,36]). One of the most noteworthy "pointers" of activation of macrophages has been held to be the ability to produce active oxygen species upon stimulation. Thus, macrophages activated via a lymphokine are indeed cytocidal and, particularly, tumoricidal [4,36,39]. On the other hand, elicited, i.e., inflammatory macrophages, which are superior in their ability to produce superoxide [6], are inferior to activated macrophages in their cytocidal powers [4,29,39]. Thus, there must be an involvement of factors other than oxygen radicals per se. This matter constitutes an interesting puzzle that has recently been examined by measuring the appropriate enzyme kinetics in a number of differently treated mouse macrophages. It was not the amount of enzyme activity (reduced pyridine nucleotide oxidase) that was responsible for the spectrum of abilities to produce oxygen radicals (i.e., V_{max}), but rather K_m, or the affinity of the enzyme for the NAD(P)H [39]. Whether the entire answer to the riddle of what constitutes "activation" of macrophages will emerge from such studies, or whether more complex immunologic factors are involved, remains to be explored.

Active Oxygen Radicals in the Function of Lymphocytes

The only noteworthy case of the involvement of oxygen radicals in lymphocyte function occurs in the case of the cytolytic activity of NK cells. It was shown that these cells respond to the presence of appropriate target cells with increased chemiluminescence and an increased superoxide-sensitive reduction of cytochrome *c* [33]. This was true only for target cells that were actually susceptible to the NK cells. Furthermore, antibodies to the effector cells, fixation with glutaraldehyde, or the presence of superoxide dismutase in the system eliminated all three functional activities mentioned, while α and β interferons enhanced these properties modestly. Catalase had no effect, raising questions as to whether the hydroxyl radical, which results from interaction of peroxide and superoxide, is indeed the key factor here (see Table 1, reaction 5). A further development in this context [34] is a recent observation that these "large granular lymphocytes" produce interleukin-1, characteristic of macrophages, as well as interleukin-2 and α and γ interferons, characteristic of T lymphocytes. The earlier very fascinating report stimulated an article that asks the question of whether the NK cell is "a phagocyte in lymphocyte's clothing" [3], that has even more force now.

Danger of Oxygen Radicals to the Host

Since stimulation of granulocytes to produce superoxide, etc., in the presence of bacteria has been shown to cause genetic change in the latter (reviewed in [4,16]), and since the idea has been advanced that release of oxygen radicals may, for example, affect endothelial cells adversely [4,16], it is clear that some thought must be given to effects of the phenomena on the host itself. Increasing information is accumulating on this aspect of the oxygen radical as a double-edged sword [16].

Role of Bacterial Cell Wall Monomers in Stimulation of Phagocytic White Blood Cells and in Protection of the Intact Organism

Muramyl peptide monomers have been determined to be capable of replacing whole mycobacteria in Freund's complete adjuvant [1, 27]. They have been shown, using pure synthetic compounds, to be important immunostimulants, i.e., to be responsible for increased antibody production when administered with antigen. They have also been demonstrated to be pyrogenic, in the main, and in some cases to have a direct influence on macrophages [1,12, 27,37]. It has been shown that macrophages, for example, exposed to muramyl dipeptides exhibit increased oxygen radical production after a short time in culture [32]. Thus, there is clear evidence that these bacterial components have important host-protective properties.

Recently, it has been noted that they may also be somnogenic; that is, they increase the proportion of time spent in slow-wave sleep, and the depth of the latter, in rabbits, cats, and rats [24,26]. A long list of synthetic and natural compounds has been examined and the compounds compared for their somnogenicity, immunoadjuvanticity, and pyrogenicity. The degree of overlap of these functions was greater than 90% [26]. Examination of tissues from normal rats has demonstrated that muramic acid, presumably as a muramyl peptide, is normally present in liver, kidney and brain [41]. Muramyl components have been shown to be released by macrophages "fed" with labeled bacterial cell walls [40]. There is little doubt that mammalian tissues cannot synthesize muramic acid, to judge from the weight of opinion and the author's exhaustive efforts to test the matter. They should therefore be considered as essential exogenous substances that contribute to physiologic control processes, in mammals at least.

In studying the effects of muramyl peptides already mentioned, one must include the question of their mode of contact with cells. There are indeed specific binding sites for such compounds on murine macrophages, as indicated in Table 5, contrary to earlier reports that were based on inadequate levels of radioactivity [38]. Within the limits of the number of compounds so far examined, there is complete correlation between somnogenicity and binding to macrophages in this test.

Table 5. MDP binding sites of murine macrophages[a]

Macrophages	Class of binding sites	
	Minor K_d (p*M*)	Major K_d (μ*M*)
Resident	~ 50	
Elicited	~ 300	3.5
Activated	~ 500	
Sites per cell	200-500	~ 2×10^6

[a]MDP is *N*-acetyl-*D*-muramyl-*L*-alanyl-*D*-isoglutamine. The labeled ligands used were iodinated MDP-*L*-tyrosine methyl ester or iodinated *N*-*p*-hydroxyphenylpropionyl-MDP-*L*-lysine. (The K_d values cited were obtained with the former. Those for the latter are 3-5 times higher.) For binding to occur, the alanine linked to muramyl must be *L*- and the isoglutamine must be *D*-. Peptides longer than MDP exhibit enhanced binding. An additional amide group (e.g., on diaminopimelic acid of longer muramyl peptides) is not tolerated.

In reaching the conclusion of this paper, the following facts should be added: (a) muramyl peptides induce release of interleukin -1 (or endogenous pyrogen) by macrophages (reviewed in [1, 11,31]); (b) a monoclonal antibody to muramyl dipeptide linked to a polypeptide cross-reacts with interleukin-1 [11], as well as with the sleep-promoting factor (a muramyl peptide); (c) interleukin-1 itself induces slow-wave sleep [25]. These observations stimulate one to consider the possibility that over evolutionary time, immunoadjuvanticity, pyrogenicity, and somnogenicity were linked in a positive mechanism against bacterial infection, and that the phenomenon of slow-wave sleep might be viewed as closely allied to immune and antibacterial mechanisms in protecting higher organisms.

Acknowledgments. The author acknowledges with gratitude the contributions of all his colleagues, listed in work from this laboratory and cited in the Bibliography. He especially acknowledges D. Silverman's prosecution of the unpublished studies of macrophage binding sites for muramyl peptides. The original work in this paper was supported by Grant AI-03260 from the United States Public Health Service, N.I.H.

References

1. Adam A, Lederer E (1984) Muramyl peptides: Immunomodulators, sleep factors and vitamins. Med Res Rev 4:111-152
2. Babior BM, Crowley CA (1983) Chronic granulomatous disease and other disorders of oxidative killing. In: Stanbury JB, Wyngaarden JB, Fredrickson DS, Goldstein JL, Brown MS (eds) Metabolic basis of inherited disease. McGraw-Hill, New York, pp 1956-1985
3. Babior BM, Parkinson DW (1982) The NK cell: a phagocyte in lymphocyte's clothing. Nature 298:511
4. Badwey JA, Karnovsky ML (1980) Active oxygen species and the functions of phagocytic leukocytes. Annu Rev Biochem 49:695-726
5. Badwey JA, Curnutte JT, Robinson JM, Lazdins JK, Briggs RT, Karnovsky MJ, Karnovsky ML (1980) Comparative aspects of oxidative metabolism of neutrophils from human blood and guinea pig peritoneum: magnitude of the respiratory burst. Dependence upon stimulating agents and localization of the oxidases. J Cell Physiol 105:541-551
6. Badwey JA, Robinson JM, Lazdins JK, Briggs RT, Karnovsky MJ, Karnovsky ML (1983) Comparative biochemical and cytochemical studies on superoxide and peroxide in mouse macrophages. J Cell Physiol 115:208-216
7. Badwey JA, Curnutte JT, Robinson JM, Berde CB, Karnovsky MJ, Karnovsky ML (1984) Effects of free fatty acids on release of superoxide and on change of shape by human neutrophils: reversibility by albumin. J Biol Chem 259:7870-7877
8. Bainton DF (1980) Changes in peroxidase distribution within organelles of blood monocytes and peritoneal macrophages after surface adherence *in vitro* and *in vivo*. In: van Furth R (ed) Mononuclear phagocytes: Functional aspects. Martinus Nijhoff, The Hague, pp 61-86
9. Briggs RT, Drath DB, Karnovsky ML, Karnovsky MJ (1975) Localization of NADH oxidase on the surface of human polymorphonuclear leukocytes by a new cytochemical method. J Cell Biol 67:566-586
10. Bromberg Y, Pick E (1983) Unsaturated fatty acids as second messengers of superoxide generation by macrophages. Cell Immunol 79:240-252
11. Chedid L, Bahr GM, Modabber FZ, Dinarello CA, Wolff SM (1983) Mise in evidence d'une structure bacterienne dans deux mediateurs humains; un facteur favorisant le sommeil et une monokine. CR Acad Sci Paris 297: 209-212
12. Cummings NP, Pabst MJ, Johnston RB (1980) Activation of macrophages for enhanced release of superoxide anion and greater killing of *Candida albicans* by injection of muramyl peptide. J Exp Med 152:1659-1669

13. Daems WTh, van der Rhee HJ (1980) Peroxidase and catalase in monocytes, macrophages, epithelioid cells and giant cells of the rat. In: van Furth R (ed) Mononuclear phagocytes: Functional aspects. Martinus Nijhoff, The Hague, pp 43-60
14. Drath DB, Harper A, Gharibian J, Karnovsky ML, Huber GL (1978) The effect of tobacco smoke on the metabolism and function cf rat alveolar macrophages. J Cell Physiol 95:105-113
15. Fridovich I (1975) Superoxide dismutases. Annu Rev Biochem 44:147-159
16. Fridovich I (1983) Superoxide radical: An endogenous toxicant. Annu Rev Pharmacol Toxicol 23:239-257
17. Hammarstrom S (1983) Leukotrienes. Annu Rev Biochem 52:355-377
18. Jones HP, Gai G, Petrone WF, McCord JM (1982) Colmodulin dependent stimulation of the NADPH oxidase of human neutrophils. Biochim Biophys Acta 714:152-156
19. Kakuichi S, Sobue K (1983) Control of the cytoskeleton by calmodulin and calmodulin-binding proteins. TIBS 8:59-62
20. Karnovsky ML, Badwey JA (1983) Determinants of the production of active oxygen species by granulocytes and macrophages. J Clin Chem Clin Biochem 21:545-553
21. Karnovsky ML, Lazdins JK (1978) Biochemical criteria for activated macrophages. J Immunol 121:809-813
22. Klebanoff SJ (1980) In: van Furth R (ed) Mononuclear phagocytes: Functional aspects. Martinus Nijhoff, The Hague, p 1105
23. Klebanoff SJ, Clark RA (1978) The neutrophil: Function and clinical disorders. North Holland, Amsterdam
24. Krueger JM, Pappenheimer JR, Karnovsky ML (1982) The composition of sleep-promoting factor isolated from human urine. J Biol Chem 257:1664-1669
25. Krueger JM, Walter J, Dinarello CA, Wolff SM, Chedid L (1984a) Am J Physiol 246:R994-999
26. Krueger JM, Walter J, Karnovsky ML, Chedid L, Choay JP, Lefrancier P, Lederer E (1984b) Muramyl peptides. Variation of somnogenic activity with structure. J Exp Med 159:68-76
27. Lederer E (1982) Immunomodulation by muramyl peptides: Recent developments. Clin Immunol Newsletter 3:83-86
28. McPhail LC, Clayton CC, Snyderman R (1984) A potential second messenger role for unsaturated fatty acids: Activation of Ca^{2+}-dependent protein kinase. Science 224:622-625
29. Nathan CF (1982) Secretion of oxygen intermediates: Role in effector functions of activated macrophages. FASEB 41:2206-2211
30. Nishizuka Y (1984) The role of protein kinase C in cell surface signal transduction and tumour promotion. Nature 308:693-698
31. Oppenheim JJ, Togawa A, Chedid L, Mizel S (1980) Components of mycobacteria and muramyl dipeptide with adjuvant activity induce lymphocyte activating factor. Cell Immunol 50:71-81
32. Pabst MJ, Johnston RB Jr (1980) Increased production of superoxide anion by macrophages exposed in vitro to muramyl dipeptide or lipopolysaccharide. J Exp Med 151:101-114
33. Roder JC, Helfand SL, Werkmeister J, McGarry R, Beaumont TJ, Duwe A (1982) Oxygen intermediates are triggered early in the pathway of human NK cells. Nature 298:569-572
34. Scala G, Allavena P, Djeu JY, Kasahara T, Ortaldo JR, Herberman RB, Oppenheim JJ (1984) Human large granular lymphocytes are potent producers of interleukin-1. Nature 309:56-59
35. Simmons SR, Karnovsky ML (1973) Iodinating ability of various leukocytes and their bactericidal activity. J Exp Med 138:44-63

36. Soberman RJ, Karnovsky ML (1981) Biochemical properties of activated macrophages. In: Pick E (ed) Lymphokines. Academic, New York, pp 11-13
37. Takemura R, Werb Z (1984) Secretory products of macrophages and their physiological functions. Am J Physiol 246(Cell Physiol 15):C1-C9
38. Tenu J-P, Roche A-C, Yapo A, Kieda A, Monsigny M, Petit J-F (1982) Absence of cell surface receptors for muramyl peptides in mouse peritoneal macrophages. Biol Cell 44:157-164
39. Tsunawaki S, Nathan CF (1984) Enzymatic basis of macrophage activation: Kinetic analysis of superoxide production in lysates of resident and activated mouse peritoneal macrophages and granulocytes. J Biol Chem 259: 4305-4312
40. Vermeulen MW, Gray GR (1983) Glycopeptides released by macrophages after ingestion of bacterial cell walls. Fed Proc 42:1221
41. Zhai Sen, Karnovsky ML (1984) Qualitative detection of muramic acid in normal mammalian tissues. Infect Immunity 43:937-941

Discussion

(pp. 351-363)

In response to questions from *Blake*, bearing on localization of release of oxygen radicals, *Karnovsky* stated that such radicals really are located on the outside of the macrophage plasmalemma, this view being reinforced by experiments using a nonpenetrating inhibitor that blocks H_2O_2 formation and release. Even when using phorbol myristate acetate as a stimulus, if some oxygen radicals enter the cytosol, the number must be below the level of cytochemical detection. No definite answer can be offered on the degree of dissociability of oxygen radical release and breakdown of intracellular granules; the research groups led by *Weissman*, *Babior*, and others have reported some experiments indicating that degranulation and release of oxygen radicals are not absolutely linked.

In commenting on queries from *McGhee* concerning muramyl peptides, *Karnovsky* indicated that breakdown of gut bacteria may, of course, be one means whereby muramyl peptides are absorbed, enter the body, and turn up in mammalian tissues. An important experiment to be done in the future will utilize germ-free animals on a synthetic diet. *Adam* and *Lederer* make many matters clear in their recent overview of muramyl peptides (*Med Res Rev* 4:111-15, 1984) concerning these substances, produced by bacteria. With respect to the cross-reactivity between the anti-muramyl dipeptide monoclonal antibody and interleukin-1 (Il-1), and whether the antibody conceivably is targeted against an epitope associated with a cell surface receptor for Il-1, *Karnovsky* summed up experiments only just completed indicating high affinity saturable binding characteristics of the system. Planned experiments using *Chedid's* monoclonal antibody and Il-1 prepared by *Dinarello* should clarify the situation.

Joiner referred to a recent paper by *Snyderman's* group and inquired whether the arachidonic acid findings might be mediated via the protein kinase C system. *Karnovsky* commented that he was aware of the paper mentioned and noted that the paper by *Pick* of Israel dealing with macrophages, published a couple of years ago, also is supportive of the notion. Both investigative groups believe that polyenoic fatty acids could be a "potential" second messenger. He emphasized that these groups used concentrations of arachidonic acids which were four or five times higher than those mentioned in his presentation at this Symposium. Returning to the subject of O_2^- release, *Karnovsky* related some interesting experiments his group has conducted using *cis*- and *trans*-parinaric acids to determine "fluidity" of membranes, i.e., the proportion that is liquid crystalline versus the proportion that is gel-like. The results of this work are consistent with O_2^- release reflecting "fluidity" of the membrane.

The focus of thinking shifted back to metabolic triggering mechanisms with a question from *Quie*, pertaining to chronic granulomatous disease (CGD). *Karnovsky* expressed the view that CGD is, in all probability, not a single entity representing a solitary error in the oxidase system. For example, *Segal*, *Owen-Jones*, *Borregard*, and others have shown that there may be an abnormality of the special cytochrome *b* in some patients and a problem with the enzyme that reduces the cytochrome *b* in other patients. And what about other sites where the triggering event may be defective? For example, a higher gel-like bilayer lipid content, that prevents the initial signal acting as an effective trigger for releasing peroxide and superoxide, is possible.

Final questions, from *Morrison* and *Sparling*, respectively, related to mechanisms explaining how added albumin leads to shutoff of response to polyenoic fatty acids and to a potential role of iron in intracellular killing via the Haber-Weiss reaction. *Karnovsky* emphasized the very low affinity binding or dissolution of the fatty acids within the cell membrane lipid bilayer. Thus, albumin can readily pull them out. By way of clarifying the situation, he indicated that if one compares binding to cells of palmitic acid, inactive with respect to induction of O_2^- release, vis-à-vis binding of linoleate, which is an active stimulus, the *cis*-polyene starts off with a very rapid uptake component and then follows a linear, nonsaturable binding curve. In contrast, the palmitic acid pattern exhibits a linear, nonsaturable binding component right from the first. It turns out that the linear rate of palmitate uptake parallels the linear component of linoleate binding. If one subtracts the nonsaturable linear rate from the total binding of *cis*-polyenoic fatty acid, one gets the rapid saturable component. When the rapid saturable binding component is plotted as a percentage of maximum uptake, and the O_2^- release is plotted as a percentage of maximal release (both on the ordinate) against fatty acid concentration on the abscissa, the two curves are found to superimpose without any difficulty at all.

With respect to the iron and Haber-Weiss reaction question, *Karnovsky* said that, even though it is a very complicated reaction, a wild guess seemed appropriate in view of the type of company he was enjoying during the Symposium. If the "killer oxygen" radical is a hydroxyl radical and it follows the Haber-Weiss reaction, as modified by *McCord* and *Fridovich*, iron could be an essential component indeed. Changes in availability of iron might translate to changes in the manner killing took place, remembering that the cell has different killing mechanisms and that, even under optimal conditions, hydroxyl radical production is two orders of magnitude lower than superoxide release.

Concluding Remarks to Sessions 1–4

Closing Remarks of the Schloss Gracht Conference

Z. A. McGee

Most of us were drawn here by either a direct or indirect interest in pathogenic mechanisms of infection. Our interests probably derive from very different sources. As scientists we are interested in pathogenic mechanisms because we like to experience that most noble of all pleasures, the joy of understanding. As individuals concerned with the health of other humans, we also want to develop new approaches to the prevention and treatment of infectious diseases.

Unfortunately (to use the language of conflict management) we have adopted a very confrontational stance with regard to pathogenic microorganisms. They cause disease and we aim antibiotics at them to try to kill them. We are polluting the environment with antibiotics, and we give the organisms no alternative but to evolve mechanisms of resistance. We are, in other words, forcing evolution. I have great concerns about this. It is not simply that the microorganisms are evolving more resistance to antibiotics. Rather, my major concern is that they are evolving more effective means of genetic change. It is quite possible that the genetic changes will result not only in resistance to a greater number of antibiotics but also in the more ready acquisition of virulence factors which can make the organisms a greater threat to life. The virulence factors that can be acquired as extrachromosomal DNA range from diphteria toxin to pili that aid attachment of bacteria to mucosal surfaces.

It seems to me that in dealing with pathogenic bacteria we ideally want to avoid confrontation and avoid forcing evolutionary change. Instead, we should seek to fully understand the various steps in the pathogenic process the microorganisms induce and seek immunologic or other means to block critical, preferably early steps in that process. In other words, we should not try to destroy bacteria, but to alter their behavior, to change them from pathogens to commensals. To make this possible we are seeking during the course of this meeting to define and focus on the various steps in microbial pathogenic processes and the molecular mechanisms by which these steps are mediated.

It is clear that attachment is an early step in the pathogenic process and that it is important in disease caused by many pathogens. Pili and other surface factors are important to that initial pathogen-host cell interaction. The sort of strategy that Dr. Schoolnik is pursuing in mapping the pilin subunits of gonococci is being brought to maturity as we test the function not only of the pilin subunits but also various subunit fragments of known amino acid sequences. In order to design an optimally effective vaccine, we are testing in collaboration with Dr. Schoolnik the pilin subunit fragments to determine whether they are accessible to antibody when they are in native pili on viable gonococci.

On the one hand I am very impressed with the logic and systematic nature of Dr. Schoolnik's approach and the approach being taken in a similar manner with gonococci and other bacteria by other investigators. On the other hand I know that we are dealing in many cases with obligate human pathogens which have for eons successfully avoided our immunologic attempts at ridding ourselves of them. It is unlikely that these organisms could have so successfully eluded our immune systems and still have common antigens that are important in the pathologic process and are readily accessible to antibodies. The organisms may avoid host immunity by having a large array of antigens which differ from strain to strain. In addition, a number of bacteria have apparently evolved the capacity to change the antigens they display to the host from time to time. This may serve the purpose of an immunologic disguise. Alternatively, some organisms may have to change their surface factors in order to successfully move from one step in the pathogenic process to another, getting rid of those factors that impede them as they move to the next step.

In order to develop a strategy for interrupting the attachment of bacteria to host cells, a process mediated by the interaction of ligands on bacteria with receptors on host cells, it is important to identify the receptors as well as the ligands. For instance, the receptors for gonococcal pili appear to have a very restricted distribution in the animal kingdom. Gonococci do not attach to the genital epithelium of any animals except humans and chimpanzees. Unless we believe in the vengeful god theory of the presence of receptors for gonococci in humans, we must ask what those receptors are doing in human genital epithelium. Do the receptors perform a normal function which has been subjugated by gonococci in a form of successful biologic mimicry? What does the body think it is seeing when it is seeing a gonococcus? These questions are especially important to answer before any attempts are made to block attachment by the use of decoy ligand molecules or by directing antibodies toward the receptor. If the receptor is critical to a normal function, such strategies could result in harm to the host.

Through carefully performed genetic manipulations of bacteria coupled with the study of the interaction of the altered bacteria in animals or intact human mucosa in organ culture, we have begun to determine some of the bacterial surface factors and other factors which play a critical role in the disease processes caused by gonococci, meningococci, and *H. influenzae*. For instance, we have heard during the meeting about studies of this sort that have been carried out with gonococcal strains genetically altered so that they are deficient in IgA protease and also strains of *H. influenzae* that have had structural lesions made in their lipopolysaccharide (LPS). As Dr. Braun mentioned, approaches such as there are going to be very powerful tools in determining the role in pathogenesis of certain microbial molecules.

One cannot help but be impressed with the various roles we have heard about for LPS in the disease process. LPS molecules induce toxic damage to human fallopian tube mucosa in the absence of complement. They may also serve as the target of bacteriolytic antibodies or of antibodies that block the serum bactericidal reaction. They also serve as an immunoregulator and, I suspect, they may well have other functions. The fact that both lipopolysaccharide and peptidoglycan molecules are immunoregulators and both damage human fallopian tube mucosa suggests the possible involvement of secondary messenger molecules in the damage they induce.

The "invasion" step, transgression of the mucosal barriers by micro-organisms, is also an important part of the pathogenic process. The intriguing findings of Dr. Blake - the translocation of protein 1 (the porin protein) from the membranes of gonococci into the membranes of mammalian cells - have generated the provocative hypothesis that porin protein translocation may, in analogy to the action of porin-like Fc receptors in macrophages, result in internalization of bacteria or possibly in tissue damage. Dr. Moxon mentioned a caveat with regard to thinking that the process by which micro-organisms pass across the epithelial barrier occurs rapidly and without residual bacteria in the cells. His point is well taken. If one goes back into the literature on the pathology of gonococcal infections, it is quite clear that the pathologists around the turn of the century who examined a great deal of gonococcal-infected mucosa were completely convinced that the microorganisms spent prolonged periods (up to years) harbored in the genital epithelium. In the words of one pathologist of that day, the gonococci, "once firmly established in these spots [the epithelium] are like the garrison of a bomb-proof fort, which in spite of a fierce attack from all sides, can go on quietly existing, ready to sally forth whenever a suitable occasion arrives." The possibility that microorganisms reside for varying periods within mucosal cells has some other circumstantial evidence to back it up. We frequently see people successfully treated with ampicillin for *H. influenzae* infections who are still carriers of *H. influenzae* in the oropharynx. This may be because ampicillin does not enter epithelial cells well. Eradication of those *H. influenzae* is most successfully carried out with rifampin, an antimicrobial that does enter cells well. Clearly, we need to know more about molecular mechanisms of transgression of mucosal barriers by pathogenic bacteria and the possible persistence of bacteria in mucosal cells.

Although we glibly talk about targeting immune reactions to mucosal surfaces, I think it is fairly clear that we are only beginning to learn about the mucosal immune system and how we can manipulate it to help achieve our goals. I was delighted that Dr. Jerry McGhee took the opportunity to talk about the trafficking of immune cells. We have discussed how we might be able to induce immune reactions at one mucosal surface that result in protective immunity of another mucosal surface to which it is less easy to deliver antigens. It is possible that the microbial molecules that result in transport of bacteria across cells of the epithelial barrier will prove useful in more effectively delivering antigens to the cells that process them as one of the first steps in the immune reaction. We must, if we are to elicit optimally protective mucosal immunity, learn how to deliver antigens in a form which will produce immune reactions that will be more long lasting and will be comprised of antibodies of high affinity.

There are many problems; there are many opportunities. To paraphrase Dr. Tony Allison, most scientists, in whatever age they live, think that theirs is the most exciting of times. The events of this meeting have convinced me that this is the most exciting of times. It has been a delight to have you, the participants in this conference, share ideas with each other and with me. I want to thank Dr. Jackson for his vision in constructing a meeting of this type, one in which people in different disciplines can hear what each other are thinking and can use the various tools and strategies to move all of us forward. I would also like to thank Dr. Thomas and his staff who have made the meeting both an intellectual treat and a personal pleasure.

Statement

W. Opferkuch

The intention of Session 2 was to learn more about what enables microbes to circumvent defense mechanisms, thus gaining an advantage in the invasion of the host. It is necessary to learn more about these mechanisms in order to develop new strategies for treatment. The mechanisms known or proposed are listed in Table 1. They can be divided into two groups. One group concerns the inability of the host to react against the challenge of an invading microbe. The second group are the microbial factors which paralyze host defense mechanisms.

Table 1. Avoidance of host defense mechanisms

A. Inability of host defense

1. No recognition of the invader
2. Defense not yet developed
3. Genetically determined deficiency
4. Immunosuppression

B. Microbial factors

1. Antigenic variation
2. Disturbance of antibody formation
3. Serum resistance
4. Resistance to phagocytosis
5. Resistance to T cell-dependent defense mechanisms

The inability of the host can be either because it is not able to recognize the invader, or because it has not yet developed a defense system, as can be observed in children. Genetically determined deficiency can be divided into deficiency of the complement system, immunoglobulins, phagocytic cells, and T cell-dependent deficiency. It is very important to learn more about the defense mechanisms and the mechanisms by which bacteria invade the host from these experiments of nature. Immunosuppression can be caused by drugs and also by microbial products or infections.

Let us focus now on the second group, the microbial factors. The first mechanism is antigenic variation, a mechanism known from influenza virus or streptococcal infections. Some microbes such as *Borrelia recurrentis*, are able to vary their antigens within a single infected host. Antigenic variation is also suggested with respect to pili.

The second mechanism concerns the disturbance of antibody function. This can be caused by the induction of ineffective antibodies, as known from *Mycobacteria* or *Treponema pallidum* infections. Other microbes neutralize antibodies while releasing circulating antigens. Some microbes do not elicit antibody formation at all.

Third, serum resistance is an important virulent factor of gram-negative bacteria, although the molecular changes in bacteria which lead to serum resistance are still not clear. Three possibilities are under discussion. The first concerns the lipopolysaccharides, the second the capsule, and the third the traT protein. These different mechanisms and others we do not know can react by blocking either the alternative pathway or the classical pathway, either at the C3 level or the C5-9 level.

A fourth very important mechanism to circumvent the host defense consists of avoiding phagocytosis. There are different possibilities which have been mentioned during this Symposium: proteolytic enzymes which are able specifically to degrade immunoglobulins, or complement components. Non-opsonin-mediated phagocytosis, due to bacterial adherence has not yet been sufficiently studied. C3 binding is a more complex reaction than has hitherto been thought. It is known now that activation of C3 does not necessarily lead to binding to the cell surface and that it can also bind nonfunctionally.

The last category of resistance is the resistance to T cell-dependent mechanisms. Whether molecular mimicry is important remains unclear. Another mechanism is the induction of antigen-specific immune suppression either at the T cell level or with suppressor macrophages. Lately, in connection with AIDS, the eradication of helper cells has come under discussion. Humoral factors, like certain prostaglandins which can impair T cell-dependent defense mechanisms, should also be considered. Finally, hiding from immune response by entering a certain cell population, for instance macrophages, must also be mentioned as a possible mechanism.

Following this rather systematic outline of the possible mechanisms, we shall now turn to a discussion of those areas where our knowledge is still limited. Looking through the literature, one can find many reports about phagocytosis, opsonization, and serum resistance, although there are many questions still open in these fields. Both mechanisms are surely important for defense in the preimmune phase, but little is known about other possibilities for microbes to circumvent host defense mechanisms. There is a big gap in our understanding, especially with respect to cellular immune defense mechanisms or at the cellular level of host defenses. We know something about the stimulation of lymphocytes by LPS or peptidoglycan, but we know little about whether bacterial products or their surface components increase or decrease suppressor T cells, reduce helper cells, or lead to release of lymphokines. In addition, our knowledge is restricted as to how bacteria influence the character of immune response. Moreover, questions of local immunity or chronic infectious diseases still remain to be solved.

Perspectives

V. Braun

The papers in Session 3 were examples of the very successful application of sophisticated genetic and biochemical methods to problems regarding mechanisms of microbial pathogenicity. Genetics permits one to dissect the multifactorial cause of disease into single events and to put them together again.

By this means it is possible to resolve complex problems into single factors and to study their individual contributions separately and in various combinations. Cloning techniques, interspecies shuttle vectors, and expression vectors are most useful. However, one has to be aware of the possibility that the total may be more than the sum of the individual factors. Mixed infections are exceedingly complex. Research should be concentrated on a single well-defined model system for which all relevant parameters can be defined.

The use of advanced biochemistry will further unravel the mode of action of toxins and the regions on the biopolymers which are important for their toxicity. Genetically tailored toxins that are still immunogenic, but no longer toxic, will certainly be used for protection. Surface structures such as pili are essential for adhesion, others such as capsule for the avoidance of host defense reactions. The knowledge of the role they play in pathogenicity is not only relevant for the understanding of disease processes, but will also be important for the development of vaccines. One goal is to obtain synthetic peptides tailored for particular applications. Other possibilities are opened by the use of safely attenuated organisms which have deletions in virulence genes. Vaccines can also be produced by fusing a specific protein to another readily available protein. Other proteins, for example the IgA protease, offer the potential for development as a carrier system by which proteins of interest can be secreted. Furthermore, the proteins do not have to be made in the original strains which may be difficult to handle, but in strains more suitable for production. DNA hybridization probes containing virulence genes will in the future find wide diagnostic application since they identify pathogenic factors directly.

The mechanisms responsible for the high versatility in gene expression, as has been found for example in gonococci, borreliae, and trypanosomes, may become suitable targets for drugs to interfere with the environmental adaptability of such organisms. Knowledge of the factors that determine the permeability of membranes will aid in devising drugs that enter cells, preferably by an active transport system. The recent finding of a polymyxin B derivative that has lost most of its antibacterial activity, but still renders gram-negative bacteria susceptible to otherwise weakly active antibiotics shows another way to increase the efficiency of antibiotics. Other drugs may be developed that inhibit synthesis of siderophores which are essential for a sufficient iron supply and thus for growth. Although enterochelin occurs only in enterobacteria, it may still be worth searching for inhibitors of its biosynthesis which is achieved by about six specific steps. Of broad interest are the hydroxamate-type siderophores which are synthesized by many bacteria and fungi. They all contain *N*-hydroxy groups. Drugs interfering with *N*-hydroxylation would affect growth of a large group of microorganisms by iron deprivation. One such compound, Desferal, is used for an entirely different purpose. Its administration relieves iron overload caused by frequent blood transfusions, hemochromatosis, and other hyperferremia. Moreover, synthetic analogs of enterochelin are available that strongly bind iron, but are no longer iron donors for enterobacteria.

It is beyond doubt that the study of microbial diseases has entered a new era, perhaps a second golden age, 100 years after the time of Robert Koch. This has been brought about by the application of modern experimental techniques developed in the last 10 years.

Symposium Summary. Current Status, Forefront, and Future: Immunologic Determinants

Ph. Y. Paterson

Orientation and Personal Perspective

I want you to be sure where I'm coming from before I share my thoughts with you. Many of these thoughts, especially those pertaining to immunology and the future, will be upsetting to some of you. But please bear with me and reflect upon what I say in the light of my personal perspective of the present and future [1].

I believe all disease of all kinds is primarily or initially infectious in nature. I mean *all* disease affecting humans. For example, juvenile diabetes, at least in large part, appears to be caused by a well-known, conventional virus which appears to trigger a secondary autoimmune host response against islet cell immunodeterminants [2,3]. Efforts to develop a vaccine and render identified susceptibles "immune" to diabetes are underway.[1] Many progressive degenerative disorders of the central nervous system clearly are caused by conventional viruses or unconventional virus-like agents, capable of replicating and transmissible from one host to another [4,5]. I suspect Alzheimer's disease will follow suit, now that it has attracted our attention. After learning how to identify the infectious agents responsible for cancer, cardiovascular disease, and psychiatric disorders, and how to control them, we will find ourselves face to face with the most vexing infectious disease process of all: the aging process. At present, this is the major restrictive determinant on life expectancies routinely exceeding 100-150 years.

I believe that occurrence of each and every disease represents a transitory or persistent-irreversible breakdown in the ordinarily silent, carefully balanced microbe-host relationship which translates to clinical well-being. When this symbiotic system is working well, as it usually does, we remain well, continue to evolve from an evolutionary standpoint and enjoy a "win-win" situation as it applies to both our microbial parasites and ourselves. I believe that rupture of this essential

---

[1] Strong support has recently been provided for the view that the process of rheumatoid arthritis is initiated by or associated with parvovirus infection [3a].

relationship more often occurs through weakening of host immune defense pathways than through a chance encounter with a microbe endowed with particular virulence and invasive properties. Whatever the cause, when the breakdown occurs it is a "lose-lose" situation for the parasites in and on us and for ourselves, since both parties are threatened with premature extinction.

If the foregoing lines of thinking should be found valid with passing time, it then follows that major advances in treatment and control of infectious diseases will result from our learning more about host immune responses, and how to strengthen or replace them, than through direct attack on the infecting microbe. Already, one discerns that current programs in new drug development are and will continue to be more oriented toward different ways the host's immunologic armamentarium can be modified selectively; search for novel antimicrobial agents that impact directly on the infecting parasite will occupy less and less attention [1].

Immunology 1984

Immunology has come a long way in the last 100 years, most of this progress in a relative sense having occurred in the last 20 years. In many different ways, immunology was forced to wait for the flowering of cell and molecular biology before it, in turn, could come into bloom. And it's surely blooming, and booming, now.

An abbreviated recap of where we are at present is set out in Table 1. Up front is the importance of basic and clinical research of increasing momentum. The "spin-off" has been remarkable: understanding intracellular communication from knowledge of DNA and the workings of the genetic code; rudimentary insights into how genes may be, or are, expressed by cells with know-how concerning detection-quantitation of the endless array of gene products; meaningful animal disease models for studying microbe-mediated and immunologically mediated tissue damage stimulating disorders of human beings; and, finally, clinical research, extending through the clinic to the physicians's office, such research drawing directly on the light shed by basic research involving molecules, cells, and animals.

Real headway has been made in disease prevention (Table 1). Effective vaccines now crowd the marketplace, poliomyelitis being the most dramatic example. Initial efforts to develop immunoreagents beyond the limited scope of gamma-globulin are beginning to appear. The apparent efficacy of anti-lipopolysaccharide (LPS) or anti-endotoxin immune serum as a supplemental therapeutic modality for treating patients with gram-negative bacterial sepsis, especially those patients who present with collapsing peripheral circulation, is a good illustration [6].

Disease diagnosis and treatment has leaped forward with discovery of monoclonal antibody technology (Table 1), once the importance of identification of marker epitopes on microbes and host cells/tissues was appreciated [7]. Monoclonal antibodies also

Table 1. Immunology 1984

Category	Specific examples
Basic and clinical research	Molecular "breakthroughs": the genetic code Cell biology: gene expression Animal model disease systems Correlative clinical research
Disease prevention	Vaccines: poliomyelitis Immunoreagents: anti-core glycolipid (LPS) serum
Disease diagnosis and treatment	Monoclonal antibodies Immunologic supplementation

occupy considerable attention as therapeutic modalities [8]. We have touched on this subject at this meeting. Isn't it strange, however, that the voluminous literature describing monoclonal antibodies is conspicuously silent with respect to their affinity binding properties. Dr. Madeleine Devey should scold all of us! If we go to the lengths of producing these "pristine silver bullets", the least we can do is pay attention to some of their qualitative characteristics, affinity binding properties being high on the list. After all, how can we expect monoclonal antibodies to be therapeutically useful until we have determined that they possess medium-high to high affinity binding for the epitope against which they are directed with "electron beam" accuracy? But using monoclonal antibodies therapeutically, even those of high affinity binding, presents awesome problems. I suggest interested parties contact Dr. Denis Burger who has a closet full of woeful tales to tell. We certainly are making progress in immunologic supplementation in the form of cellular/ tissue transplants. But our histocompatibility skills leave many of our efforts far short of specific, selective, and enduring immunologic reconstitution, the ultimate goal.

Pressing Problems

Extracellular and Intracellular Parasitism

Do you realize we've spent more than two days focusing mainly on microbes that are "obligate" extracellular parasites? These are the "easy ones" where tremendous amounts of knowledge already exist [9]. Only Dr. Helmut Hahn deliberately considered facultative intracellular parasites and the cell-mediated host immune responses, so crucial in dealing with intracellular parasitism. And did you notice, despite Dr. Hahn's lucid presentation, how uneasiness or frank confusion permeated our meeting room? And what about obligate intracellular parasites, where the going gets even rougher?

T Cell Receptor and T Effector Cells

Lack of knowledge about these facets of immunology has been the main reason for our not being able to come to grips with host cell-mediated immunity. Good news! The forces of molecular genetics and immunology have ripped away the shroud which so long has prevented us from clearly perceiving what the T cell receptor is and how it works. In the last year, different laboratories have cloned part of the T cell receptor [10-12]. The other half of the receptor has recently been cloned by another research group [12a]. From a molecular standpoint, the T cell receptor looks very similar to an immunoglobulin light chain. It is just possible that we will be able to draw directly on the store of knowledge already on tap concerning immunoglobulin synthesis, assembly, and function in getting a handle on the T cell receptor. A common thread will now link together humoral (antibody) immunity and cell-mediated immunity. And how urgently immunology needs common threads in becoming the basic scientific discipline we know it will become.

Resolution of the T cell receptor controversy and the ability to study T cell binding sites as we have studied B cell surface receptors will permit insights concerning T cell receptor modulation. Based on functional studies of cloned effector T cells, there already are strong hints that a single T cell may express cytotoxic helper or delayed-type hypersensitivity activities [13]. Wouldn't it be wonderful if it turned out that all of the various subpopulations of T cells, which make cellular immunology so complicated, merely represent phenotypic/functional variations reflecting straightforward surface modulation, i.e., cell-signal/receptor display? I have a hunch it may go that way because nature, when eventually understood, invariably turns out to utilize the most simple modus operandi.

No one here has discussed in detail how T cells actually depart from the systemic circulation and "home" toward their extravascular targets. Dr. Burger gave us important clues as to how the T cells "get set" to leave, but left it at that. We could profit by applying information concerning egress of metastatic cancer cells [14]. I am referring to the production of endoglycosidase by cancer cells which appears to facilitate their penetration of the subendothelial extracellular matrix, representing yet another barrier to easy exit. Production of this enzyme appears to be an important marker for cancer cells capable of establishing metastatic cell colonies at distant anatomic loci. Work at the Weizmann Institute in Israel [15] indicates that activated T cells resemble metastatic cancer cells by expressing a 10- to 15-fold increase in endoglycosidase. It's worth looking at this aspect of immune cell "targeting" in detail.

Natural Killer Cells

Although only discovered about a decade ago, NK cells are now "coming of age" [16]. Initially thought to be host effector cells programmed specifically for dealing with cancer cell targets, it now is apparent that NK cells may exert a variety of effector cell functions, including the formidable task of eradicating obligate intracellular parasites. Morphologically, they are classified as large granular lymphocytes. At first glance they look like monocytes: large, granule-ladden cytoplasm and a nucleus with a kink in one aspect of its surface. Increasing evidence suggests that NK cells are members of the monocyte-macrophage line. Biochemically, they appear to utilize similar metabolic pathways, even to the extent of generating free hydroxyl ions [17,18]. So, it seems, Dr. Manfred Karnovsky's fantastic exhibition of monocyte-macrophage biochemistry-function may be extended with little effort to NK cells.

Immunology 1999

Where are we going? Where are we going to be by 1990 or at least by 1999? Immunologic research is going along at an ever-increasing speed, and soon will acquire the molecular undergirding to move it, once and for all, from a cell-descriptive exercise to a true basic science discipline. It can't happen too soon, in terms of the "spin-off" which will positively impact on the clinical arena.

An abbreviated statement of where we should be by 1999 is set out in Table 2. "Immuno-orchestration" will supersede the rudimentary notion embodied in the contemporary phrase, "immunomodulation". Synthetic peptides with single epitope specificity, and virtually free of clinically significant untoward reactions will be the vaccines of common use [19]. Drugs and synthetic products, and their congeners, will be available for altering host immune responses in predictable ways, i.e., upregulating (immunopotentiation) or downregulating (immunosuppression) activities of specific immune effector cells [20]. Histocompatibility testing will include specific antigens distinct from major histocompatibility complex antigens so that "perfect donor-recipient matches" can be recognized. This will permit immunologic reconstitution involving specific cell types, i.e., bone marrow stem cells differentiating to NK cells.

I have a strong conviction that the next major "biological breakthrough" will occur when be begin to understand how cells talk with each other (Table 2). Of course they do! The problem is that they use a very private, barely audible form of conversation and we haven't been smart enough to get the hang of it yet. Our capability of fully grasping the conversation between cells will allow us to begin addressing and solving the major enigmas of contemporary biomedical science, e.g., cellular differentiation, gene expression vs gene repression, and the molecular aspects of cellular transformation. I can envision our giving lectures to our students which are supplemented with tapes representing the "talk" between identical vs different cell types and cell lines.

To return to one of my initial concepts, host immune deficiency will be defined in genetic terms and specific immune cells and functions (Table 2). Knowing now that fetal cells are present in the mother's circulation and possessing a library of between 1000 and 10 000 monoclonal antibody probes binding to products

Table 2. Immunology 1999

Category	Specific examples
Immuno-orchestration	Synthetic peptide vaccines Immuno-altering reagents Specific cellular reconstitution
Cell-cell communication	Decoding, translation, and recording-amplification
Genetic engineering	Identification and correction of gene-determined immune functions

of genes encoding the most relevant and specific immunologic host responses, it should be easy to detect genetic immunodeficiency of any of a hundred or more different types by the third month of gestation. Prenatal diagnosis of serious immune deficiency already has been described [21]. In all likelihood, the genes corresponding to all of these different phenotypic immunodeficiencies will be available for use in therapy. Specific pinpointing of one genetic defect will allow insertion into the fetus of that particular gene, thereby treating and correcting the specific immunodeficiency in utero, months before it ever would have manifested itself by clinical criteria [22]. To recognize and correct a genetic disorder before the host harboring that genetic disorder has an opportunity to express it may be standard preventive medicine of the 1990s. Of course, there will be protest and public outcry. But that is the preordained and predictable overture to any major, enduring scientific "leap forward". We or those coming after us, will have the task of finding solutions to the new and larger ethical, moral, and social issues that surely will surface in concert with the immunologic advances, however breathtaking they may be. We can and will do it! The future, in terms of host immune defenses, is bright and exhilarating! It's a particularly good time to be alive [23].

References

1. Paterson PY (1985) Introduction to infectious diseases. In: Youmans GP, Paterson PY, Sommers HM (eds) The biologic and clinical basis of infectious diseases, 3rd edn. Saunders, Philadelphia, pp 1-7
2. Yoon J-W, Austin M, Onodera T, Notkins AL (1979) Virus-induced diabetes mellitus. Isolation of a virus from the pancreas of a child with diabetic ketoacidosis. N Engl J Med 300:1173-1179
3. Baekkeskov S et al. (1982) Autoantibodies in newly diagnosed diabetic children immunoprecipitate human pancreatic islet cell proteins. Nature 298:167-169

3a. Simpson RW, McGinty L, Simon L, Smith CA, Godzeski CW, Boyd RJ (1984) Association of parvoviruses with rheumatoid arthritis of humans. Science 223:1425-1428

4. Choppin PW (1981) Measles virus and chronic neurological diseases. Ann Neurol 9:17-20
5. Prusiner SB (1982) Novel proteinaceous infectious particles cause scrapie. Science 216:136-144
6. Ziegler EJ et al. (1982) Treatment of gram-negative bacteremia and shock with human antiserum to a mutant *Escherichia coli*. N Engl J Med 307:1225-1230
7. Goding JW (1980) Antibody production by hybridomas. J Immunol Methods 39: 285-308
8. Ritz J, Schlossman SF (1982) Utilization of monoclonal antibodies in the treatment of leukemia and lymphoma. Blood 59:1-11
9. Youmans GP (1985) Host-bacteria interaction: external defense mechanisms. In: Youmans GP, Paterson PY, Sommers HM (eds) The biologic and clinical basis of infectious diseases, 3rd edn. Saunders, Philadelphia, pp 8-17
10. Yanagi Y et al. (1984) A human T cell-specific cDNA clone encodes a protein having extensive homology to immunoglobulin chains. Nature 308:145-149
11. Hedrick SM et al. (1984) Isolation of cDNA clones encoding T cell-specific membrane-associated proteins. Nature 308:149-153
12. Chien Y-h et al. (1984) Somatic recombination in a murine T-cell receptor gene. Nature 309:322-326
12a. Saito H et al. (1984) Complete primary structure of a heterodimeric T-cell receptor deduced from cDNA sequences. Nature 309:757-762
13. Dennert G, Weiss S, Warner JF (1981) T cells may express multiple activities: Specific allohelp, cytolysis, and delayed-type hypersenstivity are expressed by a cloned T-cell line. Proc Natl Acad Sci USA 78:4540-4543
14. Vlodavsky I, Ariav Y, Atzmon R, Fuks Z (1982) Tumor cell attachment to the vascular endothelium and subsequent degradation of the subendothelial extracellular matrix. Exp Cell Res 140:149-159
15. Naparstek Y, Cohen IR, Fuks Z, Vlodavsky I (1984) Activated T lymphocytes produce a matrix-degrading heparan sulfate endoglycosidase. Nature 310:241-244
16. Heberman RB (1981) Natural killer (NK) cells and their possible roles in resistance to disease. Clin Immunol Rev 1:1-66
17. Roder JC et al. (1982) Oxygen intermediates are triggered early in the cytolytic pathway of human NK cells. Nature 298:569-572
18. Suthanthiran M et al. (1984) Hydroxyl radical scavengers inhibit human natural killer cell activity. Nature 307:276-278
19. Shinnick TM, Sutcliffe JG, Green N, Lerner RA (1983) Synthetic peptide immunogens as vaccines. Ann Rev. Microbiol 37:425-446
20. Parant MA et al. (1980) Immunostimulant activities of a lipophilic muramyl dipeptide derivative and of desmuramyl peptidolipid analogs. Infect Immun 27:826-831
21. Linch DC et al. (1984) Prenatal diagnosis of three cases of severe combined immunodeficiency: Severe T cell deficiency during the first half of gestation in fetuses with adenosine deaminase deficiency. Clin Exp Immunol 56:223-232
22. Cline MG (1984) Gene therapy. Mol Cell Biochem 59:3-10
23. Paterson PY (1979) Infectious diseases: Into the 1980's and beyond. J Infect Dis 140:125-126

Session 5

Research Perspectives

Chairman: G. G. Jackson

Introduction

The presentations reported in Sessions 1-4 provide an interdisciplinary view of the state of the art and knowledge about the pathogenesis of bacterial infections in the systems considered. As in every successful conference, new questions deserving a forum were generated. Also, it was known that important parts of ongoing investigations with valuable experiences could not be fitted into the formal presentations. Sometimes an unpublished new method or very recent observations can provide a stimulus or helpful technique for critical new data and future research. Toward meeting these goals, the short presentations in Session 5 aroused discussion and enriched the perspective of pathogenesis, prevention, and treatment of bacterial infections.

New Approaches to Evaluate Microbial Macromolecules as Potential Vaccines: Studies of the Surface of *Neisseria gonorrhoeae* Using Antibody-Gold Sphere Immunological Probes

E. N. Robinson, Jr., Z. A. McGee, M. E. Hammond, J. T. Poolman, Th. M. Buchanan, G. K. Schoolnik, and M. S. Blake

Introduction

The effectiveness of a bacterial vaccine is predicted on its ability to elicit antibodies which can (a) attach to epitopes on the surface of bacteria or on molecules elaborated by bacteria and (b) interfere with the molecular mechanisms by which bacteria cause disease. A large number of extracted, purified or synthesized gonococcal proteins are presently being examined with regard to their pathogenic role in the disease process and their potential use as vaccines [1-3]. Until recently, the immunologic tests to assess the ability of antibodies to bind to bacterial antigens have used either purified antigens or structurally altered organisms [4-6]. However, the binding of antibody to purified antigens or structurally altered organisms does not predict the binding of antibody to native antigens on the surface of viable bacteria. To determine which gonococcal antigens are indeed accessible on the surface of whole intact gonococci and to assess the cross-reactivity of vaccine-elicited antibody with various gonococcal isolates, a new method of constructing immunological probes was developed [7]. These probes consist of gold spheres linked to specific anti-gonococcal antibodies via a staphylococcal protein A intermediary. The gold spheres are electron dense and can be easily detected on the surface of either whole gonococci on electron microscopy grids or embedded and thin-sectioned gonococci examined with transmission electron microscopy [7-10]. The probes can thus detect the accessibility to antibody of antigens on the surface of intact microbes.

Method for Constructing Gold Sphere Immunological Probes

The methodology for rapidly constructing these immunological probes has been recently described in detail [7] but will be briefly outlined here. The reduction of the gold in gold chloride to its elemental form with heat and mild acid results in the formation of electron dense gold spheres [11] (see Fig. 1). Varying the initial concentration of acid results in gold spheres of different sizes (15 nm to 40 nm or greater) (see Fig. 1). Staphylococcal protein A added to the suspensions of gold coats the surface of the spheres due to electrostatic forces [12] (see Fig. 2). The resultant gold sphere-protein A (GpA) com-

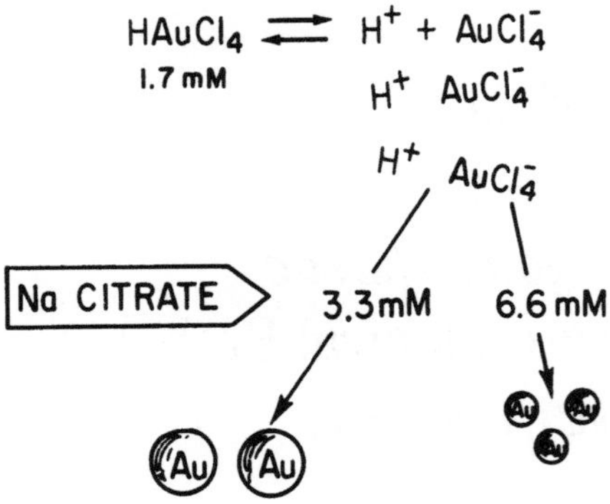

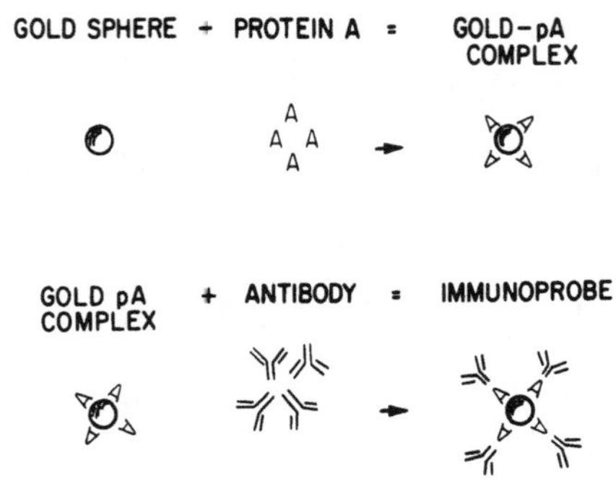

Fig. 1. Schematic diagram of gold sphere production. Note the versatility of sphere size provided by varying the initial concentration of acid. The use of a double label – small gold spheres conjugated to antibodies with specificity for one macromolecule and larger gold spheres conjugated to antibodies with specificity for another macromolecule – allows the simultaneous localization of two antigens [7,11,15,16]

Fig. 2. Schematic diagram of complexing gold spheres to staphylococcal protein A (*top*) and the conjugation of the resultant gold-protein A complex to antibody (*bottom*). (For procedural details, see [7].)

plexes are then purified and concentrated using repetitive ultracentrifugations [7]. The GpA complexes then can be stored at 4°C for at least six months with no apparent instability or loss of affinity for immunoglobulin G.

Suspension of GpA complexes (100 μl) are then ultracentrifugated at 50 000 xg for 2 min. The resultant pellets are resuspended with(100 μl)of either polyclonal antisera, purified IgG, or mouse ascites fluid containing monoclonal antibodies. After 30 min incubation at room temperature, the resulting GpA-antibody conjugates are purified using repetitive washings and ultracentrifugations (see Fig. 2).

Use of Gold Sphere Immunological Probes to Detect Surface Antigens on Bacteria

Gonococcal organisms are harvested directly from the surface of agar plates and suspended in a drop of HEPES-buffered MEM using a platinum wire loop and gentle aggitation. Carbon stabilized formvar coated copper electron microscopy grids are floated on the suspensions of gonococci [13]. The organisms attach to the surface of the grids and can be exposed to immunologic reagents while on the grid. The electron microscope grids with attached intact organisms are transfered to drops of 1% bovine serum albumin in HEPES-MEM to diminish nonspecific binding of the immunoprobe to the formvar surface. The grids are then exposed to the specific gold sphere antibody conjugate, washed vigorously in phosphate buffered saline and negatively stained with 1% phosphotungstic acid. Once dry, all specimens can be examined immediately with a transmission electron microscope, and the binding of the GpA-antibody conjugates to the surface structures of bacteria assessed visually.

With this technique, the gold immunoprobes have been used to detect the ultrastructural localization of gonococcal pilus antigens of whole gonococci and the degree of antigenic cross-reactivity of native gonococcal pili on organisms of different strains [7]. Antibodies elicited in rabbits against purified gonococcal pili were complexed to the gold spheres, and the resultant GpA-antibody conjugates were used to mark whole gonococcal organisms (see Fig. 3). The conjugates were specific in marking pili and did not mark the surface or the outer membrane blebs of the gonococci. The antibody conjugates were highly selective in marking the gonococcal pili of the strains used to elicit the antibody; there was no significant antigenic cross-reactivity of native gonococcal pili among several gonococcal strains tested [7]. The gold immunoprobes therefore allow the determination of the surface accessibility of antigens to antibody, the ultrastructural localization of antigens on whole organisms, and the degree of antigenic cross reactivity of surface macromolecules.

Future Use of Gold Sphere Immunological Probes

Gold spheres are excellent probes for the detection of antigens in embedded and thin sectioned specimens. One can use Lowicryl K4M ([14], Chemische Werke Lowi, Waldkraiburg, West Germany), a hydrophilic methacrylate polymer, as a matrix with which to embed whole gonococcal organisms and experimentally infected tissues. This polymer facilitates antigenic preservation and accessibility of antigens to immunoprobes while maintaining ultrastructural detail. The simultaneous examination of thin-sectioned and whole bacteria marked with GpA-monoclonal antibody conjugates will allow the localization in three dimensions of macromolecules in the outer membrane of bacteria. The same immunoprobes should also allow the ultrastructural localization of bacterial macromolecules thought to be virulence factors in naturally or experimentally infected tissues preserved and embedded in Lowicryl K4M.

Acknowledgments. These studies were supported by research grants AI-20265 (Z.M.), AI-18637 (M.S.B.), and AI-10615 (M.S.B.), from the National Institute of Allergy and Infectious Diseases, U.S. Public Health Service, by a grant from the R.J. Reynolds Foundation (M.E.H.), by a grant from Institut Merieux (T.M.B.), and by a grant from the Veterans Administration (G.K.S.). Dr. Robinson is the recipient of a Venereal Diseases Research Fellowship from the American Social Health Association. Dr. Schoolnik is a Fellow of the John A. Hartford Foundation. Dr. Poolman is the recipient of an international Fogarty Fellowship, grant 1-F05-TW03147-01. Dr. Blake is the recipient of an Irma P. Hirsche Fellowship.

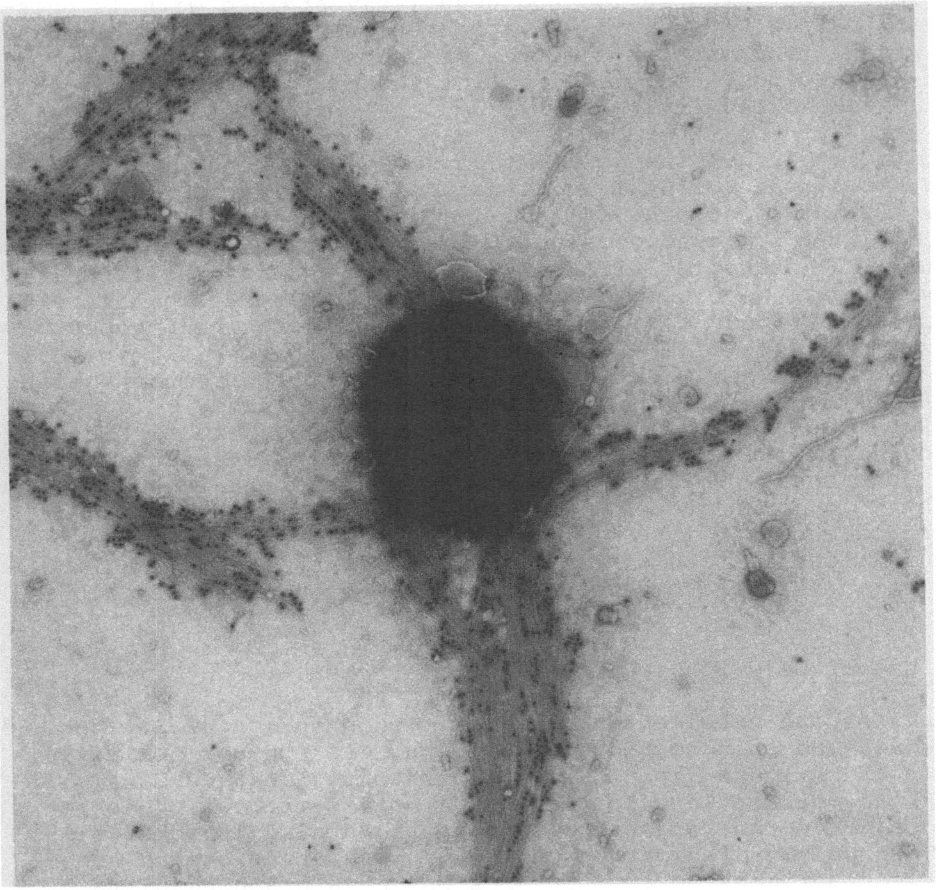

Fig. 3. *Neisseria gonorrhoeae*, strain MS11, P+ (piliated) transparent clone, exposed to gold spheres conjugated with antisera against purified pili from gonococcal strain MS11. Note heavy marking by gold spheres of pilus structures and absence of marking of the outer membrane blebs or the formvar background. Negative stain. × 21 600

The second author is particularly grateful to Dr. Jayne Clark, Ms. Jan Aprin, Ms. Carol Bowcutt, Ms. Holly Shurtleff, and Ms. Connie Drenker for their caring and skill which made his participation in the writing of this manuscript possible. The authors are also grateful to Dr. Loren Hoffman of Vanderbilt University for his help in developing the technique for using gold immunoprobes with thin-sectioned material.

References

1. Gotschlich EC (1984) Gonorrhea. In: Germanier R (ed) Bacterial vaccines. Academic Press, Orlando, Florida, pp 353-371
2. Schoolnik GK, Tai JY, Gotschlich EC (1983) A pilus peptide vaccine for the prevention of gonorrhea. Prog Allergy 33:314-331
3. Blake MS, Gotschlich EC (1983) Gonococcal membrane proteins: Speculations on their role in pathogenesis. Prog Allergy 33:298-313
4. Sandstrom EG, Knapp JS, Buchanan TM (1982) Serology of *Neisseria gonorrhoeae*: W antigen serogrouping by coagglutination and protein I serotyping by enzyme linked immunosorbent assay both detect protein I antigens. Infect Immun 35:229-239
5. Rothbard JB, Fernandez R, Schoolnik GK (1984) Strain-specific and common epitopes of gonococcal pili. J Exp Med 160:208-221
6. Tam MR, Buchanan TM, Sandstrom EG, Holmes KK, Knapp JS, Siadak AW, Nowinski RC (1982) Serological classification of *Neisseria gonorrhoeae* with monoclonal antibodies. Infect Immun 36:1042-1053
7. Robinson EN, McGee ZA, Kaplan J, Hammond ME, Larson JK, Buchanan TM, Schoolnik GK (1984) Ultrastructural localization of specific gonococcal macromolecules with antibody-gold sphere immunological probes. Infect Immun 46:361-366
8. Goodman SL, Hodges GM, Livingston DC (1980) A review of the colloidal gold marker system. Scanning Electron Microsc II:133-146
9. Horisberger M, Rosset J (1977) Colloidal gold, a useful marker for transmission and scanning electron microscopy. J Histochem Cytochem 25:295-305
10. Roth J, Bendayan M, Orci L (1978) Ultrastructural localization of intracellular antigens by the use of protein A-gold complex. J Histochem Cytochem 26:1074-1081
11. Frens G (1973) Controlled nucleation for the regulation of the particle size in monodisperse gold suspensions. Nature Physical Science 241:20-22
12. Romano EL, Romano M (1977) Staphylococcal protein A bound to colloidal gold: A useful reagent to label antigen-antibody sites in electron microscopy. Immunochemistry 14:711-715
13. McGee ZA, Gross J, Dourmashkin RR, Taylor-Robinson D (1976) Nonpilar surface appendages of colony type 1 and colony type 4 gonococci. Infect Immun 14:266-270
14. Roth J (1983) Application of lectin-gold complexes for electron microscopic localization of glycoconjugates on thin sections. J Histochem Cytochem 31:987-999
15. Geuze HJ, Slot JW, van der Ley PA, Scheffer RCT (1981) Use of colloidal gold particles in double-labeling immunoelectron microscopy of ultrathin frozen tissue sections. J Cell Biol 89:653-665
16. Roth J (1982) The preparation of protein A-gold complexes with 3 nm and 15 nm gold particles and their use in labeling multiple antigens on ultra-thin sections. Histochem J 14:791-801

Activity of Macrophage Processed Endotoxin

R. L. Duncan, Jr. and D. C. Morrison

The difference in relative biological activity between isolated chemically purified endotoxic lipopolysaccharide (LPS) and endotoxins generated in situ with intact bacteria used in models of pathogenic infection is an important consideration for interpretation of experimental studies of pathogenesis. We have addressed this problem by establishing an in vitro model in which endotoxins are generated in their normal state following phagocytosis of intact bacteria. These studies have been facilitated by labeling specifically the LPS component of *E. coli* with tritiated galactose by growing an expimerase deficient strain of this organism in the presence of ^{3}H-galactose. Macrophages are allowed to phagocytose the organisms for several hours followed by removal of unphagocytosed *E. coli*. This procedure results in more than 90% of the macrophage associated labeled bacteria being internalized. After 48-72 h of subsequent incubation, the radiolabeled material is harvested from the culture supernatant and from macrophage lysates. A partially purified LPS is obtained by phenol-water extraction. As a control in these studies, *E. coli* organisms are incubated with culture medium and then subjected to phenol-water extraction. The extracted LPS is purified by isopycnic density gradient ultracentrifugation to obtain LPS free from the majority of non-LPS-associated components. Approximately 50% of the radiolabel can be found in culture supernatants after 48 h in culture. The majority of the macrophage released LPS bands at a density in the gradient consistent with a lipid association. The remaining LPS that is found in the macrophage lysate shows a major peak of radioactivity with a density intermediate to the density of the LPS released into the medium of the macrophage cultures and LPS isolated from untreated *E. coli* (Fig. 1). Purified LPS from the native *E. coli* has two components, whereas both the cell lysate and the culture supernatants appear to have single components which are relatively homogeneous.

Determination of the biological activity of the macrophage processed LPS is limited, in part because of the small amount of material which can be isolated and purified. Thus, it is practical to assay only small amounts of macrophage "processed" LPS (e.g., 100-250 ng/test). A standard measurement of endotoxic activity is Limulus lysate gelation. Table 1 gives the results of five experiments using either phenol extracted LPS, lysates from macrophages, or culture supernatants. In the first three

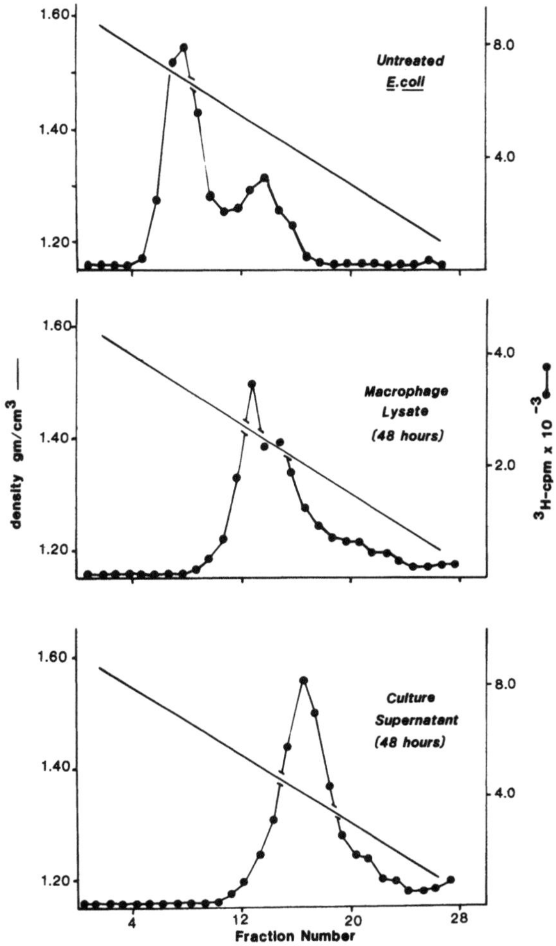

Fig. 1. Density of LPS which was phenol and water extracted from radiolabeled *E. coli* (*top*), macrophage lysates (*middle*), or culture medium (*bottom*). *E. coli* were added to macrophage monolayers derived from 5×10^6 peritoneal exudate cells, centrifuged (800 × G for 10 min), incubated 90 min, 37°C, 5% CO_2 in air), then washed to remove free *E. coli*. Fresh medium was added to the macrophage monolayers and they were cultured (37°C, 5% CO_2 in air). After 48 h the medium was collected and concentrated by Amicon filtration with a 5 ym filter. Macrophages were disrupted by distilled water and sonication. The LPS contained in the macrophage lysates, culture medium concentrate, and intact radiolabeled *E. coli* (suspended in distilled water) were extracted by the phenol-water procedure of Westphal and Jann. After extensive dialysis, the phenol-extracted material was mixed with CsCl (2.8 g/4.8 ml) and a density gradient was established by centrifugation (20 000 × G at 4°C for 48 h). Fractions (170 µl) were collected from the bottom of the gradient. The density of each fraction was determined by a refractometer (*straight line*) and the radioactivity (*full circles*) by liquid scintillation counting

Table 1. Biological activity[a] of ^{3}H-galactose labeled LPS isolated from *E. coli* J5[b] or from macrophage cultures[c] 48 h after the phagocytosis[d] of *E. coli* by macrophages

Experiment	CPM/ml contained in the last dilution of material which facilitated the clotting of Limulus amebocyte lysate[e]		
	Phenol extract	48 h macrophage lysates	48 h culture supernatants
1	2.50	1.00	1.25
2	0.60	0.60	6.00
3	N.D.	0.83	0.85
4	0.34	0.42	0.42
5	0.42	0.39	0.26

[a]Measured by determining the last dilution of material which clotted Limulus amebocyte lysate.
[b]LPS recovered from *E. coli* J5 by phenol extraction and isolated by CsCl isopycnic gradient.
[c]Macrophage cultures were obtained by incubating peritoneal exudate cells from female C3Heb/FeJ mice at 1.5×10^{6} cells/ml (in RPMI 1640 with 2% fetal calf serum) for 2 h at 37°C, then removing the non adherent cells by washing.
[d]^{3}H-galactose labeled *E. coli* J5 (2×10^{7} in 20 1) were added to each 1 ml culture, centrifuged, and cultures were incubated at 37°C. After 90 min *E. coli* not taken up by macrophages were removed by several washings and fresh medium was added back to the culture. Cultures were incubated for an additional 48 h after which supernatants were removed and concentrated 5× by Amicon filtration (ym 5 membrane). Adherent cells in each culture were disrupted by distilled water and sonication and were pooled. In experiments 1-3 the radioactive peak obtained from CsCl isopycnic gradients of the macrophage lysates or culture supernatants were tested. In experiments 4 and 5 the culture material was tested without further purification.
[e]Samples were adjusted to have the same number of CPM. Serial 10-fold dilutions in pyrogen-free water were carried out to determine the last dilution of material which would clot an equal volume of Limulus amebocyte lysate (50 1 sample + 50 1 of Limulus amebocyte lysate) (after 1 h incubation at 37°C). Serial 2-fold dilutions were likewise carried out on the last 10-fold dilution to clot. The CPM/ml in the last dilution to clot was determined by dividing the starting CPM by the dilution factor.

experiments, the LPS was phenol extracted; in the last two, it was not, but rather it remains in putative association with whatever molecular complexes may be formed in macrophages. With the exception of one experiment in which the supernatants were less active, there appear to be no distinguishable differences in comparison to phenol-water extracts, although our isopycnic density gradient analyzes clearly indicate that the LPS was asso-

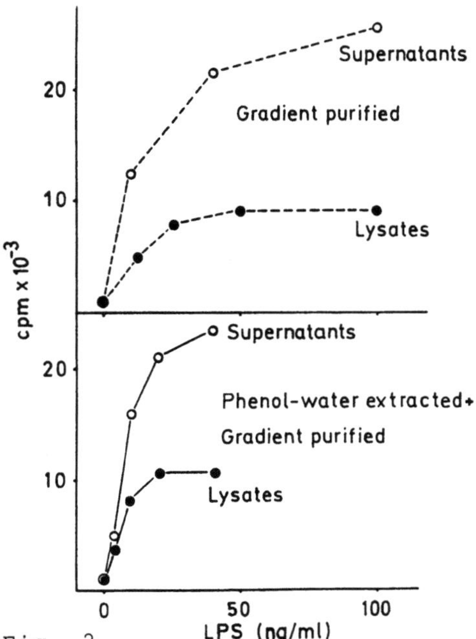

Fig. 2

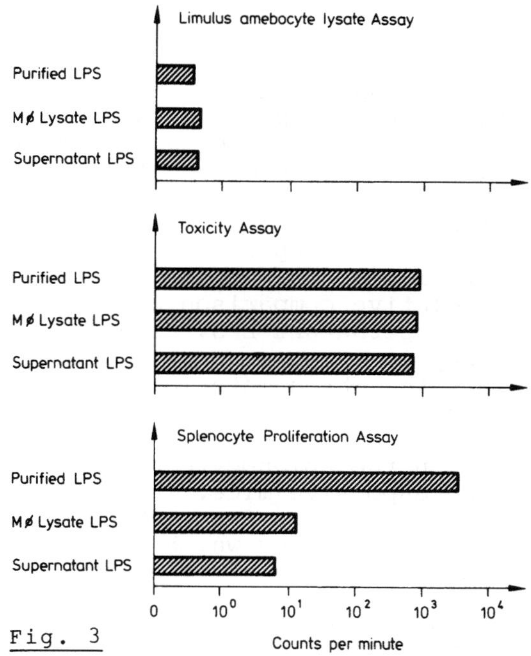

Fig. 3

Fig. 2. Induction of murine splenocyte proliferation by macrophage "processed" LPS. LPS exocytosed from macrophages which had ingested *E. coli* (supernatant LPS, *open circles*) or the LPS retained by macrophages (macrophage lysate LPS, *full circles*) was added to C3Heb/FeJ murine splenocyte cultures (2.5×10^6 cells/ml in 200 µl) at the LPS concentrations indicated. ^{3}H-thymidine was added to cultures during the last 16 h of a 48 h incubation period. Cells were harvested on glass fiber filters and ^{3}H-thymidine uptake was determined by liquid scintillation counting. Each point represents the mean for triplicate cultures. In all experiments the standard deviation from the mean was less than 10%

Fig. 3. Biological activities of macrophage "processed" and control lipopolysaccharides. The Limulus amebocyte lysate assay was carried out as described in the legend to Table 1. Toxicity of ^{3}H-galactose labeled LPS was tested in 6-8 weeks old actinomycin D-treated C3Heb/FeJ mice. Mice were sensitized to the lethal effects of LPS by an i.p. injection of 20 µg of actinomycin D (Sigma Chemical Co.) in water. LD_{50} values were calculated according to the method of Reed and Muench, based on the number of mice that died in a 72 h period. Results are expressed as the CPM associated with the amount of LPS which resulted in an LD_{50}. The lymphocyte proliferation assay was carried out as described in Fig. 2. Results are expressed as the CPM associated with the amount of LPS required to induce a stimulation index of 10 (stimulation index = experimental - background ÷ control - background)

ciated with some very lipophilic components. In contrast, if biologic activity is measured by induction of murine B lymphocyte proliferative activity, both macrophage lysates and culture supernatants manifest considerable mitogenic activity, although the culture supernatants appeared to be somewhat more active. Nevertheless, there is no detectable difference in mitogenicity between the macrophage "processed" LPS before or after phenol-water extraction (Fig. 2) which should liberate the LPS from other macrophage or bacterial constituents. These data suggest that the macrophage processed LPS rather than LPS associated material contributes to the mitogenic activity. Figure 3 shows a relative comparison of purified LPS, macrophage lysate LPS, and supernatant LPS, using a Limulus lysate assay, a toxicity assay in mice, or a cell proliferation assay. It is noteworthy that the three materials are identical for relative in vitro endotoxic activity, and equal for in vivo toxicity, but the macrophage processed material is 100-fold more active as a mitogen in the splenocyte proliferation assay using splenocytes from LPS responsive mice. These materials remained poorly mitogenic for splenocytes from LPS hyporesponsive mice suggesting that the mechanism by which macrophage "processed" LPS stimulates mitogenesis has not been altered.

The data presented are from preliminary experiments and subject to multiple interpretations, but they provide provocative information about the form of biologically active endotoxin which may be released from macrophages.

Discussion

Q: Do you know what is changed chemically on the LPS by the macrophages?

A: The lipid A is probably intact, because of the unchanged activity with respect to the Limulus assay, although that is certainly weak chemical evidence. Further, lipid A dissociated from macrophage "processed" LPS by mild acid hydrolysis retains its mitogenic activity. There probably are not major changes in the core and O antigens, because the galactose label is contained in both. We have preliminary data suggesting that the dideoxy terminal hexose, specifically colitose, has been modified or degraded. The evidence in support of this conclusion is that the thiobarbituric acid assay of the processed LPS allows detection of KDO, where this is not possible in the native *E. coli* LPS (due to the presence of high concentrations of colitose). Therefore, the preliminary information suggests that there is a modification in the terminal O-side chain sugars, and that is the only biochemically detectable change.

Q: Were the nanogram values for comparison calculated from radioactivity, or how did you get them?

A: Because of the limited amount of material available, we have made the implicit assumption that the specific activity calculated for the native phenol extracted LPS approximates that in the processed LPS. The indirect evidence in support of that would be the fact that in at least two distinct assay systems there is a precise relationship between the three preparations (lethality and Limulus lysate responses). The probability that the specific activity would change in such a way that both of these parameters would be altered in the same way seems unlikely, but I am open to the suggestion that the exactitude of the nanogram measurement is weak. A more precise comparison would actually be counts per minute, but if that is used, people confuse it with the results of assays that also are expressed in counts per minute (i.e. mitogen assays).

Q: Macrophages have an alkaline phosphatase. Have you looked for the production of phosphates?

A: We do not have enough material to do biochemical assays. One would have to use a label. Currently, we are using a double label with tritiated acetate to preferentially enrich lipid A labeling and then examining the macrophage-processed material for ratios of lipid to carbohydrate by observing the tritium to ^{14}C ratio.

Laboratory Characterization of Lipopolysaccharides (LPS)

R. E. W. Hancock

There are two types of LPS that can coexist in one strain: smooth and rough. This has been observed in *Pseudomonas aeruginosa* and *Salmonella typhimurium* as well as many other organisms.

Two methods have been used to isolate LPS. Phenol-water extraction has been used for the smooth strains and anhydrous phenol/chloroform/petroleum ether for the rough strains. Both of these techniques are selective in the species of LPS that they isolate. Both provide rather low yields; with some organisms, the yields are impossibly low. Included among these species are *Agrobacterium*, *Bacteroides*, many strains of *Pseudomonas aeruginosa* and *Pseudomonas fluorescens*. In addition, the methods are selective. For example, with the phenol/chloroform/petroleum ether procedure, the rough core LPS cannot be isolated from a strain of *P. aeruginosa* that contains 80% rough LPS. When the O-polysaccharide is extracted with the phenol-water technique, the O-side chains are enriched.

We have used a technique that is simple. Basically, cells are dissolved in SDS and the LPS precipitated (Darveau and Hancock, J. Bacteriol. 155:831-838, 1983). Yields are about 60%-80% and the LPS is pure by all criteria. Advantages in using the SDS technique are a 50-fold higher yield of some LPSs and the detection of O-side chain-containing LPS in strains previously thought to have only rough LPS.

A purely technical comment concerns the method of running an SDS polyacrylamide gel with LPS in it. A typical artifact that can appear is in the restricted heterogeneity observed. Multiple clusters of O-side chain containing LPS can be caused by hydrophobic interaction between adjacent molecules of LPS or by divalent cation binding of the adjacent LPS molecules. On a purely technical basis, there are three things that can be done to eliminate these problems: addition of EDTA to the gel which removes divalent cations and removal of hydrophobic bonds either by having urea in the gel or by increasing the SDS concentration to 0.5%. Although these are purely technical points, they are important because LPS gels are becoming a major method of documenting the character of LPS in the literature.

Bacterial Growth on Biomaterials

J. W. Costerton

A device was developed to replace the test tube in determining the adherence, growth, and inhibition of growth of bacteria on biomaterials (Fig. 1). The fluids of interest include serum, synovial fluid, urine, or another body fluid or secretion. The test sample with bacteria is allowed to flow through the device. The build up of the mass of organisms on the surface occurs in a short period of time (Fig. 2). The discs can then be removed and put into a system to test for phagocytosis of the attached organisms, for serum killing, for specific antibody effects, or for the determination of the efficacy of antibacterials against bacteria that are adherent to a surface.

Discussion

Q: In the interpretation of the effect of subinhibitory concentrations of an antibiotic in modifying microbial attachment and susceptibility, is it not possible that the presence of serum is modifying the results?

A: We could find no influence of serum on the resistance or susceptibility of the bacteria against the antibiotics tested. The only change is if the bacteria are lysed by the serum.

Comment: The way to do the experiment is to grow the organisms in the presence of subinhibitory concentrations of an antibiotic, wash the bacterial cells, then add them to the serum in the absence of an antibiotic. Only then is it possible to monitor antibiotic induced cell surface changes that have occurred.

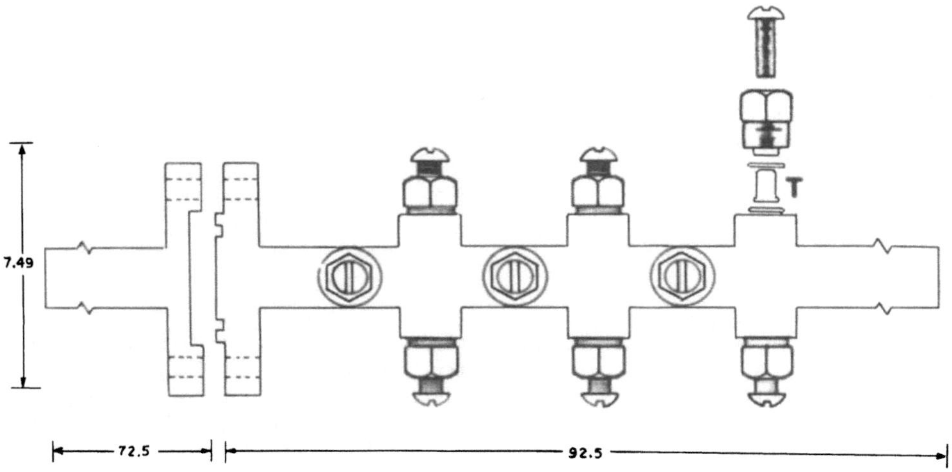

Fig. 1

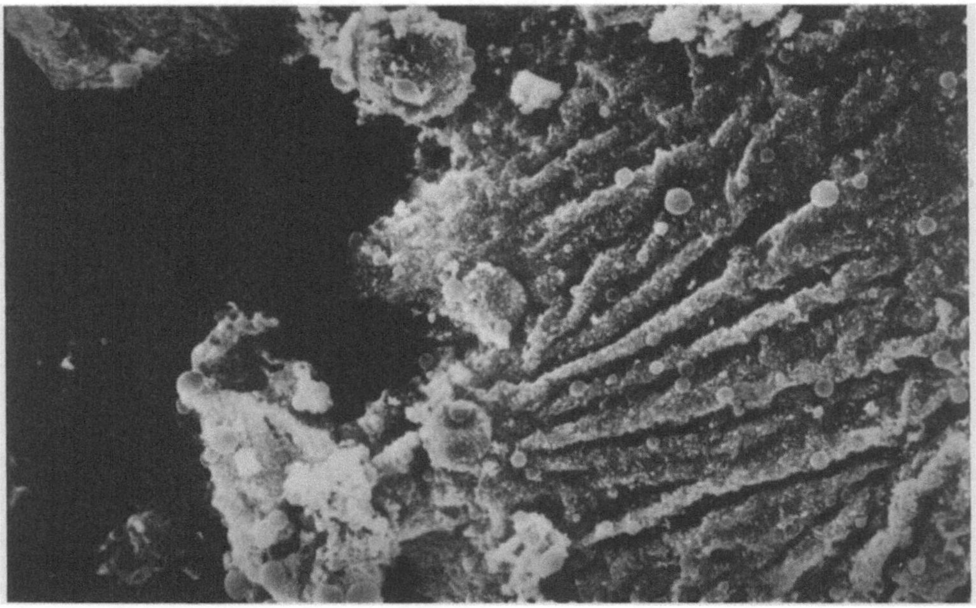

Fig. 2

Iron Utilization and Invasiveness of *Hemophilus influenzae*

P. F. Sparling

Hemophilus influenzae classically has been defined as a heme-requiring microorganism. Many species of microorganisms use heme in vitro, but there probably is not very much unbound heme available in vivo. It is known that free heme is bound in the serum to hemopexin and is rapidly removed to an intracellular location. Free hemoglobin is similarly bound to haptoglobin and rapidly removed from serum. The most abundant (and most persistent) iron source in serum is iron-transferrin. The question investigated was, can a microbe that by definition requires heme for growth in vitro actually use other iron sources such as transferrin that might be more readily available in vivo?

We grew *H. influenzae* with protoporphyrin instead of heme which allows one to test specifically whether the strains can use transferrin as a sole source of iron. Some results are shown in Table 1. Each of four tested *H. influenzae* isolates had a normal doubling time in iron-depleted broth medium supplemented with 20% iron-saturated human transferrin. Most pharyngeal or respiratory *H. influenzae* isolates used transferrin as a source of iron in plate bioassays, whereas none of a small sample of non-pathogenic *H. parainfluenzae* could do so. All (28/28) systemic isolates of *H. influenzae* could use transferrin as a sole source of iron. Thus, there may be novel unrecognized mechanisms of iron transfer that can differentiate pathogenic capability among strains of Hemophilus. Similar systems may apply to other pathogenic species, but little has been done with some of the very common organisms.

Discussion

Q: About 5% of invasive *H. influenzae* infections are caused by organisms that do not have a capsule (non type b). Do these invasive strains have a high correlation with transferrin binding or utilization as an iron source?

A: I hope that will be determined by others who have the strains, interest, and capability to do so.

Table 1. Ability to use transferrin as a source of iron was tested on enriched medium containing protoporphyrin IX and the iron chelator EDDA, which prevented growth in the absence of a useable source of iron. (Data of D.A. Herrington and P.F. Sparling)

Isolate	Ability to use Fe^{3+}-TF
H. influenzae (b)	
(meningitis, bacteremia)	28/28
H. influenzae	
(pharyngeal, respiratory)	28/35
H. parainfluenzae	
(pharyngeal, respiratory)	0/10

Complement Resistance and the *tra-T* Gene

R. P. Levine

It has been reported that plasmid R-100 confers serum resistance on laboratory strains of *E. coli* K12. The resistance is correlated with the presence of the plasmid-borne *tra-T* gene. Subsequent investigations using a *tra-T* probe and with *E. coli* isolated from children with systemic infections have shown that of the *E. coli* isolated from either the blood or cerebral spinal fluid from 12 children, nine of the isolates carried the *tra-T* gene. One of the strains spontaneously lost its plasmid and became serum sensitive. Since the reinsertion of a plasmid carrying the *tri-T* gene produced meager serum resistance, it appears that *tra-T* alone is not responsible for complement resistance.

Discussion

Q: A puzzle about the *tra-T* gene is that it is made in only about 100 000 copies of the cell, which is low for an outer membrane protein. Do clinical isolates have larger numbers of the plasmid?

A: I do not know.

Comment (Opferkuch): We did similar experiments and also obtained an inconclusive increase in serum resistance after plasmid insertion of the resistance gene. Studies by DNA homology indicated that we had isolated a mutant of *E. coli* that had chromosomal absence of serum resistance.

Antibiotic Alteration of Bacterial Membranes

W. Opferkuch

Subinhibitory concentrations of beta lactam antibiotics on bacteria can influence the interaction with the serum bactericidal activity. Serum resistant strains of gram-negative bacteria recently isolated from blood cultures were treated with different beta lactam antibiotics and then tested for changes in resistance to lysis by serum (Table 1). The bacteria used in the experiments grew in serum concentrations of more than 20%; with the exception of two strains of *Serratia*. The only antibiotic that influenced the serum resistance was imipenem. Five of 12 strains changed in susceptibility to serum lysis, in two the change was of major degree and in three the change was minor. *Enterobacter aerogenes* when pretreated with imipenem was killed immediately with 20% serum and even with 5% serum (Fig. 1). The effect was dependent on drug concentration. Serum resistant strains of *E. coli* have been reported to become serum sensitive after treatment with mecillinam, but none of the strains we studied did so (Fig. 2). It is assumed that the reaction must be strain specific.

Changes in the membrane proteins of the bacteria that might reflect the change in serum resistance were investigated. No changes of the outer membrane proteins could be identified after treatment with moxalactam, piperacillin, ticarcillin, or imipenem. Also, no changes in the LPS were identified as characterized by the western blot technique. In another experiment, a quantitative and qualitative examination of the membrane vesicles of the outer and inner membrane was performed. The vesicles were prepared by osmotic shock of plasmalysed bacteria, digested by lysozyme and the remaining vesicles were subjected to sucrose density gradient centrifugation. With this method, a reduction of recoverable cytoplasmic membrane protein could be detected especially after pretreatment with imipenem. Whether these changes are related to the decreased serum resistance needs further experiments.

Discussion

Comment (Hancock): Most things that disrupt outer membranes act at a single locus on the outer membrane, which is where LPS is cross linked by divalent cations. Complement binds to the lipid A and is inhibited by divalent cations. The characterization of

Table 1. MIC of thienamycin against 12 enterobacteriaceae; maximum serum concentration in % tolerated by the bacteria before and after treatment with 1/4 MIC thienamycin

Strains		MIC µg/ml	Serum resistance in % before and after treatment with 1/4 MIC thienamycin	
			before	after
WF 52	*Escherichia coli*	0.125	20	15
BK 615	*Escherichia coli*	0.25	20	3
BK 28	*Enterobacter aerogenes*	0.5	20	15
BK 319	*Enterobacter aerogenes*	0.5	20	3
BK 383	*Enterobacter cloacae*	0.25	20	20
BK 967	*Enterobacter cloacae*	0.5	20	20
BK 177	*Klebsiella pneumoniae*	0.25	20	20
BK 1171	*Klebsiella pneumoniae*	0.25	20	20
BK 1435	*Proteus mirabilis*	4	20	15
BK 74	*Proteus morganii*	2	20	20
BK 31	*Serratia marcescens*	1	8	8
BK 1292	*Serratia marcescens*	0.5	8	8

LPS as different or not different on the basis of gel mobility can be highly artifactual and partially dependent on the technique used for isolation of the LPS. LPS is a heterogeneous molecule and the chemical analysis of it is very difficult. To say that the LPS patterns are the same is not sufficient.

Comment (McGee): Subinhibitory concentrations of antibiotics cause changes in the protein 2 on gonococci and a similar protein on the outer membrane of meningococci. At subinhibitory concentrations of tetracycline, the organisms do not have pili; with penicillins the number is diminished, but there are whole pili in the background that appear as if they had lost their anchor. It is very a provocative finding that deserves further examination.

Reply: We have examined the influence of beta lactam antibiotics on pilation in *E. coli* by EM and could not find any loss of pili. In addition, we examined non-opsonin mediated phagocytosis by macrophages. Beta lactam antibiotics that produce filament formation increased the effect, but there was no effect from the drugs that induce round cell formation like imipenem.

Comment (Costerton): One-quarter of an MIC inhibits adherence of *Staphylococcus aureus* to bone surfaces and one tenth MIC has an

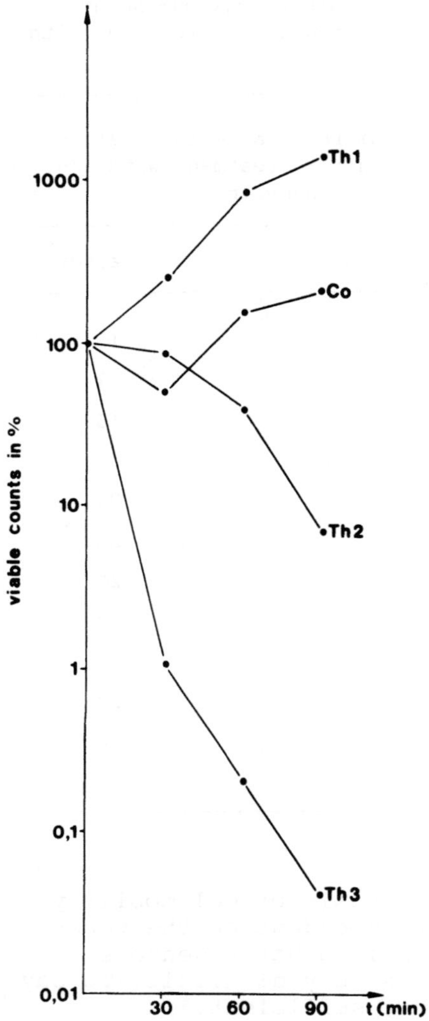

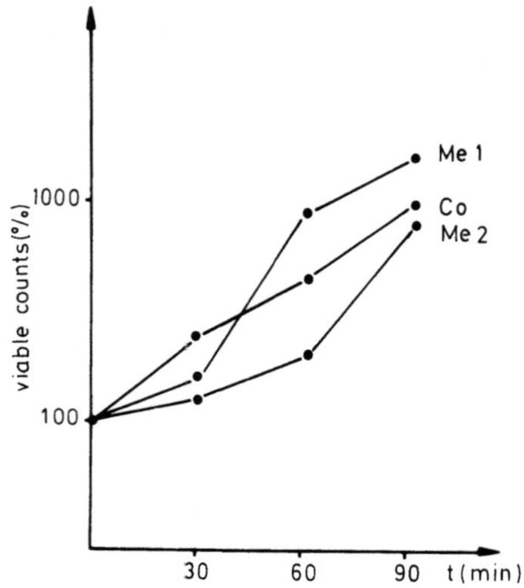

Fig. 2. The influence of Mecillinam on the serum bactericidal activity to *E. aerogenes* BK 319. The bacteria are grown in the presence of: Co = 20% human serum, Me 1 = 1/4 MIC Mecillinam, Me 2 = 1/4 MIC Mecillinam + 20% human serum

◄ Fig. 1. The influence of Imipenem on the serum bactericidal activity to *Enterobacter aerogenes* BK 319. The bacteria are grown at 37°C in the presence of: Co = 20% human serum, Th 1 = 1/4 MIC Imipenem, Th 2 = 1/4 MIC Imipenem + 5% human serum, Th 3 = 1/4 MIC Imipenem + 20% human serum

inhibitory effect. There may be some usefulness of these subinhibitory concentrations of the beta lactam antibiotics.

Reply: The effects are strain specific and drug dependent. One cannot draw valid general conclusions from the various observations that are presently published.

Persistent Bacterial Meningitis: Lyme Disease

A. G. Barbour

The tick-borne disorder of Lyme disease was probably first described in Northern Europe in the early part of the century. A prominent feature of the disease, especially in Europe, is a form of chronic meningitis. When accompanied by a radiculitis, the meningitis is known as Bannwarth's syndrome. In both the United States and Europe another common and characteristic manifestation of Lyme disease is erythema chronicum migrans (Fig. 1) [1]. Spirochetes have been isolated from the blood and from the periphery of the skin lesions of patients with erythema chronicum migrans (ECM). Identical spirochetes have also been recovered from the cerebrospinal fluid of patients with Lyme disease meningitis. Using these spirochetes as antigens, we and other investigators have found that some European and American patients with chronic meningitis, either with or without a preceding ECM skin lesion, have high antibody titers in both the serum and cerebrospinal fluid. Examination with the Western blot procedure of cerebrospinal fluid from these patients with persistent meningitis revealed antibodies to a number of components of the spirochetes. The persistence of this bacterial infection in the presence of high concentrations of spirochete-specific antibody

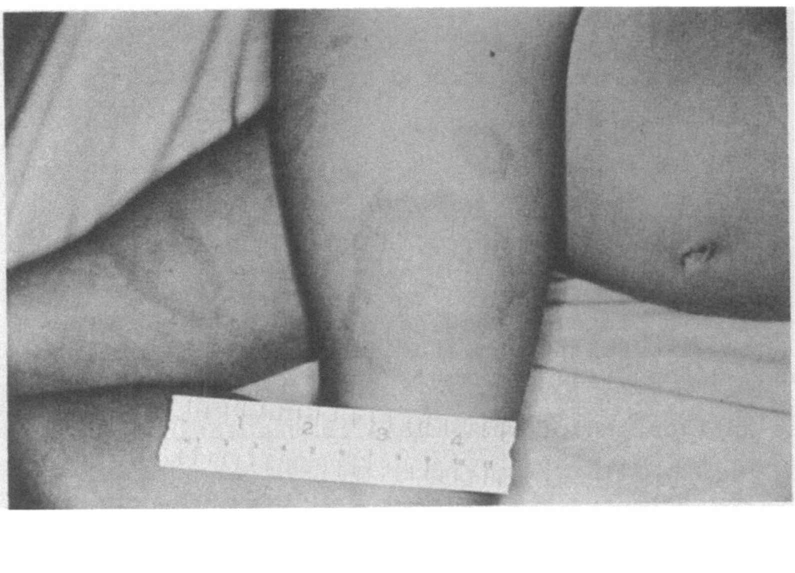

Fig. 1

raises questions about the pathogenesis of both this manifestation of Lyme disease and also the chronic arthritis that can occur as a sequela of ECM.

One advantage to working with the Lyme disease spirochete, in contrast to work with *Treponema pallidum*, the agent of another persistent spirochetal disease, is that we can serially passage the organism in the laboratory without co-cultivation. Interestingly, when the Lyme disease spirochete is first isolated from patients or from other mammals, it usually grows as a large aggregate (Fig. 2). With prolonged passage in vitro, the organisms stop clumping and grow free in the medium.

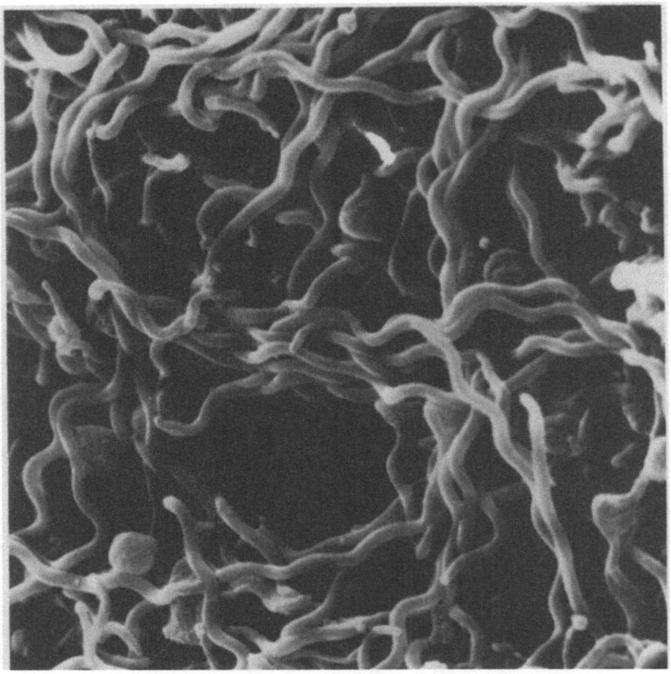

Fig. 2

Discussion

Q: Do the spirochetes in tissues grow in masses as they do in vitro?

A: There are some skin biopsies showing that. Also liver biopsies from patients with Relapsing Fever, another tick-borne spirochetal disease, often will show small colonies of organisms.

Q: Against what antigen and of what class is the antibody in the spinal fluid?

A: Many patients have antibodies that bind to the axial filament protein. The antibodies are of both IgG and IgM classes.

Q: Is the elevated IgM a specific antibody, is it polyclonal and does it react as rheumatoid factor?

A: It is not a rheumatoid factor. It is polyclonal but there may also be oligoclonal peaks in the spinal fluid.

Q: Spirochetes are avidly phagocytized by human neutrophils in vitro. Are the organisms located in macrophages of patients intracellularly when the skin lesions are biopsied?

A: The tissue location of the organisms does not seem to be intracellular, but instead they are found in the extravascular spaces. There is a paradox here. How can the spirochetes in vivo persist apparently extracellularly when they seem to be so easily opsonized and phagocytized in vitro?

Reference

1. Steere AC, Malawista SE, Hardin JA, Ruddy S, Askenase PW, Andiman WA (1977) Erythema chronicum migrans and Lyme arthritis: The enlarging clinical spectrum. Ann Intern Med 86:685-698

Antiadhesive Properties of Monoclonal Antibody Against Type 1 Fimbriae of *E. coli*

E. H. Beachey and S. N. Abraham

Bacteria bind specifically to receptors on epithelial cells by ligand (adhesin) molecules on the surface of bacteria. We believe that adhesin-receptor interactions are responsible for tissue tropism and for the binding of bacteria to specific tissues where they cause infections. We have investigated the possibility of nullifying the adhesion-receptor reaction both by producing antibodies to the adhesin on the bacteria and to the receptor on the epithelial cells. As a model the mannose receptor and type 1 fimbriae were used.

Table 1. Immunological properties of hybridoma antibodies against type 1 fimbriae

Hybridoma antibodies	IgG class	Agglutination of fimbriated *E. coli*	Immuno-precipitation of fimbriae	ELISA titers against isolated fimbriae
CD3	1	+	+	409 000
AA8	1	-	-	819 000
GG1	2a	-	-	409 600
IIG1 (control)	1	-	-	<200

Table 1 shows some properties of three monoclonal antibodies against whole type 1 fimbriae, one (CD3) of which agglutinated *E. coli* and precipitated a preparation of fimbriae. The other two (AA8 and GG1) did not, but they had a high titer of activity by ELISA against the isolated fimbriae. The latter two antibodies reacted with the subunits of the fimbriae in a Western blot, whereas the antibody that precipitated the fimbriae, did not. It was observed that the CD3 agglutinating antibody reacted only with polymers that were greater than 102,000 molecular weight, which represents six subunits of the fimbriae. In EM, the CD3 antibody was observed to arrange itself in a spiral manner around the fimbriae (Fig. 1A,B). Figure 1C shows the

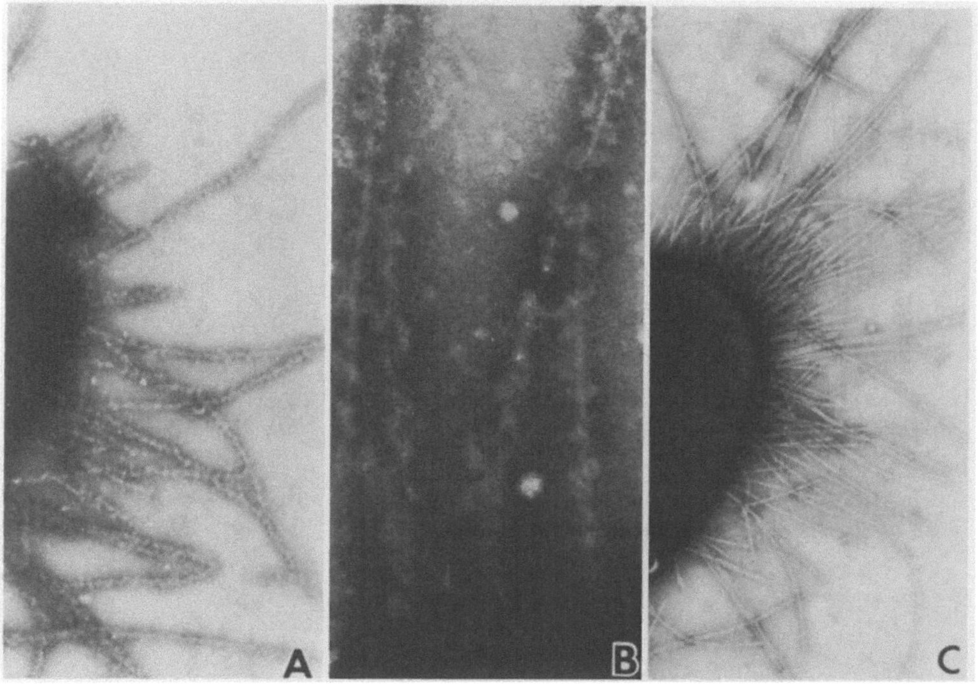

Fig. 1

nonreactivity with one of the antibodies that did not agglutinate the organisms and is a subunit specific antibody.

The specific reactivity was shown immunochemically by use of purified fimbriae to which all of the antibodies reacted. However, the nonagglutinating clones reacted only with the filtrate of purified fimbriae that contained subunits smaller than 50,000-100,000 molecular weight. In contrast, the agglutinating clone reacted with the retentate but not with the filtrate. With CD3, the quarternary structure-specific antibody, the isolated fimbriae competitively inhibited the binding of the antibody to fimbriae in an ELISA reaction whereas fimbrial subunits prepared by exposing fimbriae to boiling acid and to saturated guanidine hydrochloride were noninhibitory. Fimbriae reassembled from the subunits by addition of magnesium chloride again inhibited the antibody reaction. If the fimbrial subunits II (Fig. 2) were again dissociated, the antibody reactivity was lost once again. The reaction with the nonagglutinating subunit specific monoclonal antibody was just the opposite. The subunits were inhibitory in an ELISA reaction, whereas the intact fimbriae or reassembled fimbriae had no activity. Figure 3 shows the isolated fimbriae (panel A), the dissociated fimbriae (panel B), and reassembled fimbriae (panel C). These reassembled fimbriae regained their original structure and reacted with CD3 antibody (panel D).

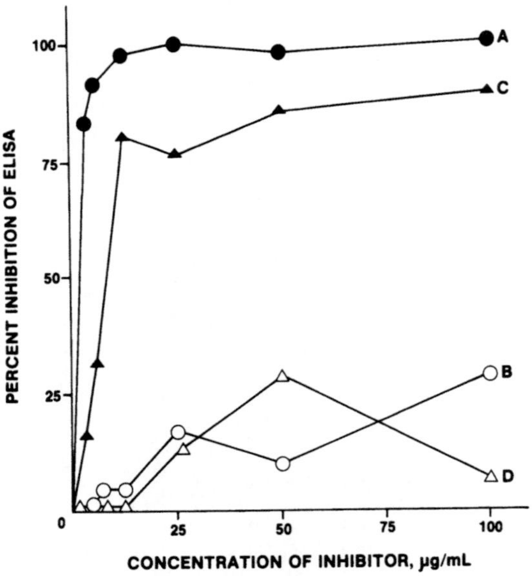
PERCENT INHIBITION OF ELISA
CONCENTRATION OF INHIBITOR, µg/mL
A
B
C
D
0
25
50
75
100

Fig. 2

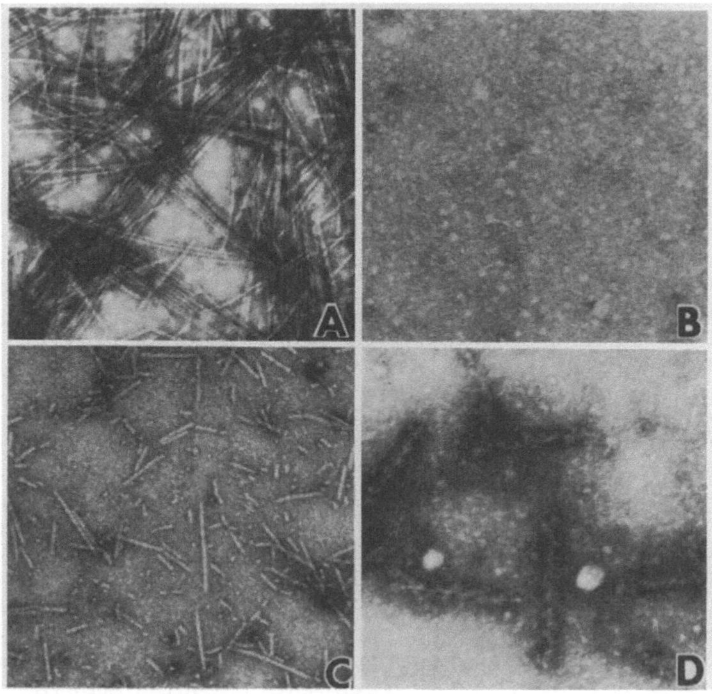
A
B
C
D

Fig. 3

By passive immunization in a mouse model of ascending pyelonephritis, the structure-specific antibody was protective in 13 of 16 animals and decreased the mean number of bacteria in the kidney and bladder, whereas there was no protection by the antibody against the fimbrial subunit. Use of another antibody against the D-mannose specific receptor of uroepithelial cells also was partially protective, but an N-acetylgalactosamine specific antibody directed against a different receptor had no protective activity.

The results demonstrate the principle that protection against bacterial infections can be mediated by antibodies directed against either the adhesin of the bacterial cell or the receptor on the host cell.

Reference

1. Abraham SN, Hasty DL, Simpson WA, Beachey EH (1983) J Exp Med 158:1114-1128

Molecular Basis of Host Tissue Specific Pathogenesis of Enterobacteriaceae

G. K. Schoolnik and D. L. Lark

A fundamental concept of infection is that molecular interactions determine events in pathogenesis. I will address the molecular basis for three events that are related in specifying the phenomenon of host range of infection. One is the molecular basis for the species specificity of infection. A second is the molecular basis for tissue tropism, the basis by which organisms invade some and not other tissues. The third is the molecular basis for one individual being receptive to infection, whereas other members of the same species may not be so predisposed.

These events can be presented at the molecular level in terms of the adhesins that an organism expresses and the complementary molecules at the host cell surfaces to which they bind. Anti-receptor antibodies are a means of mapping the topography of receptors on human tissues (Table 1). One could describe the surface of *E. coli* as being comprised of common pili or a common adhesin. It is recognized by the agglutination of guinea pig erythrocytes, a process that is inhibited in the presence of mannose. With regard to human cells, this process seems to mediate the adherence of *E. coli* to buccal epithelium and to a protein in urine, the Tamm-Horsfall protein. Also, there are fimbriae on the bacterial surface that agglutinate human erythrocytes in which the minimal receptor is alpha galactose 1,4 beta galac-

Table 1. *E. coli* chromosome-encoded pili

Type	Agglutination	Minimal receptor	Human target
Common	Guinea pig	Mannose	Buccal epithelium (Tamm-Horsfall protein)
Gal-Gal	Human	αGal 1-β4Gal	Uroepithelium (P-blood group)
X_1	Human	NAN(2-3)lac	Urcepithelium
X_2	Human	Unknown	Urcepithelium

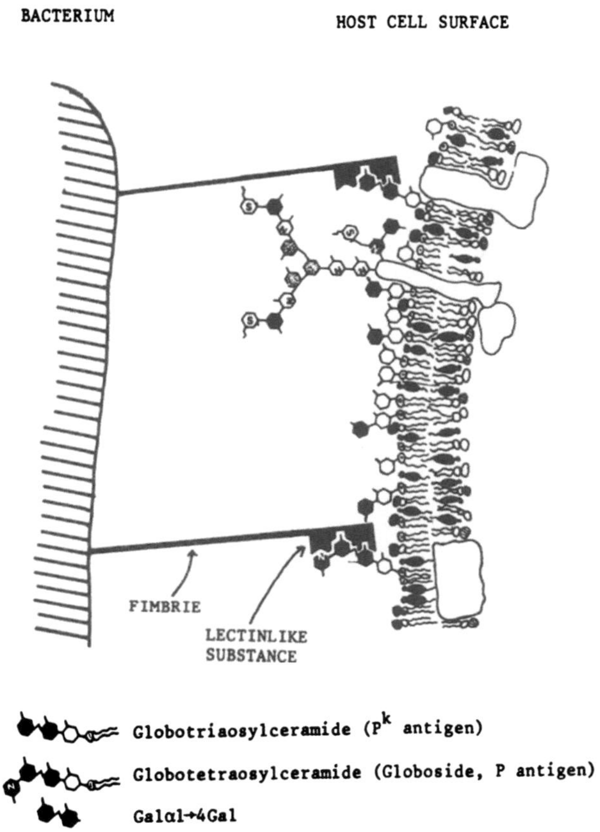

Fig. 1. The adherence of an uropathogenic *E. coli* bacterium to Galα1→4Gal containing glycolipids of the uroepithelial surface. (Adapted from Leffler et al. 1984)

tose, and that adhesin mediates the adherence of the organism to uroepithelium, to substances that are part of the p blood group system. There are other adhesins as well, but I will concentrate on the human tissue receptors for these two adhesins.

There are glycoconjugates on the surface of cells that are complementary to specific receptor binding domains on the adhesins (Fig. 1). In this case, the specific complementary interactions are shown for the p adhesin. Using artificial receptor antigens, it is possible to elicit antibodies that are specific for the receptors (Fig. 2). In this case, alpha mannose 1,2 alpha mannose was synthesized with a linker group and a reactive group that allowed it to be conjugated to serum albumen. Alpha gal 1,4 beta gal was created in the same way. These were used as a bovine serum albumen (BSA) conjugate to elicit antibody in rabbits. It was purified by affinity chromatography in which the same receptor material was linked to a solid phase. A polyclonal but monospecific reagent was thereby prepared. Tests showed that the antibody to the alpha gal 1,4 beta gal was specific for that disaccharide and for no other. Competitive inhibition assays with heterologous disaccharides showed no inhibition, indicating that the reagent was specific for the isomeric linkage as well as the monosaccharide content.

Fig. 2

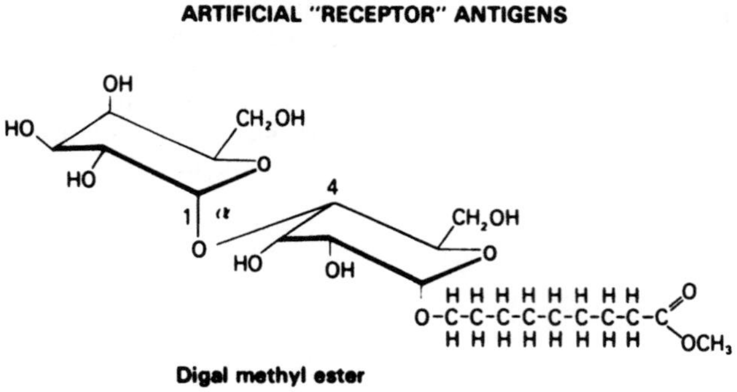

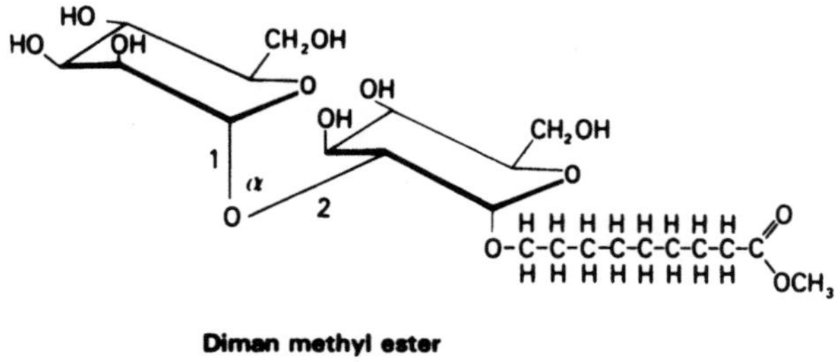

Examination of naturally occurring glycosphingolipids, which in some cases contain the alpha gal 1,4 beta gal moiety, showed that the curve of inhibition was specific for the trihexoside in which galactose was in the terminal position at the nonreducing end. In contrast, gangliosides showed very little inhibition. Therefore, only when the alpha gal 1,4 beta gal moiety is at the terminal end, can it be recognized by this antibody.

The same kind of analysis was performed on the alpha man 1,2 alpha man moiety antibody. This reagent is specific for the isomeric linkage; mannose, even alpha man 1,6 alpha man, was not bound by the antibody. Thus, the particular sugars, their isomeric linkage, and the location in the terminal position of glycosphingolipids can be deduced. These antibodies were used to examine human tissues with an immunoperoxidase assay to determine the location of receptors for bacterial lectins. In human kidney, the reagent specific for the receptor of p fimbria is found only in the collecting ducts and proximal tubular cells. In the renal papilli where pyelonephritis is initiated, the presence of the receptor is readily visualized.

It is possible to construct a map of the distribution of the specific receptors in human tissues and therefore address the question of tissue tropism in this particular infection (Table 2). The alpha gal 1,4 beta gal and alpha man 1,2 alpha man receptors were apparent in most of the tissues of the genitourinary tract, except the glomerulus and lamina propria. This indicates that there is a molecular basis in these tissues for

Table 2. Immunoperoxidase detection of Syn Man-Man and Syn Gal-Gal pilus receptors in human urogenital tissue

Tissue/Cell	Intensity of pilus disaccharide receptor[a]	
	Syn Man-Man[b]	Syn Gal-Gal[c]
I. Vagina		
Squamous epithelium	+3	+3
II. Bladder		
Transitional epithelium	+3	+2
Lamina propria[d]		
Fibroblasts	O	O
Smooth muscle	+2	+2
Endothelial cells	+3	+3
III. Ureter		
Transitional epithelium	+3	+2
IV. Renal pelvis		
Transitional epithelium	+3	+2
V. Kidney		
Glomerulus	O	O
Proximal tubular cells	+2	+2
Loop of Henle cells	+1	+/-
Collecting ducts	+3	+3

[a] Intensity of pilus disaccharide receptor - graded 3+ (intense brown) to O (no brown reaction product).
[b] Mannose pilus receptor was assessed by monospecific, affinity-purified rabbit antibody to synthetic αD-Man(1→2)αD-Man.
[c] Gal-Gal pilus receptor was assessed by monospecific, affinity-purified rabbit antibody to synthetic αD-Gal(1→4)βD-Gal.
[d] The distribution of pilus receptors in the lamina propria of the bladder were the same throughout the urogenital tract.

their receptivity to these bacterial adhesins. However, the significance of the alpha man 1,2 alpha man tissue receptor can be nullified by the presence in urine of the Tamm-Horsfall protein which binds common pili and blocks their ability to associate with the tissue receptor. The alpha gal 1,4 beta gal receptor however, is free to interact with the p adhesin. These findings provide a molecular explanation for the observation that the p adhesin is significantly associated with pyelonephritogenic *E. coli*. Use of antireceptor antibodies to examine the distribution of the adhesin receptors should be useful for other organ systems.

Discussion

Q: Can the number of specific receptors be modulated up or down?

A: The control of receptor exhibition and density on cell surfaces relates to the proposal that receptor-dense people are predisposed to recurrent infections of the urinary tract. This hypothesis has not yet been proven, but there does seem to be a predisposition for people of the p1 blood group for recurrent urinary tract infections and it has been proposed that these individuals might exhibit more receptors on urogenital epithelial surfaces. We anticipate testing for relevant glycosyl transferases in serum to see if the number of receptors on epithelial surfaces can be estimated with a simple blood test.

Q: Is there cyclicity of receptor expression in the same host during the diurnal, menstrual, or other biocycles?

A: The receptivity of cells harvested from the urogenital tract at different times in the menstrual cycle varies for a variety of bacterial adhesins in a reproducible way.

Q: Are receptor-specific antibodies better for finding the sugars in tissues than lectins that are specific for the sugars?

A: It might be more appropriate to use the bacterial adhesin, i.e., lectin, because antibodies might be too specific. However, adhesins can bind tissues readily by mechanisms that are not entirely specific, although there are specific mechanisms as well. Thus, in practice they are more difficult to work with.

Reference

1. Leffler H, Svanborg-Eden C, Schoolnik G, Wadström T (1984) Glycosphingolipids as receptors for bacterial adhesion: Host glycolipid diversity and other selected aspects. In: Boedeker, EC (ed) Attachment of organisms to the gut mucosa, VII. CRC Press, Boca Raton, Florida

Enhanced Antibody Responses to the Capsular Antigen of *Hemophilus influenzae* Type B in Infants Vaccinated with Oligosaccharides Coupled to a Protein Carrier

P. W. Anderson

The invasiveness of *H. influenzae* type b (Hib) comes from its ability to evade the nonspecific host defenses. Unlike the other capsular types, the type b fails to engage the alternate pathway of complement fixation, and the capsular polymer (PRP) by itself fails to activate C3, but antibody permits classical activation of complement [4, 5; Levine, this volume]. Infants, after the catabolism of maternal IgG, have a period of about two years with little of no anti-PRP, during which time they are highly susceptible to infection with Hib. Purified bacterial capsular polymers have been used successfully as vaccines in adults, but will not work in babies. Injection of such polymers appears to trigger antibody synthesis in previously primed B lymphocytes, but it does not elicit a secondary, memory response: a second injection does not raise antibody levels higher than the first.

It has been shown that antibody to pneumococcal capsular polysaccharide could be induced by the disaccharide determinant coupled as a hapten to a protein carrier. We adapted this approach to present the determinants of PRP in a form that would act as a primary and memory-inducing immunogen without the addition of potentially toxic or mutagenic linker molecules [1]. The carrier was CRM197, a missense mutant protein derived from diphtheria toxin, which is antigenically identical to the toxin but nontoxic [3]. The strategy was to take advantage of the carrier-specific priming created by the routine vaccination of infants with diphtheria toxoid in DPT vaccine. Figure 1 shows the geometric mean serum anti-PRP levels in three groups of babies [2]. One group received only the routine DPT vaccine at ages 2, 4, and 6 months of age. The second received the purified PRP polymer simultaneously with DPT. In both of these groups the antibody levels declined throughout the period of test to practically undetectable levels at a rate expected for catabolism of maternal IgG antibody. The third group received the carrier-oligo-PRP conjugate and also DPT injected in a separate site. Their levels likewise declined after the first injection, but after the second the titers rose and after the third rose still further. At age nine months, ordinarily the time of highest susceptibility to Hib, the mean titer was about 30-fold higher than that in the other groups. Data not shown indicate that the antibodies included IgG and were bactericidal to Hib in the presence of complement.

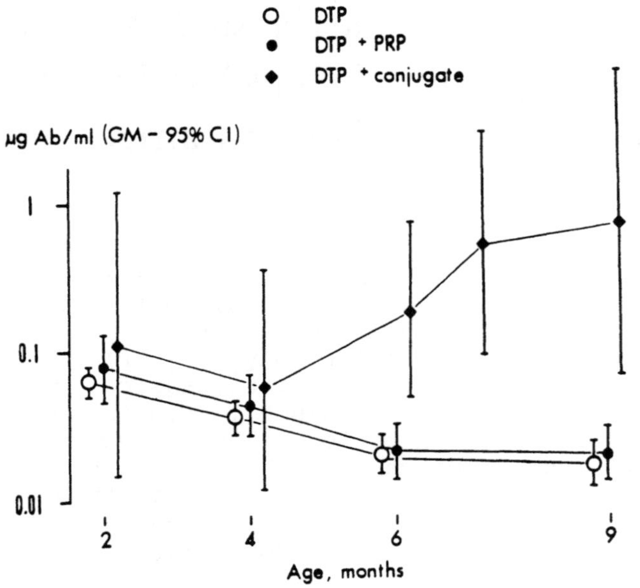

Fig. 1. Anti-PRP antibody response induced by the Dcr-PRP^{vs-1} conjugate vaccine administered at 2, 4, and 6 months of age as measured by the RIA. All the antibody classes are detected by this assay. Geometric means (GM) and 95% confidence intervals (CI) are displayed. *Open circles*: 200 infants who received no Hib vaccine but only routine DTP; *full circles*: 30 infants who received unconjugated PRP vaccine simultaneously with DTP in a 2, 4, and 6 months schedule; *diamond*: 7 infants vaccinated with conjugate

Thus, the previously noted failure of infants to make antibody after vaccination with PRP is not an inherent unresponsiveness to the antigenic determinants, and the lag in maturation of immunologic responsiveness to PRP can be overcome by presentation of the determinant coupled to the carrier protein.

Discussion

Q: Is it possible to use the vaccine in mothers before delivery in order to passively cover the infant for two to four months before the child can respond?

A: In adults the capsular polysaccharide alone is immunogenic. About two-thirds of mothers will have IgG-containing antibody to PRP after a single injection of PRP alone which is probably adequate to protect their babies for six to seven months. The other third do not have such a response and they might be candidates for immunization with a vaccine that would overcome their block. We are just beginning to study women who were poor responders to PRP vaccine to see whether they might have a response to the PRP-conjugate vaccine.

Q: Is it the maternal antibody that is suppressing the immune response in the infants who do not respond?

A: The unresponsiveness to the capsular antigen persists for about 18 months which is much longer than maternal antibody. As was shown, it is not just the presence of antigen that elicits the antibody response but the form in which it is presented.

References

1. Anderson P (1983) Antibody Responses to *Haemophilus influenzae* Type b and Diphtheria Toxin Induced by Conjugates of Oligosaccharides of the Type b Capsule with the Nontoxic Protein CRM_{197}. Infect Immun 39:233-238
2. Anderson P, Pichichero ME, Insel RA (1985) lmmunization of two-month-old infants with protein-coupled oligosaccharides derived from the capsule of *Haemophilus influenzae* type B. J Pediatrics (accepted for publication)
3. Pappenheimer AM, Uchida T, Harper AA (1972) An immunological study of the diphtheria toxin molecule. Immunochemistry 9:891-906
4. Quinn PH, Crosson FJ, Winkelstein JA, Moxon ER (1977) Activation of the alternative complement pathway by *Haemophilus influenzae* type b. Infect Immun 16:400-402
5. Sutton A, Schneerson R, Kendall-Morris S, Robbins JB (1982) Differential complement resistance mediates virulence of *Haemophilus influenzae* type b. Infect Immun 35:95-104

Monoclonal Antibody Protection Against *Pseudomonas aeruginosa*

R. E. W. Hancock

Biotechnology companies are isolating monoclonal antibodies against various bacterial products with the aim of utilizing them in prevention and therapy of infection. One that has received attention is the anti-lipid A monoclones for all gram-negative bacteria. Unfortunately, the early results have been quite disappointing. Our investigation was to see if some outer membrane proteins which are functionally conserved were also antigenically conserved and would provide a candidate antigen for a vaccine.

We have isolated monoclonal antibodies against two distinct surface epitopes of protein F of *P. aeruginosa*. Figure 1 is a Western blot that shows that all of the strains representing the serotypes of *P. aeruginosa*, which differ on the basis of different O-antigenic composition of their LPS have a single protein, protein F, of the same molecular weight, which interacts with a single monoclonal antibody against protein F. This result differs from other gram-negative organisms like *Neisseria* and *Hemophilus*. Both classes of antibodies we have studied interact with this protein. An indirect immunofluorescence assay using the monoclonal antibodies suggests that it is surface epitopes with which the monoclonal antibodies are reactive.

To test whether the antibody gave protection the monoclonal antibody was given in the tail vein of mice, either two hours or 24 hours prior to an intraperitoneal challenge. The challenge strains were PA103 or M2. Both produce large amounts of extracellular products that kill mice within 2-12 hours after the intraperitoneal challenge. The results obtained with one of the two challenge strains is shown in Fig. 2 as the per cent survival after 24 hours. The test group (upper line) received 0.1 mg of purified monoclonal antibody. The control group were given a monoclonal antibody that does not react with surface proteins. The number of surviving mice are shown at each inoculum and the differences between the groups are statistically significant by the Fisher exact test.

The results suggest that there is the potential for a vaccine component for passive protection against severe infections with *P. aeruginosa*. However, there are about 200,000 postulated vaccines in the literature and it is arguable whether or not monoclonal antibodies will become the commercial vaccines of the

Fig. 1

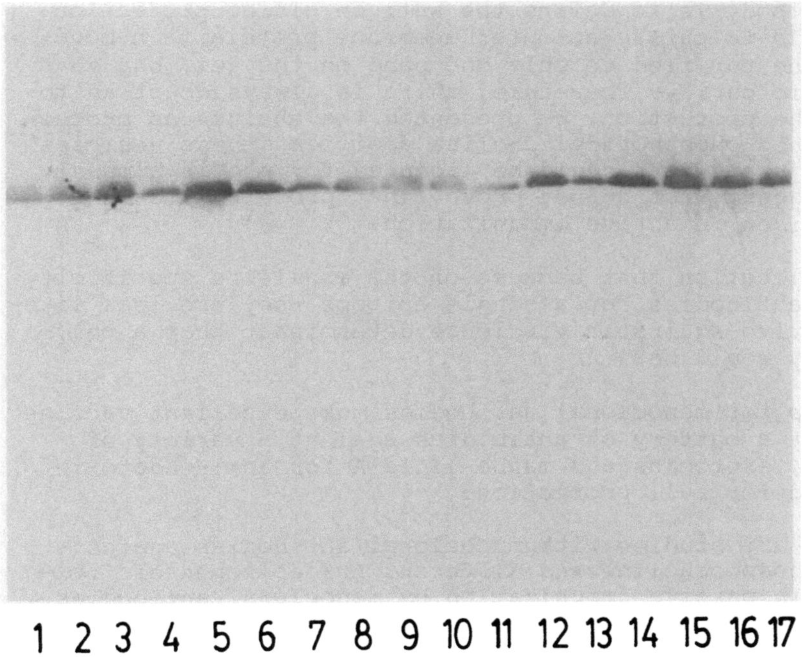

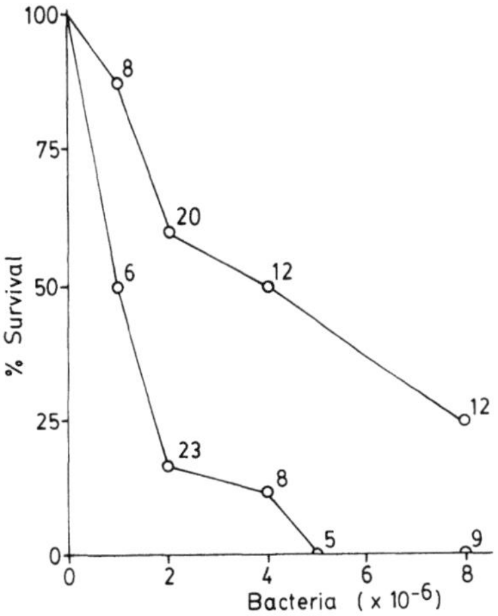

Fig. 2

future. Millions of dollars are going into their development and discussion is necessary about whether physicians and scientists believe it is a proper and practical direction for therapy.

Discussion

Q: Have the mice in which the anti-protein F antibody was produced been challenged?

A: Yes, active immunization is protective. The reason to study monoclonal antibody is to define the antigen giving protection. It is impossible to purify an outer membrane protein to homogeneity. It can be purified to only one band on the gel, but that is not antigenic purity. Therefore, there is always doubt as to the basis of the protection. We presented the antigen as protein incorporated into phosphotidyl choline vesicles (these vesicles serve as an adjuvant that could be licensed for use in humans). Our results suggest, but do not prove, that protein F was the protective antigen in active immunization.

Q: Is your implication that because of the exquisite specificity of monoclonal antibodies for a single epitope they are less likely to be effective against a virulence determinant than a polyclonal antibody would be?

A: No. Antigens for monoclonal antibodies make excellent vaccine candidates, but a battery of antibodies against a variety of porin proteins, exotoxins and maybe lipid A for anti-endotoxin may be required for full protection.

Comment: There are studies with monoclonal antibodies against pneumococcal phosphocholine and different LPS epitopes of *Salmonella* for use in passive immunization by monoclonal antibodies rather than as a basis for active immunity.

A: The major issue is whether enough of a monoclonal antibody preparation can be made to allow it to be used therapeutically or prophylactically for all of the patients who are at risk of severe infections with *Pseudomonas*. Also, antibody has a limited half-life in vivo. Such use is perhaps logistically impossible for infections of long duration. As therapy for bacteremias of short duration, monoclonal antibodies could be effective. However, few researchers have succeeded in making monoclonal antibodies of human origin in any significant amount and the dangers of using mouse immunoglobulins in man, especially if used repeatedly, must be remembered. In contrast, the use of the specific antigen that has elicited the protective monoclonal antibody could be a highly efficient form of prophylaxis.

Antibody Responses in Patients with Cystic Fibrosis

B. H. Iglewski

There is a mistaken belief that patients with cystic fibrosis (CF) respond to only a selected few antigens of *P. aeruginosa*. It is necessary to recognize, however, that virtually everything that is known about the immune response in these patients is from observations in people who have had substantially long term colonization with *P. aeruginosa*. There are no published data on the specificity of the antibody response from the first episode of colonization. After exposure to the antigens of *P. aeruginosa*, for many years CF patients have antibody against virtually all of the known antigens of the species including LPS, toxin A, alkaline protease, and elastase.

We have examined the serum of CF patients and found enormously high titers of antibodies to all of the antigens noted. Human monoclonal antibodies against the products of *P. aeruginosa* have been obtained by the fusion of cells from CF patients. In a single screen, human monoclonal antibodies can be selected against at least four pseudomonal antigens. Thus, patients with CF have a very active antibody response to the persistent infection with *P. aeruginosa*. Some reports suggest an inverse relation between the antibody titers and the clinical status of the patient. Circulating immune complexes have been measured and there is a concern that they participate in the pathogenesis of the disease complications. What is still unknown is information about the secretory antibodies in the respiratory tract and especially the immunoresponsiveness of secretory immunoglobulins to the initial infection.

Discussion

Q: Is the size of the circulating immune complexes in CF large or small?

A: They are of varying sizes and contain immunoglobulins G and M.

Comment: In contrast to immunocompromised patients who have bacteremias with *P. aeruginosa*, an immunologic defect in patients with CF has never been convincingly shown. The incidence of immune complexes is as high as 90% in CF patients in the terminal phases of the disease. These complexes are enriched 20-30 times with antibody against exotoxin A or LPS. Antibody surplus rather than antibody deficiency may be the problem. In one clinical trial, immunosuppressive therapy was given because of an observed correlation between hypogammaglobulinemia and good prognosis of CF. The role of antibody in the course of the disease must be carefully distinguished from that in patients with burns, allograft transplant recipients, and others who are immunosuppressed.

Cell Mediated Immunity Against Bacterial Abscess Formation

K. A. Joiner

Subcutaneous injection of mice with certain bacteria produces an abscess (Fig. 1). In histologic cross section the necrotic center is encased by a well defined capsule developed by the host response (Fig. 2). When the abscess volume in nude mice was compared with conventional mice at various times after inoculation of *B. fragilis* or *S. aureus*, it was smaller in nude than in normal mice (Fig. 3) [1]. Also the abscesses were smaller by a number of other parameters such as smaller areas of leukocyte infiltration and smaller collagen capsules. The results suggested a role for cell mediated immunity in bacterial abscess formation.

Recently, it has been shown by other workers that T-lymphocytes were required for protection against experimental intra-abdominal abscesses with *B. fragilis* species [2, 3]. This was established by observing the protection of animals against the development of an induced intra-abdominal abscess following the trans-

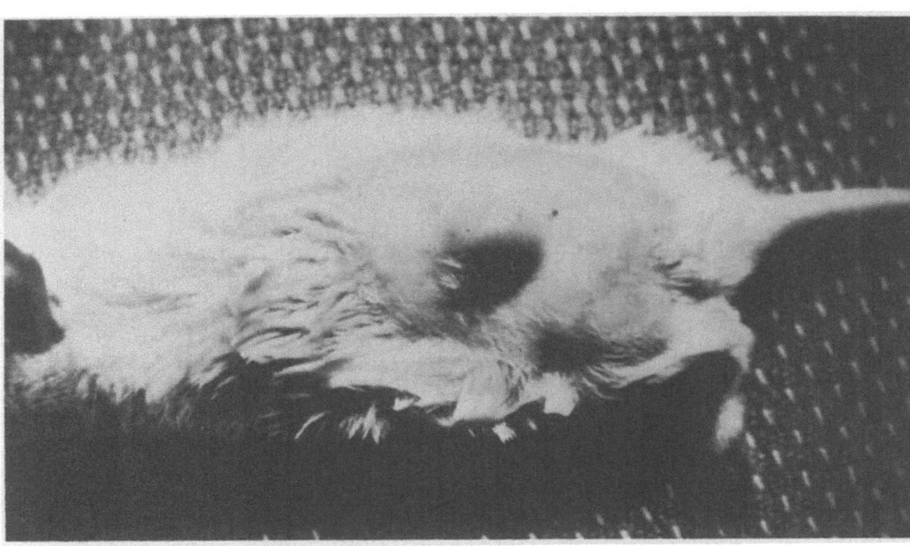

Fig. 1

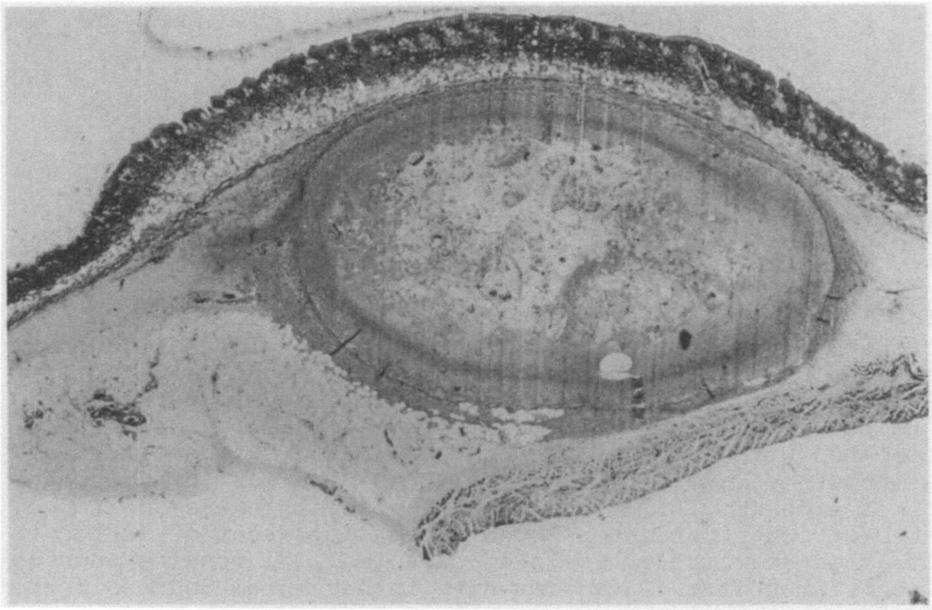

Fig. 2

fer of T-cells from animals that had been immunized with the capsular polysaccharide of *B. fragilis*. Passive immunization with high titer antibody against the capsular polysaccharide of *B. fragilis* was not protective. The protection with T-cells was antigen specific, but it was not restricted by the H2 gene locus. The protective cells were Thyl positive and Lyl negative, Ly 2-3 positive. A heat stable factor elaborated by the T-cells was lytic for *B. fragilis* in the presence of complement [4]. It is proposed that the observed cytohumoral mechanism of T-cells mediates an effect in preventing abscess formation.

Discussion

Q: If the complement dependent T-cell function is non-H2 restricted, it mimics antibody dependent bacteriolysis which in this model was not effective. How was it shown that the complement was the effector of a unique T-cell factor, what is the nature of this non-antibody bacteriolysin and how does it activate the complement cascade effecting bacteriolysis?

A: I can not comment about the uniqueness of non-haplo type restriction of a complement dependent T-cell function. The protection against abscess formation was clearly shown to be T-cell dependent, and in complement depleted mice the effect could not be obtained. In vitro, the semipurified component from the T-cells is not bacteriolytic against *B. fragilis* in the absence of complement. Further characterization of the material is in progress [D.L. Kasper, personal communication].

Fig. 3

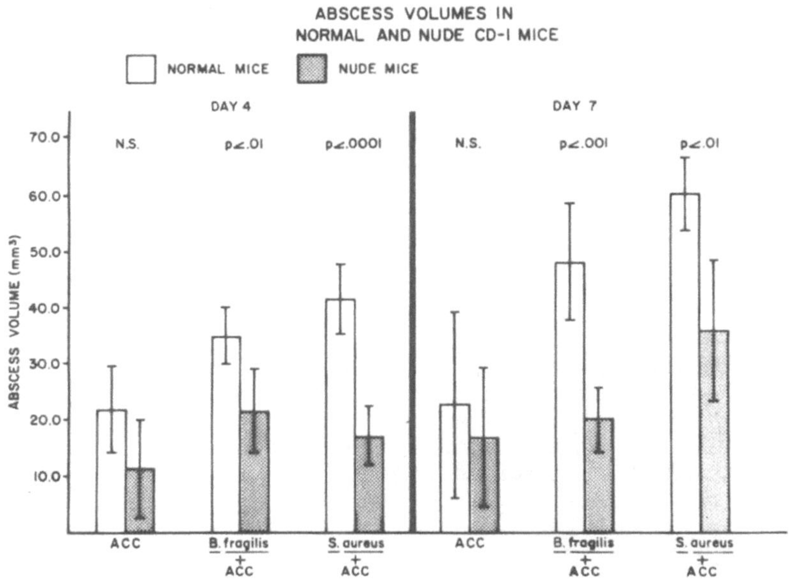

Q: Is it a synergistic effect of a complement-dependent factor and a cytotoxic natural killer (NK) T-cell?

A: The entire protection can be obtained with the elaborated factor alone and does not seem to require NK activity.

Q: Then it is a complement-dependent T-cell immune lymphokine?

A: Yes.

References

1. Joiner KA, Gelfand JA, Onderdonk AB, Bartlett JG, Gorbach SL (1980) Host factors in the formation of abscesses. J Infect Dis 142:40-49
2. Onderdonk AB, Markham RB, Zaleznik DF, Cisneros RL, Kasper DL (1982) Evidence for T Cell-Dependent Immunity to *Bacteroides fragilis* in an Intraabdominal Abscess Model. J Clin Invest 69:9-16
3. Shapiro ME, Onderdonk AB, Kasper DL, Finberg RW (1982) Cellular Immunity to *Bacteroides fragilis* Capsular Polysaccharide. J Exp Med 154:1188-1197
4. Zaleznik DF, Finberg RW, Lally KP, Onderdonk AB, Kasper DL (1983) Cooperation of T-Cells and Complement in Immunity to Intraabdominal Abscess Formation. Clin Research 31:379A

Induction of the Common Mucosal Immune System

J. R. McGhee

Work with *Streptococcus mutans* vaccine toward the prevention of dental caries is an approach that might apply to any type of vaccine. The cell wall of *S. mutans* has the usual types of streptococcal cell wall antigens. After isolation of these antigens, their oral administration induces a very poor response of the secretory IgA immune system. Living antigens are better, and some non-living particulate antigens induce a good IgA response. A conventional approach to vaccine development would be to make the purified antigens particulate. For dental caries, this is being done by constructing multilamilar liposomes, placing the purified antigen in the liposome and using an adjuvant such as lipophilic muramyl dipeptide (MDP). The material is placed into the stomach by intubation (of mice or rats). Induction of immunity through the common mucosal immune system can be assessed in several ways.

A more long range plan for vaccine development is to use recombinant DNA techniques. Again using the *S. mutans* model, the strategy is to isolate *S. mutans* DNA and with a cloning vector insert it into either *E. coli*, an avirulent *Salmonella*, or a selected hybrid strain. The property being sought in the carrier bacterial strain is that it selectively colonizes the Peyer's patches in the intestine. The bacterial adherence and proliferation releases antigen to the lymphocytes comprising a part of the common mucosal immune system. Through stimulation and recruitment of immunosensitized cells, the secretory IgA response is induced. Although the genetic construction of a purified antigen placed in a suitable carrier for oral administration is a more long range approach to the development of vaccines, mutants that selectively colonize the intestinal tract are already available.

Thus, there are two current approaches to vaccine development that seem very promising for eliciting immunity to infections of the mucosa and secretory lumenal surfaces by oral vaccines that will stimulate a common secretory IgA response.

Discussion

Q: Are the antigen associated liposomes stable in the gut and are they taken up as a complex?

A: Initial investigation indicates that the liposomes containing antigen are selectively taken up by the cells of the intestinal tract. They are taken up by specialized epithelial cells over the Peyer's patches.

Q: Can a booster type response be obtained and is there a need to give parental antigen simultaneously?

A: Multiple oral doses of the particulate *S. mutans* antigen vaccine are given. This involves two or three oral immunizations initially and then at weekly intervals.

Q: What ist known about the ability ot immunize in order to get a response at a specific site?

A: We still do not fully understand all aspects of induction of the mucosal immune response. We know the most about inducing a response in the gut associated lymphoreticular tissues (GALT). The first step is to have purified particulate antigen that will penetrate into the Peyer's patches. There is some evidence that local antigen is important, but whether it is processed by macrophages and induces T-helper cells or directly stimulates B-cells to undergo differentiation to IgA synthesis, is unknown. In order to induce a significant local response, it is probably necessary to have the antigen present locally.

MIX
Papier aus verantwortungsvollen Quellen
Paper from responsible sources
FSC® C105338

If you have any concerns about our products,
you can contact us on
ProductSafety@springernature.com

In case Publisher is established outside the EU,
the EU authorized representative is:
Springer Nature Customer Service Center GmbH
Europaplatz 3, 69115 Heidelberg, Germany

Printed by Libri Plureos GmbH
in Hamburg, Germany